HERBAL COMPANION

AHFS DI

2001

EDITORIAL STAFF

Lynn Forget, R.PH., J.D.
Managing Editor, Reference, IMC

Julia Goldrosen, M.S.P.H.
Director of Research, IMC

Jacqueline A. Hart, M.D.
Senior Medical Editor, IMC

Tommy Hyun, M.S.
Research Associate, IMC

Denis Meacham
Editorial Director, IMC

Tricia Tyler
Executive Editor, Reference, IMC

Leonard A. Wisneski, M.D., F.A.C.P.
Medical Director, IMC

PRODUCTION STAFF

Ray Auen
Graphic Designer, ASHP

Johnna Hershey
Director, Publications Production Center, ASHP

Gerald K. McEvoy, Pharm.D.
Assistant Vice President, Drug Information, ASHP

Lisa Shannon
Project Manager, Drug Information and Database Services, ASHP

Jeff Shick, R.Ph.
Director, Database Information Services, ASHP

Table of Contents

Preface *p. v*

Notices and Disclaimers *p. vii*

Advisory Board *p. viii*

Herbals *p. 1*

Supplements *p. 107*

Index *p. 175*

© Copyright, 2000

by the American Society of Health-System Pharmacists, Inc.
7272 Wisconsin Avenue
Bethesda, MD 20814
All Rights Reserved.

All materials distributed as part of *Herbal Companion to AHFS DI*™ is copyrighted. Reproduction, storage in a retrieval system, or transmission of this material or any other part thereof in any form or by any means without the express written permission of the American Society of Health-System Pharmacists is prohibited.

Printed in the United States of America.

INTERNATIONAL STANDARD BOOK NUMBER (ISBN):

1-58528-017-8

For Ordering Information

Write
American Society of Health-System Pharmacists
Customer Service Dept.
7272 Wisconsin Ave.
Bethesda, MD 20814

Phone
301-657-4383

Fax
800-665-ASHP

Payments to ASHP are not deductible as charitable contributions for federal income tax purposes. However, they may be deductible under other provisions of the Internal revenue code.

Preface

The *Herbal Companion to AHFS DI*™ is published by the American Society of Health-System Pharmacists (ASHP) as an adaptation of information from Integrative Medicine Communications' (IMC) database on complementary and alternative therapies. IMC, in partnership with the American Botanical Council, is responsible for publishing the English translation of the *Complete German Commission E Monographs* and remains the exclusive publisher of the English version of this well-respected reference. The German Commission E Monographs were developed by the German Federal Institute for Drugs and Medicinal Devices, Germany's equivalent to the US Food and Drug Administration. The accuracy of the information available within the Commission E Monographs creates a benchmark for the safety and efficacy of phytomedicine, and the monographs are regarded as *the* authoritative compendium on therapeutic medicinal herbs for health-care professionals, representing today's highest standard in phytomedicinal evaluation. First published in 1998, the translation represents IMC's initial efforts in fostering safe and efficacious use of complementary and alternative therapies.

Subsequent to this effort, IMC set out to build an ever-expanding database that would allow healthcare professionals from various educational and philosophical backgrounds access to a complete array of approaches used to maintain health, treat disease, and manage conditions. Building such a reference requires respect for the evidence to support the use of "conventional" and "nonconventional" therapeutic modalities, and the ability to utilize the talents of advisors, researchers, writers, fact checkers, proofreaders, and project managers in synthesizing the information into a tightly formatted and well-balanced final work. It is from this database that the *Herbal Companion to AHFS DI* is derived.

The *Herbal Companion to AHFS DI* provides unbiased, science-based, reference information intended to assist clinicians in integrating conventional and alternative medicine into their patients' care. This information is aimed at bridging the gap between conventional and alternative medicine by providing comprehensive information on herbs and nutritional supplements and their integration with conventional medicine. IMC maintains the same rigorous standards of medical information development and review processes employed by conventional medical publishers, focusing on integrative medicine. A team of medical writers and health information researchers prepares the data, which are reviewed by a team of advisors from IMC's editorial board. IMC's medical director and chief medical editor govern the information development and board review processes. IMC conducts ongoing research and review of scientific and clinical data, selecting and highlighting the most important findings. Scientific review is performed by IMC's medical advisors, physicians, and other clinicians with experience in the integration of conventional and alternative therapies and recognized expertise in specific modalities.

The *Herbal Companion to AHFS DI* is intended to provide essential, accurate, practical, referenced, and formatted information—not theory—about herbs and nutritional supplements. Each monograph reflects a consistent organization and scope, aiding the familiar user who requires a quick review of the facts or the unfamiliar user who seeks an overview of the subject matter. In developing the monographs, breadth of coverage, then depth of coverage as space allowed, was the focus since each monograph was designed to fill just a few printed pages. The result is a quick review of therapeutic options, from various schools of healing and health promotion. The information is well researched, succinctly presented, and consistently formatted. References are contemporary and clinically important, tracking the relevant and excluding the irrelevant. A panel of health professionals representing the intended audience of pharmacists, physicians, nurses and nurse practitioners, nutritionists, dietitians, chiropractors, herbalists, naturopathic physicians, and other health practitioners

Preface (Continued)

continues to help shape the product and to review the information for appropriateness.

The monographs in the *Herbal Companion to AHFS DI* are objective and should not be viewed as preferentially advocating alternative versus conventional therapy. The development of this information is not supported by funding or sponsorship of any kind from complementary, alternative, or conventional therapy manufacturers, developers, or providers. A 6-step methodology is used in developing these monographs: data collection from over 3000 industry standard sources, including over 500 medical journals; data assessment by an intramural research staff that employs scientific criteria; production of evidence-based documents and databases based on this assessment; peer review by an advisory board consisting of recognized physicians, scientists, and other medical professionals; rigorous checking and cross-checking by senior editors of information included in the database; and ongoing review and updating of the information. The result is objective information about herbs and nutritional supplements that is comprehensive, authoritative, and science-based and that can be used with confidence by health-care professionals.

Currently, millions of individuals are integrating complementary and alternative therapies into the daily management of their health and wellness, often without consulting a clinician. In 1998, it was estimated that about half of adults in the US used alternative therapies and about two-thirds of these did so without consulting their clinician. Sales of herbal products and nutritional supplements are projected to exceed $6 billion in 2001, almost doubling in just 3 years. Conventionally trained health-care professionals whose patients are asking questions about integrating complementary and alternative therapies into their care should not rely on anecdotal evidence and unsubstantiated theories about the use of these therapies. The *Herbal Companion to AHFS DI* is intended to provide objective, authoritative information that can be used in counseling and caring for patients who are interested in integrating such therapies. We are confident that health-care professionals will find the *Herbal Companion to AHFS DI* a useful resource in addressing patient questions about such therapies.

NOTICES AND DISCLAIMERS

Integrative Medicine Communications (IMC) is responsible for the content in the herb and supplement monographs included in the *Herbal Companion to AHFS DI*. The content was *not* developed by the American Society of Health-System Pharmacists (ASHP), *nor* did ASHP participate in the editorial or review process for this material. As a result, ASHP makes no representations or guarantees regarding the accuracy of the information contained herein. Inquiries about specific statements included in the herb and supplement monographs in the *Herbal Companion to AHFS DI* can be directed to IMC in writing at 1029 Chestnut Street, Newton, MA 02464; by phone at 617-641-2300; by facsimile transmission at 617-641-2301; or via the internet at www.onemedicine.com.

While care has been taken by IMC to ensure the accuracy of the information presented, no reponsibility is assumed by IMC or ASHP for any injury and/or damage to any person or propery as a matter of product liability, negligence, or otherwise, or from any use or operation of any methods, products, instructions, or ideas contained in any materials herein. This publication contains information relating to general principles of medical care that should not in any event be construed as specific instructions for individual patients. The nature of medical information is that it is constantly evolving because of ongoing research and clinical experience and is often subject to interpretation and the uniqueness of each clinical situation and patient. The reader is advised to check product information (including package inserts) for changes and new information regarding dosage, precautions, and contraindications before administering any drug or compound. No claim or endorsement is made for any drug or compound currently in investigative use. Because of the dynamic nature of medical information, readers are advised that decisions regarding therapy must be based on the independent judgment of the clinician, changing information about a given therapy or modality (e.g., as reflected in the literature), and changing medical practices.

Advisory Board

Robert A. Anderson, M.D.
Bastyr University
Bothell, WA

Dennis Awang, Ph.D.
President, MediPlant Consulting Services
Ottawa, Ontario, Canada

Shiva Barton, N.D.
Naturopathy
Wellspace
Cambridge, MA

Stuart Bell, M.D.
Internal Medicine
Attending Physician, University of Maryland Hospital
Baltimore, MD

Mark Blumenthal
Herbs
American Botanical Council
Austin, TX

Lawrence J. Cheskin, M.D., F.A.C.P.
Gastroenterology
Associate Professor of Medicine
Director, The Johns Hopkins Weight Management Center
Johns Hopkins School of Medicine
Director, Division of Gastroenterology
Johns Hopkins Bayview Medical Center
Baltimore, MD

Rebecca Couris, Ph.D., R.Ph.
Nutrition and Pharmacy
Massachusetts College of Pharmacy
Boston, MA

Steven Dentali, Ph.D.
Senior Director, Botanical Sciences
Rexall Sundowne, Inc.
Boca Raton, FL

James Dillard, Ph.D.
Managed Care
Oxford Health Plans
New York, NY

James Duke, Ph.D.
Botanical Medicine
Author, *The Green Pharmacy*

Rainer Engle, M.D.
Associate Professor of Urology
Johns Hopkins Medical Institute
Maryland Urology Associates
Baltimore, MD

Constance Grauds, R.Ph.
Pharmacy
President, Association of Natural Medicine Pharmacists
San Rafael, CA

Gary M. Guebert, D.C., DACBR
Chiropractic
Login Chiropractic College
St. Louis, MO

Yan Qiu He, M.D., O.M.D., L.Ac.
Chinese Medicine and Acupuncture
American WholeHealth
Chevy Chase, MD

Peter Hinderberger, M.D.
Internal Medicine/Homeopathy
Medical Director, Ruscombe Mansion Community Health Center
Baltimore, MD

Dahlia Hirsch, M.D.
Ophthalmology
Fellow, American College of Surgeons
Associate Professor, University of Maryland Medical Center
American Holistic Medical Association
Baltimore, MD

William H. B. Howard, M.D., F.A.C.S., F.A.C.P.E.
Surgery/Sports Medicine
Attending Physician, Johns Hopkins Hospital
Baltimore, MD

ADVISORY BOARD (CONTINUED)

Joel A. Kahn, M.D.
Chief Medical Officer, InteliHealth
Blue Bell, PA

Kathi Kemper, M.D., M.P.H.
Holistic Pediatrics
Children's Hospital
Boston, MA

Vasant Lad, B.A.M.S., M.A.Sc.
Ayurveda
Ayurvedic Institute
Albuquerque, NM

Joseph Lamb, M.D.
Senior Clinician
American WholeHealth
Alexandria, VA

Lonnie Lee, M.D.
Complementary and Alternative Medicine
Kaiser Permanente Mid Atlantic
College Park, MD

Richard A. Lippin, M.D.
Internal Medicine
Southampton, PA

Bill Manahan, M.D.
Assistant Professor, Family Medicine
University of Minnesota
Mankato, MN

Anne McClenon, N.D.
Naturopathy/Midwifery
Compass Family Health Center
Plymouth, MA

Marc S. Micozzi, M.D., Ph.D.
Adjunct Professor, Department of Medicine
University of Pennsylvania School of Medicine
Philadelphia, PA

Sherif H. Osman, M.D.
President, Medical Staff
Harford Memorial Hospital
Fallston General Hospital
Bel Air, MD

Kenneth R. Pelletier, Ph.D., M.D.
Disease Management
Stanford University School of Medicine
Stanford, CA

David Perlmutter, M.D.
Neurology
Director, Perlmutter Health Center
Naples, FL

Daniel Redwood, D.C.
Chiropractic
Redwood Chiropractic and Wellness
Virginia Beach, VA

Paul T. Rogers, M.D.
Facility Medical Director
Bright Oaks Pediatrics
Bel Air, MD

Paul J. Rosch, M.D., F.A.C.P.
Bioenergetic Medicine
American Institute of Stress
New York, NY

Scott Shannon, M.D.
Integrative Psychiatry
North Colorado Medical Center
Banner Health System
Fort Collins, CO

R. Lynn Shumake, P.D., R.Ph.
Medicinal Herbs/Nutrition
American Herbalist Guild
Blue Mountain Apothecary and Healing Arts
Glenwood, MD

Pamela Stratton, M.D.
Associate Professor, Obstetrics and Gynecology
Uniformed University of the Health Sciences
Bethesda, MD

John B. Sullivan, Jr., M.D.
Associate Director, Arizona Poison Center
Associate Dean, University of Arizona Health
Sciences Center
Tucson, AZ

Advisory Board (continued)

Dana Ullman, M.P.H.
Homeopathy
Homeopathic Educational Services
Berkeley, CA

Marcellus Walker, M.D., L.Ac.
Internal Medicine, Acupuncture
Center for Lifelong Health
New York, NY

Allan Warshowsky, M.D., F.A.C.O.G.
Holistic Obstetrics/Gynecology
Long Island Jewish Medical Center
New York, NY

Eric Wellons, M.D.
Union Memorial Hospital
Baltimore, MD

David Winston
Herbalist American Herbalists Guild
President, Herbalist and Alchemist
Washington, NJ

Thomas Wolfe
Professional Member, American Herbalists Guild
Smile Herb Shop
College Park, MD

Elizabeth Wotton, N.D., L.M.
Naturopathy/Midwifery
Hanscom AFB, MA

Terry Yochum, D.C., D.A.C.B.R., F.C.C.R.(C), F.I.C.C.
Chiropractic/Radiology
Director, Rocky Mountain Chiropractic Radiological Center
Instructor, Department of Radiology
University of Colorado School of Medicine
Denver, CO

David J. Zieger, D.O., A.B.F.P
Osteopathic Medicine
American Whole Health
Chicago, IL

HERBALS 101

Aloe

Names

■ **English**
Aloe

■ **Botanical**
Aloe vera/Aloe barbadensis/Aloe ferox

■ **Plant Family**
Liliaceae

■ **Pharmacopeial**
Aloe barbadensis/capensis

Overview

Aloe vera has a long history of use as a medicinal plant, with written record going back to 1750 BC. The plant has a wide variety of uses because different parts of the plant have different medicinal properties. The mucilaginous gel that is most widely associated with aloe vera comes from the inner part of the leaf. It is separated from the pericyclic tubules, specialized cells that are under the epidermis of the leaf. Those cells have a bitter yellow latex or juice that is dried to form a pharmaceutical product called aloe latex. Aloe gel is used for wound healing, both internally and externally. It greatly speeds the healing of many skin injuries, including ulcerations, burns, frostbite, and abrasions. Aloe latex is a powerful cathartic and is used for constipation. Because it can cause painful cramping, it is not used as often as gentler herbal laxatives. Lower doses of aloe latex can be effective in preventing kidney stone formation or reducing their size. Lower doses can also be effective as a stool softener, which is particularly helpful in the case of hemorrhoids.

Aloe gel is now found in many commercial skin-care products, shampoos, and conditioners. But some studies have shown that it does not retain its healing ability when stored. There is now a stabilized form of the gel that may be able to be stored and still retain the healing action, but fresh aloe gel from the leaves is still the best option.

Aloe gel may also be taken internally, often in a liquid form called aloe juice. In this form, aloe can help heal peptic ulcers by inhibiting stomach acids that irritate ulcers. Aloe juice also improves digestion by destroying many bacteria that cause infection.

Recent studies have shown that aloe juice has important HIV-fighting properties. Its antiviral ability attacks the virus itself, but more important, it greatly enhances the action of AZT. A polysaccharide constituent of aloe, acetylated mannose, worked synergistically with AZT in vitro to inhibit HIV replication, and researchers believe the supplemental use of acetylated mannose may reduce required AZT dosage by as much as 90%.

Macro Description

A perennial plant; yellow flowers; tough, fleshy leaves grow up to 20 inches long, 5 inches across, up to 30 per plant; grows to 4 feet. Grown in most tropical and subtropical locations, including Caribbean, southern United States, Latin America, and the Middle East.

Part Used/Pharmaceutical Designations

- Leaves

■ **Constituents/Composition**

Anthraquinones, aloins, anthranoids, aglycones, polysaccharides (including glycoproteins and mucopolysaccharides), and prostaglandins

■ **Commercial Preparations**

Aloe gel is best fresh from an aloe plant. Slit a leaf lengthwise and remove gel. Aloe gel is also available commercially in stabilized form. Aloe latex is available as a powder or in 500 mg capsules for use as a laxative. Aloe juice is available in liquid form.

Medicinal Uses/Indications

- Aloe was historically used to treat burns.
- Traditional herbal actions: antibacterial, antifungal, anesthetic, antipyretic, antipruritic, moisturizer, vasodilator, anti-inflammatory, anthelmintic, cathartic, stomachic, demulcent, emmenagogue, laxative combined with carminative, vulnerary
- Clinical applications: burns (due to radiation, sunburn, and other causes), headaches, dry skin, rashes (due to dermatitis, poison ivy, or insect bites), kidney stones, hemorrhoids, hives, HIV, constipation, wound healing, peptic ulcers, immune system enhancement, diabetes, asthma

■ **Pharmacology**

Aloe vera contains vitamins C and E and zinc, which are all important for wound healing. Glycoproteins in aloe gel inhibit and break down bradykinin, a mediator of pain and inflammation. Aloe gel also inhibits thromboxane, which also causes inflammation. Aloe gel stimulates fibroblast and connective tissue formation, a healing action that most other anti-inflammatories don't have. The polysaccharides in aloe seem to stimulate skin growth and repair as well. Aloe also increases blood flow to burned tissue, which helps it heal.

Aloe gel has been particularly effective in healing diabetic leg ulcers because along with its other wound healing capabilities, it also lowers blood sugar.

Aloe gel's antibacterial and antifungal ability compares favorably with that of silver sulfadiazine, an antiseptic used regularly in treatment of extensive burns. Aloe vera extract has been shown to kill *Pseudomonas aeruginosa, Klebsiella pneumoniae, Serratia marcescens, Citrobacter species, Enterobacter cloacae, Streptococcus pyogenes, Streptococcus agalactiae, Staphylococcus aureus, Escherichia coli, Streptococcus faecalis,* and *Candida albicans.*

Aloe's active cathartic component is aloin. In small doses, it gives tone to intestinal muscle. In larger doses, it becomes a strong purgative, increasing colonic secretions and peristaltic contractions in the large intestine. It is harsher on the system than other anthraquinone laxatives, such as cascara and senna. The anthraquinones in aloe latex prevent kidney stone formation by binding calcium in the urinary tract and reducing the growth rate of urinary calcium crystals.

Aloe juice heals peptic ulcers by inhibiting pepsin when the stomach is empty, releasing it only to digest food. It inhibits the release of hydrochloric acid by preventing the binding of histamine to parietal cells. It also heals and prevents other irritants from reaching the ulcer. Aloe juice aids the digestive process by increasing gastric pH, reducing yeast infections, and improving water retention.

Acemannan, an antiviral compound of aloe juice, is a powerful immune system stimulant. It enhances macrophage activity, the function of T cells and interferon production. Acemannan has been effective for treatment of HIV, influenza, and measles. It has a direct antiviral effect on HIV by inhibiting glycosylation of viral glycoproteins. Even more promising, it enhances the action of AZT. Studies show that acemannan, combined with suboptimal noncytotoxic concentrations of AZT, acts synergistically to inhibit replication of HIV and herpes simplex virus type 1.

Dosage Ranges and Duration of Administration

- The dosage for dry aloe extract is very small (50 to 200 mg).
- For general use: dosage of gel or juice 2 tbsp. tid (the standardized aloe product measure to hydroxyanthracene derivatives is not widely available in the USA)
- For prevention of kidney stones: 2 to 3 tbsp. daily
- For laxative purposes: 500 to 1,000 mg daily (care should be taken that laxative doses of aloe are accompanied by carminative herbs to prevent griping)
- For burns or wound healing, topically: aloe vera gel applied liberally (fresh gel from aloe plant is best)
- For hemorrhoids, as a stool softener: dry aloe extract, 0.05 to 0.2 g
- For HIV: 800 to 1,600 mg of acemannan a day (equivalent to .5 to 1 liter of aloe vera juice, although amount of acemannan may vary in different products)
- For constipation: 20 to 30 mg hydroxyanthracene derivatives per day, calculated as anydrous aloin

Cautions

■ **Adverse Effects/Toxicology**

Aloe gel is safe for external use, unless it causes a rare allergic reaction. Discontinue use if it irritates the skin. It is not useful for treatment of deep, vertical wounds (e.g., cesarean incision). Aloe latex may cause severe intestinal cramps or diarrhea.

■ **Warnings/Contraindications/Precautions**

Pregnant or nursing mothers should not ingest aloe latex. It may cause uterine contractions and trigger miscarriage. Contraindicated for gastrointestinal illness, intestinal obstruction, appendicitis, and abdominal pain of unknown origin. May aggravate ulcers, hemorrhoids, diverticulosis, diverticulitis, colitis, and irritable bowel syndrome. If taken over a long time, can cause dependence or disturbance of electrolyte balance. May cause urine to turn a harmless red color. Should not be used for children under 12.

Interactions

Chronic use of aloe latex could cause potassium deficiency, which could interfere with cardiac glycoside and antiarrhythmic drugs. Potential for potassium deficiency is increased if used with thiazide diuretics, licorice, or corticosteroids.

Regulatory and Compendial Status

German Commission E approves aloe latex for chronic constipation, with certain reservations.

References

Blitz JJ, et al. Aloe vera gel in peptic ulcer therapy: preliminary report. *J Am Osteopath Assoc.* 1963;62:731–735.

Blumenthal M, ed. *The Complete German Commission E Monographs.* Boston, Mass: Integrative Medicine Communications. 1998.

Castleman M. *The Healing Herbs.* New York, NY: Bantam Books. 1991.

Danhof I. Potential benefits from orally-injested internal aloe vera gel. International Aloe Science Council Tenth Annual Aloe Scientific Semina; 1991; Irving, Texas.

Duke J. *The Green Pharmacy.* Emmaus, Penn: Rodale Press. 1997.

Fahim MS, Wang M. Zinc acetate and lyophilized *Aloe barbadensis* as vaginal contraceptive. *Contraception.* 1996;53:231–236.

Fulton JE Jr. The stimulation of postdermabrasion wound healing with stabilized aloe vera gel-polyethylene oxide dressing. *J Dermatol Surg Onco.* 1990;16:460.

Grindlay D, Reynolds T. The aloe vera phenomenon: a review of the properties and modern uses of the leaf parenchyma gel. *J Ethnopharmacol.* 1986;16:117–151.

Gruenwald J, Brendler T, Jaenicke C et al, eds. *PDR for Herbal Medicines.* Montvale, NJ: Medical Economics Company. 1998.

Heggers J, et al. Beneficial effects of aloe in wound healing. *Phytother Res.* 1993;7:S48–S52.

Murray M, Pizzorno J. *Encyclopedia of Natural Medicine.* Rocklin, Calif: Prima Publishing. 1991.

Murray M. *Healing Power of Herbs.* Rocklin, Calif: Prima Publishing. 1995.

Newall C, et al. *Herbal Medicines.* London, England: Pharmaceutical Press. 1996.

Plemmons JM, et al. Evaluation of acemannan in the treatment of aphthous stomatitis. *Wounds.*1994;6.

Saoo K, et al. Antiviral activity of aloe extracts against cytomegalovirus. *Phytother Res.* 1996;10:348–350.

Schmidt JM, Greenspoon JS. Aloe vera dermal wound gel is associated with a delay in wound healing. *Ostet Gynecol.* 1991;78(1).

Shida, T. et al. 1985. Effect of aloe extract on peripheral phagocytosis in adult bronchial asthma. Planta Med 51.

Schmidt JM, Greenspoon JS. Aloe vera dermal wound gel is associated with a delay in wound healing. *Ostet Gynecol.* 1991;78(1).

Syed TA, et al. Management of psoriasis with aloe vera extract in a hydrophilic cream: a placebo-controlled, double-blind study. *Trop Med Int Health.* 1996;1:505–509.

Tyler V. *The Honest Herbal.* New York, NY: Pharmaceutical Products Press. 1993.

Vazquez B, et al. Anti-inflammatory activity of extracts from aloe vera gel. *J Ethnopharmacol.* 1996;55:69–75.

© *Copyright Integrative Medicine Communications*

Barberry

Names

- **English**
  Barberry/Barberry bark/Barberry root/Barberry root bark

- **Botanical**
  Berberis vulgaris

- **Plant Family**
  Berberidaceae

- **Pharmacopeial**
  Berberis vulgaris/Berberidis cortex/Berberidis radix/Berberidis radicis cortex

Overview

In traditional folk medicine, barberry soothes sore throats, treats diarrhea or constipation, and eases inflammation and infection of the urinary, gastrointestinal, and respiratory tracts. It may reduce the discomfort of arthritis and rheumatism, soothe psoriasis, and treat chronic yeast infections. These uses reflect barberry's reputation as an herbal antibiotic.

Sought after as an alternative to goldenseal (a once-endangered botanical regarded as "king" of herbal antibiotics by some individuals), barberry and other herbs with similar constituents (e.g. berberine) and actions are termed mucous membrane tonics and adaptogens by herbalists. Mucous membrane tonics regulate the flow of mucous; they may increase or decrease mucous secretion. Adaptogens also allow immune factors already present within the body to stimulate antibacterial responses during illness.

The study of barberry's isoquinoline alkaloid constituents has overshadowed study of the plant as a whole. These constituents are potentially therapeutic, with bactericidal, smooth muscle, and cardiovascular effects.

Barberry was used in ancient Egypt to prevent the plague, during the middle ages in Europe as a purgative and antiseptic, and by Native Americans as tea to stimulate the appetite. It has other uses as well; the yellow color of the root and inner bark provide a semi-colorfast clothing dye, and the berries can be made into jam or sugared for cake decorations.

Macro Description

Deciduous shrub grows to nine feet. Branches, gray, bear thorns. Leaves alternate or in rosette formation, can be various colors, spiny teeth, four to five leaves per branch. Flowers, bright yellow, in $2^{1}/_{2}$ inch racemes, bloom April to June. The berries are red and grow in drooping bunches. Inner bark is yellow.

The bark of the stem and root, and the root itself, are used medicinally. Traditionally, the berries were also used as a tonic in tea, but they do not contain isoquinoline alkaloids and are more closely associated with culinary use. Barberry grows in the northeastern United States, particularly in New England, and is native to Europe.

Part Used/Pharmaceutical Designations

- Roots
- Berry
- Root bark
- Stem bark

- **Constituents/Composition**
  Isoquinoline alkaloids berberine, berbamine, oxyacanthine, jatrorrhizine, columbamine, palmatine, magnoflorine; also, resin, tannins

- **Commercial Preparations**
  Crude bark for tea or powdered in capsules; aqueous alcohol or alcohol extracts available as 1:5 tinctures or standardized fluid extracts (standardized to 8% to 12% isoquinoline alkaloids); ointment

Medicinal Uses/Indications

- Traditional: Berry as tea, diuretic, expectorant, laxative, appetite stimulant; root bark and bark as tea, anti-inflammatory, diaphoretic, astringent, antiseptic, laxative, bitter tonic, alterative (blood purifier), cholagogue (liver stimulant that promotes bile excretion)
- Conditions: chronic diarrhea, dysentery, indigestion, eye ailments, mouth sores, jaundice, hepatitis, fever, hemorrhage, arthritis, rheumatism, low back pain, stomach bacterial infections, *H. pylori*
- Clinical applications (listed as "unapproved" in German Commission E monograph): Inflammation/infection of the kidneys and urinary, bronchial, and gastrointestinal tracts; liver, spleen, and circulatory disorders; spasms; and chronic candidiasis

- **Pharmacology**

Herbalists provide much of the information available on the usage and effects of whole barberry rootbark and bark preparations. While these sources often corroborate empirical results of barberry use, scientific study tends to focus on determining the scope and application of the bactericidal activity of the isoquinoline alkaloid constituents. At least one study demonstrated superior anti-inflammatory actions of whole barberry extract, compared to single constituents. By using tissue or bacterial cultures and single alkaloid preparations, researchers have determined antimicrobial, bactericidal, anti-inflammatory, immune-stimulant, hypotensive, antifibrillatory, antiarrhythmic, sedative, anticonvulsant and smooth muscle effects.

Berberine has in vitro antibacterial activity. Actions against *Staphylococcus, spp., Streptomyces, spp., Chlamydia, spp., Corynebacterium diphtheria, Escherichia coli, Salmonella typhi, Vibrio cholerae, Diplococcus pneumoniae, Pseudomonas, spp., Shigella dysenteriae, Entamoeba histolytica, Trichomonas vaginalis, Neisseria gonorrhoeae, N. menengitidis, Treponema palidum, Giardia lamblia, Leishmania donovani,* and *Candida albicans* may be due to adhesion blockage of the streptococci to host cells through the depletion of lipoteichoic acid and fibronectin. In other studies berberine raised blood flow to the spleen; reduced fever, possibly by altering interferon response to microorganisms; stimulated bile secretion; altered bilirubin levels; inhibited brain tumor cells in rats; and was superior to sulfacetaminde against *Chlamydia trachomatis*.

In vitro studies demonstrate that oxyacanthine dilates blood vessels, modulates adrenaline, and is bactericidal to *Bacillus subtilis, Colpidium colpoda*. Palmatine is antiarrhythmic, adrenocorticotrophic, analgesic, and bactericidal. Jatrorrhizine is sedating, hypotensive, and fungicidal. In animal studies, one experiment showed a berbamine-induced immune response in mice with influenza.

These actions have not been scientifically demonstrated to occur in the human body. Berberine absorption in the small intestine is poor, and large doses obtained through excess intake of berberine-containing plant preparations cause negative side effects on the stomach and small intestines. However, because it is excreted through the urine, it may have antibiotic actions specific to that area of the body. This remains to be proven, but concurs with traditional use.

Dosage Ranges and Duration of Administration

For throat, urinary, gastrointestinal, respiratory inflammation or infection, including chronic candidiasis, any of the following can be taken for five to seven days.

- Tea: 2 to 4 g steeped dried root tid
- Tincture (1:5): 3 to 6 ml tid
- Dry extracts: 250 to 500 mg tid

For skin disorders: 10% extract of barberry in ointment, applied topically tid

Cautions

- **Adverse Effects/Toxicology**

American Herbal Products Association safety rating: 2b. Safe with appropriate use, but do not use during pregnancy. Due to a lack of scientific documentation of barberry's purported therapeutic uses, the German Commission E monograph lists barberry as an unapproved herb.

Barberry root and root bark preparations have not caused any of the toxic effects noted with excessive or lethal doses of berberine. (At doses higher than 0.5 g, berberine causes lethargy, nose bleeds, difficulty breathing, skin and eye irritation, kidney irritation, nausea, vomiting, diarrhea. Small doses stimulate respiratory system, large doses lead to respiratory paralysis. Lethal doses cause hemorrhagic nephritis.)

- **Warnings/Contraindications/Precautions**

Overconsumption of berberine-containing plant medicines may irritate mucous membranes, particularly in the stomach. Do not use during pregnancy.

Interactions

Excess berberine intake may interfere with B vitamin assimilation.

Regulatory and Compendial Status

In the United States, barberry is a dietary supplement; in Germany the Commission E does not approve therapeutic use due to lack of scientific documentation of effects.

References

Amin AH, Subbaiah, TV, Abbasi KM. Berberine sulfate: antimicrobial activity, bioassay, and mode of action. *Can J Microbiol.* 1969;15:1067–1076.

Bergner P. Goldenseal and the common cold; goldenseal substitutes. *Medical Herbalism: A Journal for the Clinical Practitioner.* Winter 1996–1997;8:1.

Blumenthal M, ed. *The Complete German Commission E Monographs.* Boston, Mass: Integrative Medicine Communications; 1998.

Foster S, Duke JA. *A Field Guide to Medicinal Plants: Eastern and Central North America.* Boston, Mass: Houghton Mifflin; 1990.

Harborn J, Baxter H. *Phytochemical Dictionary: A Handbook of Bioactive Compounds from Plants.* Washington DC: Taylor & Francis; 1993.

Ivanovska N, Philipov S. Study on the antiinflammatory action of *Berberis vulgaris* root extract, alkaloid fractions, and pure alkaloids. *Int J Immunopharmacol.* 1996;18:552–561.

Kowalchik C, Hylton W, eds. *Rodale's Illustrated Encyclopedia of Herbs.* Emmaus Pa: Rodale Press; 1998.

Leung A, Foster S. *Encyclopedia of Common Natural Ingredients Used in Food, Drugs, and Cosmetics.* 2nd ed. New York, NY: John Wiley & Sons; 1996.

McGuffin M, Hobbs C, Upton R, Goldberg A. *American Herbal Products Associations's Botanical Safety Handbook.* Boca Raton, Fla: CRC Press; 1996.

Muller K, et al. The antipsoriatic Mahonia aquifolium and its active constituents; I. Pro- and antioxidant properties and inhibition of 5-lipoxygenase. *Planta Med.* 1994;60:421–424.

Murray M. *The Healing Power of Herbs: the Enlightened Person's Guide to the Wonders of Medicinal Plants.* Rocklin, Calif: Prima Publishing; 1995.

Murray M, Pizzorno J. *Encyclopedia of Natural Medicine.* 2nd ed. Rocklin, Calif: Prima Publishing; 1998:310.

Shamsa F, et al. Antihistaminic and anticholinergic activity of barberry fruit (*Berberis vulgaris*) in the guinea-pig ileum. *J Ethnopharmacol.* 1999;64:161–166.

Sotnikova R, et al. Relaxant properties of some aporphine alkaloids from Mahonia aquifolium. *Methods Find Exp Clin Pharmacol.* 1997;19:589–597.

Sun D, Courtney HS, Beachey EH. Berberine sulfate blocks adherence of Streptococcus pyogenes to epithelial cells, fibronectin, and hexadecane. Antimicrob Agents Chemother. 1988;32:1370–1374.

© *Copyright Integrative Medicine Communications*

Bilberry

Names

- **English**
  Bilberry

- **Botanical**
  Vaccinium myrtillus

- **Plant Family**
  Ericaceae

- **Pharmacopeial**
  Myrtilli fructus/Myrtilli folium

Overview

In World War II British pilots noticed that eating bilberries or bilberry preserves before flying nightly bombing raids improved their vision. Since then, studies have shown that bilberry contains more than 15 different anthocyanosides, flavonoid compounds that not only improve visual acuity, but are important for the treatment of many eye disorders, including cataracts, macular degeneration, diabetic retinopathy, and night blindness. A botanical relative of blueberry, cranberry, and huckleberry, the anthocyanosides in bilberry are also known for their ability to stabilize collagen, rebuild capillaries, inhibit platelet aggregation, reduce hyperglycemia, relax smooth muscle, and increase gastric mucus. Dried bilberry fruit is rich in tannins and pectin, making it an effective treatment for diarrhea, both historically and in modern day European usage.

Bilberry extract contains the highest percentage of anthocyanidin content (25% compared to 0.1% to 0.25% in fresh fruit), making it the most effective means of treatment. This extract improves the delivery of oxygen and blood to the eyes, the maintenance of which is necessary to prevent cataracts and macular degeneration. The extract is also a powerful antioxidant, preventing free radical damage that can cause cataracts and macular degeneration and lead to cancer and heart disease. Bilberry extract's ability to stabilize and strengthen collagen protects the integrity of the eye tissue against glaucoma. The anthocyanosides also strengthen the area of the retina that controls vision and the adaptation between dark and light, improving poor night vision and poor day vision in particular.

The ability of bilberry extract to strengthen capillaries not only protects the eye from the hemorrhaging associated with diabetic retinopathy, but also makes it an important aid for other vascular disorders as well. Because this strengthening power is combined with the ability to reduce platelet aggregation, the extract may help prevent ischemic stroke without risking hemorrhagic stroke. It is also very effective for varicose veins and hemorrhoids and helps reduce the risk of arteriosclerosis. As an antioxidant, bilberry is able to raise the levels of intracellular vitamin C, which increases the protection to the capillary walls, improving circulation. The collagen stabilizing, antioxidant, and anti-inflammatory properties of the extract make it very helpful for treatment of arthritis.

Bilberry leaves have been used historically to treat diabetes mellitus by lowering blood glucose levels, an ability that may be related to their chromium content. Use of bilberry extract to prevent and improve diabetic retinopathy is documented. These uses are not approved, however, by the German Commission E, which refers to a lack of documented evidence for bilberry leaves' efficacy.

Anthocyanosides help protect against ulcers by stimulating mucus flow that protects the stomach lining from digestive acids. Their ability to relax smooth muscle is thought to relieve dysmenorrhea as well.

Macro Description

Deciduous shrub, grows to 16 inches. Stems are multibranched and erect; leaves are pointed and oval; flowers are small, pink, and white; berries are round and purple-black when ripe. Native to Europe, Asia, and North America. Flowers from April through June. Fruit collected July through September.

Part Used/Pharmaceutical Designations

- Fruit

- **Constituents/Composition**
  Catechins, invertose, flavonone glycosides, and anthocyanosides (particularly glycosides of malvidin, cyanidin, and delphinidin).

- **Commercial Preparations**
  Fresh or dried berries; tea made from dried leaves or dried berries; bilberry extract (standardized for 25% anthocyanidin)

Medicinal Uses/Indications

Traditional herbal actions: antioxidant, stimulates gastric mucus, breaks down plaque deposits on arterial walls, strengthens capillary walls and causes new capillary formation, vasodilator, reduces platelet aggregation, astringent, antidiarrheal, muscle relaxant, membrane and collagen stabilizing, anti-inflammatory, vascular tonic

Clinical applications: eye disorders (poor night and day vision, cataracts, glaucoma, diabetic retinopathy, macular degeneration), ulcers, ischemic stroke, angina, diarrhea, dysmenorrhea, circulation, rheumatoid arthritis, varicose veins, hemorrhoids, circulation problems, vascular disorders, diabetes, capillary fragility

- **Pharmacology**
  Research on the pharmacology of the bilberry has focused primarily on its anthocyanoside content. Anthocyanosides strengthen and protect collagen by reinforcing its natural matrix, preventing free radical damage, and inhibiting cleavage caused by inflammation and the release of compounds that cause inflammation (e.g., histamine). This protects tissue from secondary damage from inflammation and aids the regeneration of new tissue after injury.

Anthocyanosides build and strengthen capillaries by increasing intracellular vitamin C levels and decreasing capillary permeability. This aids the circulation of blood to connective tissue in the body, promoting healing after injury or damage from inflammation. Stronger capillaries prevent hemorrhage, such as the eye damage caused by diabetic retinopathy. Anthocyanosides also improve circulation in the larger arteries and veins, reducing platelet aggregation, which aids in the treatment of vascular disorders, such as varicose veins, hemorrhoids, and atherosclerosis. As well as improving circulation and blood flow in the eyes, anthocyanosides also increase the regeneration of rhodopsin in the retina. This purple pigment is crucial to the optimal functioning of the rods, cells that are important for night vision and light adaptation.

The tannins in dried bilberry are effective for treating nonspecific, acute diarrhea. Tannins act as astringents, reducing intestinal inflammation by thickening the surface protein layer of the mucous membrane. This slows the secretion process and protects against resorption of toxins. Germany's Commission E has officially recognized and positively evaluated bilberry fruit, but not bilberry leaf, for nonprescription and clinical applications.

Dosage Ranges and Duration of Administration

- For eye conditions and circulation: standardized bilberry extract (with 25% anthocyanidin) in encapsulated form, dose of 480 mg/day in two to three divided dosages. After improvement, maintenance dose of 240 mg/day for prevention.
- For dysmenorrhea or ulcer prevention: 20 to 40 mg extract tid, 1/2 cup of fresh bilberries (difficult to acquire in the U.S.), or tincture (1: 5) 2 to 4 ml tid.
- For diarrhea: 5 to 10 g crushed dried bilberry in cold water, brought to a boil for 10 minutes, then strained.
- For diabetes mellitus: Pour boiling water over 1 g (approximately $1^{1}/_{2}$ tsp.) bilberry leaf, and strain after 10 to 15 minutes. Do not continue use for long duration.

Cautions

- **Adverse Effects/Toxicology**
  There are no side effects or toxicity associated with bilberry fruit or extract. Prolonged overuse of bilberry leaf may result in severe hydroquinone poisoning, which, with continued chronic use, could be fatal.

- **Warnings/Contraindications/Precautions**
  There are no known contraindications for bilberry fruit or extract. Its use is not contraindicated during pregnancy or lactation. Prolonged overuse of bilberry leaves could result in chronic intoxication or death.

Regulatory and Compendial Status

In Germany, Commission E has approved the use of bilberry fruit and extract for treatment of diarrhea and inflammation of the mouth. Commission E has not approved therapeutic use of bilberry leaves, because efficacy has not been documented.

References

Blumenthal M, ed. *The Complete German Commission E Monographs.* Boston, Mass: Integrative Medicine Communications; 1998.

Bomser J, et al. In vitro anti-cancer activity of fruit extracts from *Vaccinium species. Planta Med.* 1996;62:212–216.

Brown D. *Herbal Prescriptions for Better Health.* Rocklin, Calif: Prima Publishing; 1996.

Detre Z, Jellinek H, Miskulin R. Studies on vascular permeability in hypertension. *Clin Physiol Bichem.* 1986;4:143–149.

Duke J. *The Green Pharmacy.* Emmaus, Pa: Rodale Press; 1997.

Gruenwald J, Brendler T, Jaenicke C et al, eds. *PDR for Herbal Medicines.* Montvale, NJ: Medical Economics Company Inc; 1998.

Havsteen B. Flavonoids, a class of natural products of high pharmacological potency. *Biochem Pharmacol.* 1983;32:1141–1148.

Morazzoni P, Bombardelli E. *Vaccinium myrtillus L. Fitoterapia.* 1996;LXVII:3–29.

Murray M. *The Healing Power of Herbs.* Rocklin, Calif: Prima Publishing; 1995.

Orsucci, PL. et al. Treatment of diabetic retinopthy with anthocyanosides: a preliminary report. *Clin Oc.* 1983;5:377.

Perossini M, et al. Diabetic and Hypertensive retinopathy therapy with Vaccinium myrtillus anthocyanosides (Tegens): Double blind placebo controlled clinical trial. *Annali di Ottalmaologia e Clinica Ocaulistica.* 1987;CXII.

Schulz V et al. *Rational Phytotherapy.* Berlin, Germany: Springer-Verlag; 1998.

Tyler V. *Herbs of Choice.* New York, NY: Haworth Press Inc; 1994.

© *Copyright Integrative Medicine Communications*

Black Cohosh

Names

- **English**
  Black Cohosh

- **Botanical**
  Cimicifuga racemosa

- **Plant Family**
  Ranunculaceae

- **Pharmacopeial**
  Cimicifugae racemosae rhizoma

Overview

Black cohosh *(Cimicifuga racemosa)* is a native American plant whose roots may provide a safe alternative to synthetic hormones in treating menopause and other female reproductive symptoms. The botanical has been widely used for more than 40 years in Europe and is approved by the German Commission E for premenstrual discomfort, dysmenorrhea, and menopausal symptoms. Black cohosh is sometimes called "black snakeroot," "bugbane," "bugwort," or "squawroot."

Although physicians widely recommend hormone replacement therapy (HRT) for menopause, only 10% to 20% of menopausal women take it. Only half of patients who receive prescriptions for HRT have them filled and fewer than 40% of those who start HRT are still taking it a year later. The primary reason women avoid HRT is fear of breast cancer. While shying away from conventional hormone treatment, Americans are embracing alternative therapies. One in three uses botanicals, herbals, or other alternative treatments at some time.

In a German study involving 629 female patients, black cohosh improved physical and psychological menopausal symptoms in more than 80% of the subjects within six to eight weeks. The botanical was well tolerated, with only 7% of patients reporting mild, transient stomach upset. A double-blind study of 60 patients showed that black cohosh relieved menopausal depression and anxiety better than both conjugated estrogens and diazepam (Valium®). Patients taking black cohosh also exhibited greater increases in the number of superficial cells in the vaginal lining. The number of daily hot flashes dropped from an average of five to fewer than one in the black cohosh group. The estrogen group reported a decrease from 5 to 3.5. More than 80% of the women taking black cohosh also reported improvements in tinnitus, heart palpitations, vertigo, and headaches.

Another significant benefit black cohosh offers over synthetic estrogen is that it does not stimulate the growth of estrogen-dependent, breast cancer cells. In vitro studies suggest it may actually inhibit growth of these cells. Studies of Remifemin brand black cohosh have shown that it enhances the effects of tamoxifen in preventing a recurrence of breast cancer.

Black cohosh relieves menopausal symptoms by suppressing the secretion of luteinizing hormone (LH) and lessening its ability to bind with receptors in the hypothalamus. Sudden bursts of LH cause hot flashes, heart palpitations, headaches, and thinning of the vaginal lining. Unlike synthetic estrogens, it does not affect follicle-stimulating hormone or prolactin release.

Although most studies have focused on black cohosh's effect on symptoms of menopause, it is also used to treat other ailments including arthritic inflammation, mild hypertension, respiratory congestion, rheumatoid arthritis, sciatica, osteoarthritis, tinnitus, muscular and neurological pain, and nervous conditions.

Macro Description

Black cohosh is a member of the buttercup family. It is a hardy perennial that grows in the shady woodlands of the United States and Canada. It grows up to five feet tall, and has a stout black rhizome and straight, dark brown roots. Small white flowers sprout from long, feathery racemes in June and July. The rhizome and roots are harvested in the fall.

Part Used/Pharmaceutical Designations

- Roots
- Rhizome

- **Constituents/Composition**
  Cimicifugin (macrotin) and isoflavone formononetin. Triterpene glycosides (principally the xylosides actein, cimicifugoside, and 27-deoxyacteine), also are present in black cohosh. Other constituents are aromatic acids (including ferulic, isoferulic, and salicylic acids) tannins, resin, fatty acids, sugars, and starch.

- **Commercial Preparations**
  The unrefined dried roots and rhizome of black cohosh are odorless and have a bitter, acrid taste. Black cohosh is available over the counter in drugstores and health-food stores in several forms. The most familiar are capsules and tablets. The botanical also is available as a liquid tincture that can be mixed in water and as a dried root that's simmered in water to make a drink similar to tea. Several natural menopause treatments are made from a combination of black cohosh and other botanicals.

Medicinal Uses/Indications

Black cohosh was traditionally used as an emmenagogue, antispasmodic, ulcerative (blood purifier), sedative, and nervine tonic. Clinical applications include the following.

- Relieves symptoms of premenstrual syndrome and painful menstruation
- Diminishes physical effects of menopause including hot flashes, heart palpitations, tinnitus, vertigo, and headaches. Tinnitus may respond best to a combination of black cohosh and the botanical Ginkgo biloba
- Eases menopause's psychological effects including depression, nervousness, and irritability
- Increases the number of superficial cells in the vaginal lining, which diminishes dryness and discomfort
- Reduces inflammation associated with arthritis and rheumatism.
- Slightly lowers arterial blood pressure by decreasing constriction of peripheral blood vessels
- Acts as an expectorant by increasing blood flow to the lungs and thinning respiratory mucus

It is unknown whether black cohosh mimics synthetic estrogen's tendency to lessen the risk of osteoporosis and heart disease.

- **Pharmacology**
  Black cohosh's estrogenic activity is associated with cimicifugin (macrotin) and the isoflavone formononetin. The botanical's antihypertensive effect is associated with actein. Ferulic and isoferulic acids give black cohosh its anti-inflammatory properties.

Dosage Ranges and Duration of Administration

The recommended dose is 40 mg per day of the crude drug. The following doses should be taken tid.

- Powdered root or as tea: 1 to 2 g
- Fluid extract (1:1): 4 ml (1 tsp.)
- Solid (dry powdered) extract (4:1): 250 to 500 ml

The following dose should be taken bid.

- Remifemin brand tablets of equivalent (containing one mg of 27-deoxyacteine per tablet): two tablets. The German Commission E had recommended administration be limited to six months. The recommendation was made before recent toxicology studies on rats, which suggest black cohosh is safe for long-term use. The U.S. FDA regulates black cohosh as a dietary supplement, providing no guidelines for dosage or duration.

Cautions

- **Adverse Effects/Toxicology**

- Rats given approximately nine times the therapeutic daily dose of two mg of 27-deoxyacteine for six months displayed no teratogenic, mutagenic, or carcinogenic effects.
- Mild gastrointestinal symptoms are the most common side effects. They include nausea, vomiting, diarrhea, and abdominal pain. Other side effects include dizziness, visual dimness, headaches, tremors, joint pain, and bradycardia.
- Although the six-month rat study attempted to replicate long-term human effects, long-term human studies have not been done.

Warnings/Contraindications/Precautions

Black cohosh is contraindicated in pregnancy, particularly during the first two trimesters because overdose may lead to premature birth. However, the botanical is often used late in pregnancy to stimulate labor. No data is available to support the use of black cohosh in women who are breastfeeding. The Germany Commission E lists no contraindications in the use of black cohosh. The botanical is appropriate for patients not suited for HRT including those with a history of breast cancer, unexplained uterine bleeding, liver and gallbladder disease, pancreatitis, endometriosis, uterine fibroids, and fibrocystic breast disease. Do not confuse black cohosh with blue cohosh, a botanical with similar properties, but less data on safety and efficacy.

Interactions

Black cohosh taken with oral contraceptives or synthetic estrogen may intensify the side effects of those drugs.

Regulatory and Compendial Status

Black cohosh has been approved by the German Commission E for the treatment of prementrual discomfort, dysmenorrhea, and menopause discomforts.

References

Beuscher N. *Cimicifuga racemosa* L. Black Cohosh. *Z Phytotherapie.* 1995;16:301–310.

Blumenthal M, ed. *The Complete German Commission E Monographs: Therapeutic Guide to Herbal Medicines.* Boston, Mass: Integrative Medicine Communications; 1998.

Daiber W. Climacteric Complaints: success without using hormones. *rztliche Praxis.* 1983;35:1946–1947.

Lieberman S. A review of the effectiveness of *Cimicifuga racemosa* (black cohosh) for the symptoms of monopause. *J Womens Health.* 1998;5:525–529.

Murray MT, Pizzorno J. *Encyclopedia of Natural Medicine.* Rocklin, Calif: Prima Publishing; 1998.

Newall CA, Anderson LA, Phillipson DJ. *Herbal Medicines: A Guide for Health-Care Professionals.* London, England: The Pharmaceutical Press; 1996.

Ringer DL, ed. *Physicians' Guide to Nutriceuticals.* Omaha, Neb: Nutritional Data Resources LP; 1998.

Schulz V, Hnsel R, Tyler VE. *Rational Phytotherapy.* Berlin, Germany: Springer-Verlag; 1998.

Stoll W. Phytopharmacon influences atrophic vaginal epithelium: Double blind-study-cimicifuga vs. estrogenic substances. *Therapeuticum.* 1987;1:23–31.

Taylor M. Alternatives to Hormone Replacement Therapy. *Comprehensive Therapy.* 1997;23:514–532.

Tyler VE. *Herbs of Choice: The Therapeutic Use of Phytomedicinals.* New York, NY: Pharmaceutical Products Press; 1994.

Warnecke G. Influencing menopausal symptoms with a phytotherapeutic agent: successful therapy with *Cimicifuga* mono-extract. *Med Welt.* 1985;36:871–874.

© Copyright Integrative Medicine Communications

Burdock

Names

- **English**
  Burdock

- **Botanical**
  Arctium lappa/Arctium minus/Arctium tomentosum

- **Plant Family**
  Asteraceae

- **Pharmacopeial**
  Bardanae radix

Overview

During the Middle Ages, burdock was valued for treating a host of ailments. English herbalists even preferred burdock root over sarsaparilla in remedies for boils, scurvy, and rheumatism. Burdock played an important role in Native American medical botany, and American herbalists have used the roots and seeds of this plant for two centuries.

Burdock root is traditionally classified as an alterative (blood purifier) and analgesic. It also acts as a diaphoretic (promoting profuse perspiration). While the leaf and root have similar pharmacological properties, most herbal remedies call for burdock root.

Burdock root is listed in the *Eclectic Materia Medica*, the *U.S. Pharmacopoeia*, and the official pharmacopoeia of several other countries. The root is used in remedies for arthritis, gout, and related inflammatory conditions. Diuretics are made from powdered burdock seeds, which yield a yellow bland fixed product called oil of lappa.

Macro Description

Burdock is a biennial common weed native to Europe and northern Asia, but now widespread throughout the United States. A member of the thistle family, it is a stout, dull pale-green plant with many spreading branches. It reaches a height of three to four feet, and its purple flowers bloom between June and October. Burdock has alternate, wavy, heart-shaped leaves that are green on the top and whitish on the bottom. The deep roots are brownish-green, or nearly black on the outside.

This plant is rarely cultivated because it easily flourishes in the wild, and it grows optimally in light, well-drained soils. The leaves are collected during the first year of growth. The roots are harvested in the fall of the first year (or in the following spring before the flowers bloom), and then air-dried.

Part Used/Pharmaceutical Designations

- Leaves
- Roots (rhizome)
- Whole herb

- **Constituents/Composition**
  Sesquiterpene lactones; polyynes (mainly trideca-1,11-dien-3,5,7,9-tetrain); caffeic acid derivatives (including chlorogenic acid, isochlorogenic acid); carbohydrates (45% to 50% inulin [fructosan], mucilages); volatile oil of complex composition (phenylacetaldehyde, benzaldehyde, 2-alkyl-3-methoxypyrazines); phytosterols, tannins.

- **Commercial Preparations**
  Commercial preparations are made from the fresh or dried underground parts (usually from Arctium lappa but sometimes from the related species Arctium minus and/or Arctium tomentosum).

Medicinal Uses/Indications

Burdock was historically used for pulmonary catarrh, arthritis and rheumatic conditions, scurvy, and venereal eruptions. It was externally applied for skin problems and applied to the forehead and soles to lessen symptoms of fever.

Burdock's traditional herbal actions are alterative, diuretic, laxative, digestive bitter, cholagogue, lymphatic cleanser, and diaphoretic. Herbalists use burdock root and leaves as a poultice for infected wounds and pimples, and it has traditionally been used as a part of blends for cancer therapy such as the Essiac formula. Herbalists warn that large doses can precipitate skin eruptions, headache, and aching joints due to excessive elimination.

Today, burdock is clinically used for a variety of skin problems, including psoriasis, eczema, contact dermatitis, skin eruptions (particularly on the head and neck), osteo and rheumatoid arthritis, and gout.

- **Pharmacology**
  Investigations conducted in the mid-1940s indicated that burdock leaf is active against gram-negative bacteria. While burdock root has only shown antibacterial activity against gram-negative strains, the leaf and flower exhibited anti-bacterial effects against both gram-negative and gram-positive strains. The roots and leaves have antifuruncalous effects and are used to treat furuncles, or boils.

Burdock reportedly has hypoglycemic properties, but the findings are contradictory. In one study, burdock extract produced a prolonged reduction in blood-sugar concentration accompanied by a rise in carbohydrate tolerance. However, in another investigation, burdock actually aggravated the diabetic condition in streptozotocin diabetic mice. In this study, burdock adversely affected parameters of glucose homeostasis, including basal glucose, basal insulin, insulin-induced hypoglycemia, and pancreatic insulin concentration.

In an in vivo experiment, both fresh and boiled burdock plant juice significantly lowered 7,12-dimethylbenz[a]anthracene (DMBA)-induced chromosome aberrations in rat bone marrow cells. DMBA usually produces chromosome aberrations of gaps and breaks, and only rarely causes more serious chromosome damage in the form of exchanges. Burdock suppressed the incidence of DMBA-induced aberrant metaphase cells (excluding cells with gaps). This suggests that burdock may block the onset of chemically induced carcinogenesis. In another investigation, burdock decreased the mutagenicity caused by *Salmonella* mutagens and toxins (both S9-metabolic-activating and non–S9-metabolic activating mutagens).

Dosage Ranges and Duration of Administration

Recommended dosage:

- Dried root 2 to 6 g in decoction tid
- Tincture (1:5) 8 to 12 ml tid
- Fluid extract (1:1) 2 to 6 ml tid
- Tea: 2 to 6 g in 500 ml water

Cautions

- **Adverse Effects/Toxicology**
  Adverse side effects have been reported for an isolated case of a patient taking burdock. However, experts eventually concluded that the adverse reaction was not due to burdock, but instead to contamination from solanaceous alkaloids (probably in belladonna leaf).

- **Warnings/Contraindications/Precautions**
  According to the German Commission E, there are no known risks associated with the use of burdock. However, skin contact with burdock root has the potential for sensitization. There is a very slight risk of contact dermatitis when using burdock root plasters. Burdock should not be taken by pregnant and lactating women since this plant has in vivo uterine stimulant effects. As a general precaution, excessive amounts of burdock root should not be consumed because the toxicology of this plant is not well understood.

Interactions

Excessive intake of burdock may interfere with hypoglycemic (antidiabetic) medications.

Regulatory and Compendial Status

The U.S. FDA classifies burdock as a dietary supplement. The root and leaf are on the General Sale List, Schedule 1, Table A [R1a] in the UK. Burdock root is sold as a nonpresription drug in France and Germany.

References

Blumenthal M, ed. *The Complete German Commission E Monographs.* Therapeutic Guide to Herbal Medicines. Boston, Mass: Integrative Medicine Communications; 1998:318.

Bradley P, ed. *British Herbal Compendium.* Dorset, England: British Herbal Medicine Association; 1992:1:46–49.

British Herbal Pharmacopoeia. 4th ed. Dorset, England: British Herbal Medicine Association; 1996:47–49.

De Smet PAGM, Keller K, Hnsel R, Chandler RF, eds. *Adverse Effects of Herbal Drugs.* Berlin, Germany: Springer-Verlag; 1997:231–237.

Dombradi CA, et al. Screening report on the antitumor activity of purified *Arctium Lappa* extracts. *Tumori.* 1966;52:173–175.

Grases F, et al. Urolithiasis and phytotherapy. *Int Urol Nephrol.* 1994;26:507–511.

Grieve M. *A Modern Herbal.* New York, NY: Dover; 1971:1:143–145.

Gruenwald J, Brendler T, Jaenicke C. *PDR for Herbal Medicines.* Montvale, NJ: Medical Economics Company; 1998:656–657

Hutchens A. *Indian Herbalogy of North America.* Boston, Mass: Shambhala Publications; 1991:62–65.

Ito Y, et al. Suppression of 7,12-dimethylbenz(a)anthracene-induced chromosome aberrations in rat bone marrow cells by vegetable juices. *Mutat Res.* 1986;172:55–60.

Lapinina L, Sisoeva T. Investigation of some plants to determine their sugar lowering action. *Farmatevt Zh.* 1964;19:52–58.

Lin CC, et al. Anti-inflammatory and radical scavenge effects of *Arctium lappa. Am J Chin Med.* 1996;24:127–137.

Millspaugh C. *American Medicinal Plants.* New York, NY: Dover Publications; 1974: 360–362.

Mowry D. *The Scientific Validation of Herbal Medicine.* New Canaan, Conn: Keats Publishing; 1986:3–6, 57–63.

Newall C, Anderson L, Phillipson J. *Herbal Medicines: A Guide for Health-care Professionals.* London, England: Pharmaceutical Press; 1996:52–53.

Swanston-Flatt SK, Day C, Flatt PR, Gould BJ, Bailey CJ. Glycaemic effects of traditional European plant treatments for diabetes. Studies in normal and streptozotocin diabetic mice. *Diabetes Res.* 1989;413:69–73.

Tyler V. *The Honest Herbal: A Sensible Guide to the Use of Herbs and Related Remedies.* 3rd ed. Binghampton, NY: Pharmaceutical Products Press; 1993:63–64.

© *Copyright Integrative Medicine Communications*

Calendula

Pot Marigold

Name

- **English**
  Calendula flower/Calendula herb

- **Botanical**
  Calendula officinalis

- **Plant Family**
  Asteraceae

- **Pharmacopeial**
  Calendulae flos/Calendulae herba

Overview

Native to southern Europe, calendula is now widespread throughout central and southern Europe, Western Asia, and the United States. This familiar garden flower has long been touted as a topical anti-infective remedy for wounds resistant to healing. Calendula is used as a therapy for a wide array of skin disorders ranging from chapped hands to lacerations.

According to the German Commission E, topical applications of calendula are safe and efficacious in decreasing inflammation and promoting granulation of wounds, burns, eczema, and other inflammatory skin conditions.

Calendula is also traditionally used to treat spasms, fever, suppressed menstruation, cancer, and a host of other ailments. Despite its varied folk medicinal uses, researchers have not been able to identify precise structure-activity relationships for the pharmacological properties of this plant.

Macro Description

Calendula is typically an annual that thrives in any soil. Its herbaceous, branching stems grow to a height of 30 to 60 cm. Its erect stem is angular, downy, and branched. A tap root averaging 20 cm in length gives off multiple, thin, secondary roots. The leaves are alternate and tomentose. Those near the ground are hairy with a spatulate base while higher-positioned leaves are smaller, with an oblong to lanceolate shape.

Calendula has a composite flowerhead situated on a well-defined green floral receptacle that crowns each stem. The inner portion of the flowerhead consists of orange-yellow, tubular florets. These ligulate florets, sometimes inappropriately called petals, are the medicinally most important part of the plant.

Part Used/Pharmaceutical Designations

- Flowers (dried flower head or dried ligulate flowers)

- **Constituents/Composition**
  Flavonoids: flavonol (isorhamnetin, quercetin) glycosides including isoquercitrin, narcissin, neohesperidoside, rutin; terpenoids, including lupeol, longispinogenin, oleanolic acid, arnidiol, brein, calenduladiol, erythrodiol, faradiol, helantriols, maniladiol, ursadiol, oleanolic acid saponins, sterols; volatile oils containing terpenoid components; bitter substance; carotenoid pigments; polysaccharides; lutein (carotenoid).

- **Commercial Preparations**
  Calendula products consist of tinctures, liquid extracts, infusions, ointments and creams. They are made from either the aerial parts or the flowers collected when the plant is flowering. The ray florets of the completely unfolded and dried capitula are used in medicinal preparations.

  Raw plant material of other genera in *Asteraceae* such as arnica and saffron are sometimes adulterated with calendula. Calendula products should be always be protected from light and moisture, and never stored for more than three years.

Medicinal Uses/Indications

External: oral and pharyngeal mucosa, wound healing, crural (leg-related) ulcers, enlarged and inflamed lymph glands, artheroma, acute and chronic skin inflammation, varicose veins, phlebitis, thrombophlebitis, dermatological conditions (wounds, furunculosis, or boils, dry dermatosis, acne, eczema, anal eczema), proctitis (rectal inflammation), conjunctivitis; also a constituent in topical preparations for dry skin, bee stings, and frostbite.

Internal: inflammatory conditions of internal organs, gastrointestinal ulcers, dysmenorrhea; liver disease, toothache, fatigued limbs, eye inflammation or degenerative eye conditions; also administered a diuretic, and diaphoretic during convulsions, fever, and obstipation (intractable constipation).

Conditions: inflammation of oral and pharyngeal mucosa; crural ulcers, skin tissue healing.

Clinical applications:

- Flower: internally for inflammation of the mouth and pharynx; externally for wounds and burns
- Herb: internally for circulatory disorders, ulcers, spasms, jaundice; externally for swelling of the hands, jaundice, wounds, eczema

- **Pharmacology**
  Calendula flower extracts have numerous pharmacological properties, including antimicrobial, antiphlogistic (treatment for fever and inflammation), immunostimulant, antitumor, estrogenic, choleretic (stimulates hepatic production of bile), and hemolytic activity.

  In an in vitro study, an organic extract of flowers from *Calendula officinalis* showed anti-HIV activity in a MTT/tetrazolium-based assay. The extract also induced a significant dose- and time-dependent decrease in HIV-1 reverse transcription activity. In other in vitro research, calendula extracts elicited an uterotonic effect in rabbit and guinea-pig preparations. Calendula also possesses trichomonacidal properties, presumably due to the terpenoid fraction of the essential oil. The volatile oil fraction has been associated with antispasmodic activity.

  Calendula extracts had antitumor activity against mouse Ehrlich carcinoma both in vitro and in vivo. The saponin-rich fraction showed the greatest amount of cytotoxic activity in vivo but not in vitro. Other research suggests that flavonoids and high molecular weight polysaccharide fractions are responsible for the immunostimulant action.

  In an in vivo study, calendula extracts exhibited topical anti-inflammatory and wound-healing activity, primarily through a mechanism involving granulatory action. In rats, calendula produced a weak anti-inflammatory effect in carrageenan-induced edema in rats. Although the constituents responsible for wound healing have not been identified, wound-healing activity is associated with a hydroalcoholic extract of calendula herb. The tissue-healing effect has been attributed to a synergism between the volatile oil and xanthophylls in calendula.

  An extract consisting of calendula and allantoin proved more efficacious than allantoin alone in promoting tissue regeneration and epithelialization of surgically induced skin wounds in rats. In other animal research, a botanical extract containing calendula was effective for burn-induced edemas and acute lymphedema. And in a clinical investigation, patients receiving a multi-plant proprietary cream containing calendula reported a decrease in post-mastectomy lymphedema-related pain. However, there were no significant clinical differences between the experimental and control groups in the reduction of edema.

  In another experiment, mice were inoculated with WAZ-2T(-SA) mammary tumor cells and then given dietary lutein extracted from calendula. Very low quantities of dietary lutein (0.002%) were more effective than higher levels in reducing mammary tumor incidence, tumor growth, and lipid peroxidation as well as in prolonging tumor latency.

Dosage Ranges and Duration of Administration

- Infusion: 1 tsp. dried florets in 8 oz. water; steep 30 to 40 minutes; drink two to three cups per day
- Fluid extract (1:1 in 40% alcohol): 0.5 to 1.0 ml tid
- Tincture (1:5 in 90% alcohol): 2 to 4 ml tid
- Ointment: 2 to 5 g crude drug in 100 g ointment

Cautions

- **Adverse Effects/Toxicology**
  Calendula is generally free of adverse side effects. However, both the flower and herb have a low potential for sensitization through frequent skin contact. Cytotoxic effects have been observed in *vitro for this plant*.

- **Warnings/Contraindications/Precautions**
  Although no major warnings are reported, calendula is known to affect the menstrual cycle. It has produced uterotonic activity in vitro presumably due to triterpenoid compounds which can act as abortive agents. In light of the limited

data on toxicology, calendula should not be used, or used with caution, during pregnancy and lactation.

Interactions

None reported.

Regulatory and Compendial Status

Commission E approves calendula flower preparations for internal use, and for external treatment of crural ulcers and poorly healing wounds.

References

Blumenthal M, ed. *The Complete German Commission E Monographs. Therapeutic Guide to Herbal Medicines.* Boston: Integrative Medicine Communications; 1998: 100.

Boucard-Maitre Y, et al. Cytotoxic and antitumoral activity if calendula officinalis extracts. *Pharmazie.* 1988; 43:220.

Casley-Smith JR. The effect of "Unguentum lymphaticum" on acute experimental lymphedema and other high-protein edemas. Lymphology. 1983; 16:150–156.

Dorland's Illustrated Medical Dictionary. 25th ed. Philadelphia: W.B. Saunders; 1974.

Fleischner AM. Plant extracts: To accelerate healing and reduce inflammation. *Cosmet Toilet.* 1985; 100:45.

Gracza L. Oxygen-containing terpene derivatives from Calendula officinalis. *Planta Med.* 1987; 53:227.

Grieve M. *A Modern Herbal.* Vol. I. New York: Dover; 1971: 517–518.

Gruenwald J, Brendler T, Christof J. *PDR for Herbal Medicines.* Montvale, NJ: Medical Economics Company; 1998: 704–706.

Isaac O. *Die Ringelblume. Botanik, Chemie, Pharmakologie, Toxikologie, Pharmazie und therapeutische Verwendung.* Wissenschaftliche Verlagsgesellschaft mbH, Stuggart; 1992.

Kalvatchev Z, Walder R, Garzaro D. Anti-HIV activity of extracts from *Calendula officinalis* flowers. *Biomed Pharmacotherapy.* 1997; 51(4):176–180.

Kioucke-Popova, et al. Influence of the physiological regeneration and epithelization using fractions isolated from Calendula officinalis. *Acta Physiol Pharmacol Bulg.* 1982; 8:83–87.

Newall C, Anderson L, Phillipson J. *Herbal Medicines: A Guide for Health-care Professionals.* London: Pharmaceutical Press; 1996: 58-59.

Park JS, Chew BP, Wong TS. Dietary lutein from marigold extract inhibits mammary tumor development in BALB/c mice. *J Nutr.* Oct 1998; 128(10):1650–1656.

Schulz V, Hansel R, Tyler V. *Rational Phytotherapy: A Physician's Guide to Herbal Medicine.* 3rd ed. Berlin: Springer; 1998: 259.

Shipochliev T. Extracts from a group of medicinal plants enhancing the uterine tonus. *Vet Med Nauki.* 1981; 4: 94–98.

Thomson WA. *Medicines from the Earth: A Guide to Healing Plants.* Alfred Van Der Marck ed. Maidenhead, England: McGraw-Hill Book company (UK); 1978: 61.

Tyler V. *The Honest Herbal: A Sensible Guide to the Use of Herbs and Related Remedies.* 3rd ed. New York: Pharmaceutical Products Press; 1993: 75–76.

Wagner H, et al. Immunostimulating polysaccharides (heteroglycans) of higher plants. *Arzneimittelforsch.* 1985; 35:1069.

© Copyright Integrative Medicine Communications

Cat's Claw

Names

- **English**
  Cat's claw

- **Botanical**
  Uncaria tomentosa

- **Plant Family**
  Rubiaceae

Overview

Used in the rainforest for over 2,000 years by indigenous tribes, cat's claw has anti-inflammatory, cytotoxic, and antiviral properties. Traditional indications include sexually-transmitted diseases, arthritis, gastritis, contraception (a reported three-year hiatus in fertility), and cancer. Purported attributes drew attention from the Westernized world: in 1997, it was on the top-ten list of herb sales in natural food stores in the U.S.

In 1989 the methods for extracting the immune-stimulant oxindole alkaloid constituents in cat's claw root bark were patented. Primarily the work of Hildebert Wagner at the Institute for Pharmaceutical Biology, Munich, and Klaus Keplinger at Innsbruck University, studies revealed that cat's claw was antiviral in the feline crown virus, the lamb Maed visna virus, human herpesvirus, and effective against neurobronchitis and allergies. Injections of the alkaloids raised T-4 lymphocyte counts, and cat's claw preparations stimulated enhanced phagocytosis, and reduced both the progression of the AIDS virus and side effects of the therapies used to treat AIDS patients. It also reduced the side effects of radiation in cancer therapy.

Today, very few studies of cat's claw in humans exist. International research institutes and manufacturing companies currently conduct studies on the pharmacokinetics and mechanisms of action for cat's claw and its isolated constituents. Results of placebo controlled, phase II trials using cat's claw in the treatment of patients with HIV and rheumatoid arthritis have not yet been published.

Macro Description

Cat's claw is a climbing shrub with woody, thick vines. Growing as high as 100 feet in the Amazon rainforest and tropical countries in South America and Central America, the vines have curved, claw-like thorns where leaves meet the stem. Inside the stem is a bitter-tasting, water-like liquid reportedly drunk as refreshment to relieve fatigue.

Two Uncaria species are called cat's claw, which are differentiated by their flowers: *U. tomentosa* has yellow-white flowers; *U. guianensis,* reddish-orange flowers. Phytochemically, *U. guinanesis* contains tetracyclic oxindoles not found in the therapeutically superior *U. tomentosa.*

The root bark is the source of medicine. Because harvesting the root destroys the plant, the inner bark of the vine may be used as well. It is unclear whether this is an equal substitute.

Part Used/Pharmaceutical Designations

- Roots
- Bark
- Vine
- Inner bark

- **Constituents/Composition**
  - Pentacyclic oxindole alkaloids (alloisopteropodine, alloteropdine, isomitraphylline, isorhynchophylline, mitraphylline, rhyncophylline)
  - Tannins (epicatechin and procyandins)
  - Quinovic acid glycosides
  - Polyhydroxilated triterpenes

- **Commercial Preparations**
  Crude bark as tea or in tablets; aqueous-alcohol extracts standardized to oxindole alkaloids, in liquid form or dried encapsulations

Medicinal Uses/Indications

Traditional: anti-inflammatory, antiviral; used for arthritis, dysentery, gastric ulcer, diabetes, cancer, menstrual disorders, convalescence, general debility, gonorrhea, cirrhoses

Conditions: acne, asthma, arthritis, bone pain, cancer, depression, fungus, fistulas, gastritis, gastric ulcer, hemorrhoids, herpes, inflammation of the urinary tract, immune system disorders, menstrual irregularities, neuralgias, rheumatism, shingles, wounds

Clinical Applications (pursuant to future research): disorders of the digestive tract; hypertension, and heart disease; HIV, AIDS, and cancers; drug or radiation side effects; allergy, herpes, shingles, arthritis, tumors, cysts, and to treat reduced physical and mental stamina

- **Pharmacology**
  Cat's claw has immune stimulant, anti-inflammatory, and antimutagenic actions.

  Pentacyclic oxindole alkaloids stimulate phagocytosis and activate T-lymphocytes and macrophages. Quinovic acid glycosides act as an antiviral against rhinovirus type 1B and vesicular stomatitis virus. The oxindoles suppress growth in tumor cell lines; five are anti-leukemic. Root and bark extracts are anti-tumor.

  In one study, mutagenic metabolites normally formed in the urine of smokers were absent following dosing with cat's claw.

  Anti-inflammatory actions may be due to the quinovic acid glycosides, which demonstrate 46% to 69% inhibition of inflammation in vivo and in vitro. The sterols beta-sitosterol, stigmasterol, and campesterol are moderately anti-inflammatory.

  Cat's claw may reduce side effects from chemotherapy, including hair loss, weight loss, nausea, secondary infections, and skin problems. Cat's claw may also have cardiovascular effects: Oxindole alkaloids rhynocophylline, hirsutime, and mitraphylline are hypotensive and vasodilative.

  Rhynophylline inhibits platelet aggregation, prevents blood clots, relaxes endothelial blood vessels, dilates peripheral blood vessels, lowers heart rate, and lowers blood cholesterol.

Dosage Ranges and Duration of Administration

Traditional use for treating conditions listed above:

- 3 to 25 g dried bark as tea or tablets
- 20 to 30 g finely chopped bark, boiled in a liter of water for 20 to 30 minutes. Take liquid tid.

Conventional use for treating mild stomach pains, sore throats, and colds; immune function; and minor injuries:

- Tea: 1 g root bark to 250 ml water, boil for 10 to 15 minutes, cool, and strain. Drink 1 cup, tid.
- Tincture: 1 to 2 ml bid to tid.
- Dry, encapsulated, standardized extract: 20 to 60 mg daily

Cautions

- **Adverse Effects/Toxicology**
  Nontoxic in traditional lore. Loose stools or diarrhea have been noted. The American Herbal Products Association (AHPA) safety rating: class 4 (indicating lack of data). Tannin content cautionary. More research could change this safety rating.

- **Warnings/Contraindications/Precautions**
  At this time, cat's claw should not be used in skin graft or organ transplant patients. Its use in patients with HIV, AIDS, and tuberculosis is controversial. Not for children under 3, or during pregnancy or breastfeeding.

Interactions

Pending further research, cat's claw should not be used with immunizations, cryoprecipitates, fresh blood plasma, or drugs that use animal protein or peptide hormones (animal sera, intravenous hyperimmunoglobulin therapy, intravenous thymic extracts, bovine/porcine insulin).

Regulatory and Compendial Status

U.S. FDA: Dietary supplement.
German Commission E: Not included in phytomedicinal monographs.

References

Aquino R, De Simone F, Pizza C, Conti C, Stein ML. Plant metabolites. Structure and in vitro activity of quinovic acid glycosides from *Uncaria tomentosa* and Guettarda platypoda. *J Nat Prod.* 1989;52:679–685.

Aquino R, De Simone F, Vincieri FF, Pizza C, Gacs-Baitz C. New polyhydroxylated triterpenes from *Uncaria tomentosa. J Nat Prod.* 1990;53: 559–564.

Blumenthal M, ed. *The Complete German Commission E Monographs.* Boston, Mass: Integrative Medicine Communications; 1998.

Blumenthal M. Herbal update: Una de gato (cat's claw): Rainforest herb gets scientific and industry attention.*Whole Foods Magazine.* 1995: 62–68, 78.

Blumenthal M, Riggins C. *Popular Herbs in the U.S. Market: Therapeutic Monographs.* Austin, Tex: The American Botanical Council; 1997.

Davis BW. A "new" world class herb for applied kinesiology practice: *Uncaria tomentosa*– a.k.a. Una de Gato (UDG). Collected Papers of the International College of Applied Kinesiology. 1992.

de Matta SM, Monache FD, Ferrari F, Marini-Bettolo GB. Alkaloids and procyanidine of an Uncaria sp. from Peru. *Farmaco* [Sci]. 1976;31:527–535.

Keplinger K, et al. *Uncaria tomentosa* (Willd.) DC.ethnomedicinal use and new pharmacological, toxicological and botanical results. *J Ethnopharmacol.*1999;64: 23–34.

Lemaire I, et al. Stimulation of interleukin-1 and -6 production in alveolar macrophages by the neotropical liana, *Uncaria tomentosa. J Ethnopharmacol.* 1999;64:109–115.

Lininger S, Wright J, Austin S, Brown D, Gaby A. *The Natural Pharmacy.* Rocklin, Calif: Prima Health; 1998:246.

McGuffin M, Hobbs C, Upton R, Goldberg A. *American Herbal Products Association's Botanical Safety Handbook.* Boca Raton, Fla: CRC Press; 1997.

Ozaki Y. Pharmacological studies of indole alkaloids obtained from domestic plants, Uncaria rhynchophylla Miq. And Amsonia elliptica Roem. et Schult. *Nippon Yakurigaku Zasshi.* 1989;94:17–26.

Sandoval-Chacon M, et al. Anti-inflammatory actions of cat's claw: the role of NF-kappaB. *Aliment Pharmacol Ther.* 1998;12:1,279–1,289.

Senatore A, Cataldo A, Iaccarino FP, Elberti MG. Phytochemical and biological study of *Uncaria tomentosa. Boll Soc Ital Biol Sper.* 1989;65:517–520.

Sheng Y, et al. Induction of apoptosis and inhibition of proliferation in human tumor cells treated with extracts of *Uncaria tomentosa. Anticancer Res.* 1998;18:3,363–3,368.

Steinberg PN. Cat's claw: medicinal properties of this Amazon vine. *Nutrition Science News.* 1995.

Wurm M, et al. Pentacyclic oxindole alkaloids from *Uncaria tomentosa* induce human endothelial cells to release a lymphocyte-proliferation-regulating factor. *Planta Med.* 1998;64:701–704.

Yepez AM, de Ugaz OL, Alvarez CM, De Feo V, Aquino R, De Simone F, Pizza C. Quinovic acid glycosides from *Uncaria guianensis. Phytochemistry.* 1991;30:1,635–1,637.

© *Copyright Integrative Medicine Communications*

Cayenne

Names

- **English**
  Cayenne (Paprika)

- **Botanical**
  Capsicum frutescens/Capsicum spp.

- **Plant Family**
  Solanaceae

- **Pharmacopeial**
  Capsicum

Overview

Cayenne, also known as red pepper, was first introduced to the world by the Caribbean Indians, who gave it to Columbus. Since then its popularity has spread, and it has become an important spice particularly in cajun and creole cooking, and in the cuisines of southeast Asia, China, southern Italy, and Mexico. Capsaicin is the most important ingredient in cayenne and gives it its spiciness. Although spiciness is associated with heat, capsaicin stimulates a section of the hypothalamus which effectively lowers body temperature. Natives of subtropical and tropical climates consume it regularly because it helps them tolerate the heat. As well as being an important spice in many ethnic cuisines, cayenne has many important medicinal properties, including supporting and stimulating the cardiovascular system, acting as a long-lasting topical analgesic, improving digestion, and acting as an expectorant, antioxidant, and antibacterial. Cayenne is very beneficial for the cardiovascular system. A study done on natives of Thailand, who ingest cayenne every day in their meals, shows that they have much lower rates of cardiovascular disease than Americans. Cayenne lowers levels of blood cholesterol. It helps prevent blood clots as well. These properties greatly reduce the likelihood of developing atherosclerosis.

The capsaicin in cayenne has very powerful analgesic properties when applied topically. It works primarily by decreasing pain transmitters in the body, making it an excellent solution for the pain caused by postherpetic neuralgia, diabetic neuropathy, toothache and trigeminal neuralgia, postmastectomy and other surgical trauma or stump pain, headaches, psoriasis, and osteoarthritis and rheumatoid arthritis. Capsaicin also reduces inflammation in joint tissues, which aggravates arthritic conditions. Use of capsaicin-laced taffy to relieve mouth pain from chemotherapy and radiation has been very effective.

Cayenne stimulates saliva and stomach secretions which promotes digestion. Its antibacterial power also fights infection in the gastrointestinal tract and can relieve infectious diarrhea. As an expectorant, it thins mucus and helps move it out of the respiratory tract, making it helpful for emphysema. Its strong antioxidants also protect lung tissue from cellular damage.

Macro Description

Shrubby, tropical perennial. Can grow up to two feet. Branches and stems are hardwood and angular. Flowers bloom in pairs or clusters, greenish or yellowish-white. Leaves broad, elliptical, puffy, wrinkled. Fruit pendulous, podlike, shiny, red, orange, and yellow when ripe. Flowers in summer. Indigenous to Mexico and Central America, but now grows in subtropical and tropical zones of Europe, Asia, Africa, and North America.

Part Used/Pharmaceutical Designations

- Seeds
- Fruit

- **Constituents/Composition**
  Capsaicin (0.1% to 1.5%), carotenoids, vitamins A and C, flavonoids, volatile oil, steroidal saponins (capsidicinsin seeds only).

- **Commercial Preparations**
  Fruit eaten raw or cooked. Fruit dried and powdered. Powder can be added to foods, stirred into juice, tea, or milk, or taken in capsule form. Capsaicin cream: Zostrix, Axsain, Capzasin-P (should contain at least 0.025% capsaicin).

Medicinal Uses/Indications

Traditional: antioxidant, expectorant, anti-hypertensive, topical analgesic, stomachic, carminative, gastrointestinal stimulant, rubefacient, antibacterial, circulatory stimulant, diaphoretic, used to strengthen integrity of veins, capillaries and arteries. Historically used to treat ulcers.

Clinical applications: emphysema, high blood pressure, rheumatoid arthritis, osteoarthritis, carpal tunnel syndrome, fever, cluster headaches, migraine, shingles, indigestion, artherosclerosis, psoriasis, flatulent dyspepsia

Can also be used topically with caution for the following: post-herpetic neuralgia, trigeminal neuralgia, post-mastectomy pain, mouth pain from chemotherapy or radiation, diabetic neuropathy, psoriasis

- **Pharmacology**
  Capsaicin is the most important pharmacological ingredient in cayenne. Cayenne contains high levels of vitamin C and A, and its carotene molecules act as an antioxidant. Cayenne supports and stimulates the cardiovascular system in several ways. It helps prevent artherosclerosis by lowering blood cholesterol and triglyceride levels, which reduces blood pressure as well. It also increases fecal excretions of free cholesterol, preventing absorption of cholesterol. It has an anti-aggregation effect on platelets and increases fibrinolytic activity.

  Cayenne contains six pain-relieving compounds and seven anti-inflammatory ones, the most important of which is capsaicin. It also contains salicylates which are similar to salicin, the herbal equivalent of aspirin. Capsaicin inhibits pain by causing an initial increase in substance P and then a depletion of it in the sensory nerves. Because of the initial stimulation of substance P, it takes several days for the pain release to become effective, but it is very helpful for chronic pain sufferers. The depletion of substance P is also thought to decrease inflammation in joint tissues affected by osteoarthritis and rheumatoid arthritis. Because cayenne is a rubefacient, it helps to increase blood flow to painful joints or cold extremities, and reduces the scaling and redness of psoriasis, although it may cause some initial burning and itching.

  The capsaicin in cayenne stimulates the cooling center of the hypothalamus, which decreases body temperature. Its salicylate content and stimulation of sweat glands help reduce fever as well.

  The gastric and duodenal mucosae have capsaicin-sensitive areas which respond to stimulation from capsaicin by increasing mucosal blood flow and vascular permeability, inhibiting gastric mobility and activating duodenal motility. This aids digestion and protects against acid- and drug-induced ulcers.

Dosage Ranges and Duration of Administration

As an external analgesic, apply capsaicin cream (0.025% to 0.075% capsaicin) directly to affected area up to qid. Also used as tincture: 1:5, 1 ml tid.

Cautions

- **Adverse Effects/Toxicology**
  Cayenne pepper is generally regarded as safe in the U.S. Topical applications may cause temporary burning sensation or redness, but this should subside without complication. Keep cayenne away from eyes, as the capsaicinoids are a strong irritant to mucosal membranes. Chronic overuse of capsaicin can be toxic.

- **Warnings/Contraindications/Precautions**
  Wash hands well after use and avoid touching the eyes. Not very soluble in water, so use vinegar to remove it best. Cream may cause skin irritation in some people. Test on small area of skin before extended use. If causes irritation, discontinue use. May cause gastro-intestinal irritation, although does not influence duodenal ulcers. Do not use for children under age 2. Safe for use during pregnancy. It is not known if the spicy compounds are transferred through breast-feeding.

Interactions

May interfere with MAOIs and antihypertensive therapy. May increase hepatic metabolism of drugs.

Regulatory and Compendial Status

On U.S. FDA list of herbs generally regarded as safe. FDA approval of capsaicin creams, Zostrix and Axsain, for chronic pain.

References

Boone CW, Kelloff GJ, Malone WE. Identification of candidate cancer chemopreventive agents and their evaluation in animal models and human clinical trials: a review. *Cancer Res.* 1990;50:29.

Chevallier A. *The Encyclopedia of Medicinal Plants.* London, England: DK Publishing Inc; 1996.

Duke J. *The Green Pharmacy.* Emmaus, Pa: Rodale Press; 1997.

Hot peppers and substance P. *Lancet.* 1983;I:1198. Editorial.

Gruenwald J, Brendler T, Jaenicke C et al, eds. *PDR for Herbal Medicines.* Montvale, NJ: Medical Economics Company; 1998.

Heinerman J. *Heinerman's Encyclopedia of Fruits, Vegetables and Herbs.* Englewood Cliffs, NJ: Prentice Hall; 1988.

Kowalchik C, Hylton W, eds. *Rodale's Illustrated Encyclopedia of Herbs.* Emmaus, Pa: Rodale Press; 1987.

Locock RA. Capsicum. *Can Pharm J.* 1985;517–519.

Munn, S.E., et al. The effect of topical capsaicin on substance P immunoreactivity: A clinical trial and immuno-hisochemical analysis [letter]. *Acta Derm Venereol (Stockh).* 1997;77:158–159.

Murray M. *The Healing Power of Herbs.* Rocklin, Calif: Prima Publishing; 1995.

Newall C, et al. *Herbal Medicines.* London, England: Pharmaceutical Press; 1996.

Tandan R, et al. Topical capsaicin in painful diabetic neuropathy. Controlled study with long-term follow-up. *Diabetes Care.* 1992;15:814.

Tyler V. *The Honest Herbal.* New York, NY: Pharmaceutical Products Press; 1993.

Visudhiphan S, et al. The relationship between high fibrinolytic activity and daily capsicum ingestion in Thais. *Am J Clin Nutr.* 1982;35:1452–1458.

Vogl T. Treatment of hunan hand. *N Engl J Med.* 1982;306:178.

Yeoh KG, et al. Chili protects against aspirin-induced gastroduodenal mucosal injury in humans. *Dig Dis Sci.* 1995;40:580–583.

© *Copyright Integrative Medicine Communications*

Celery Seed

Names

- **English**
  Celery Seed

- **Botanical**
  Apium graveolens

- **Plant Family**
  Apiaceae

- **Pharmacopeial**
  Apii fructus

Overview

Celery seed is one of the lesser-known herbs in Western herbal medicine. However, it has been known for thousands of years in other parts of the world for its varied uses. During ancient times, Ayurvedic physicians (vaidyas) used celery seed to treat people with colds, flu, water retention, poor digestion, various types of arthritis, and certain ailments of the liver and spleen. Modern research has documented that there may indeed be a pharmacological basis for most of these uses. In addition, laboratory studies on animals indicate that celery seed may be useful for treating hypertension, and even in the prevention of cancer.

Celery seed has significant diuretic properties, which may be why it decreases hypertension. (It also contains constituents that are directly hypotensive, as well as significant amounts of calcium, which also lowers blood pressure.) In addition, the diuretic action combined with the presence of bactericidal compounds in celery seed support its usefulness in treating urinary tract infection.

Scientific evidence also shows that celery seed may aid in the prevention of cancer. A number of studies have examined the ability of whole celery seed extract or its individual constituents to prevent tumor formation in animals. The results of these studies have been positive. The phthalides, which determine the characteristic odor of celery, are especially potent as anti-tumor agents.

These compounds also stimulate the production of the enzyme glutathione-S-transferase. This enzyme helps break down many toxic substances in the body and may help support the traditional application of celery seed for treating disorders such as arthritis and cancer in these cases.

Macro Description

The seed of a biennial slender plant which can grow to 60 cm in height, with three to five segmented leaves; small white flower petals; seeds are very small with a distinctive odor. Grows in northern warm or temperate zones.

Part Used/Pharmaceutical Designations

The seeds of the celery plant have traditionally been used. (The plant and roots contain many of the same active constituents, however; essential oils made from the plant have occasionally been used in traditional medicine.)

- **Consituents/Composition**

  - Volatile oils (including apiol)
  - Flavonoids
  - 3-N-butyl-phthalide
  - Alpha-linolenic-acid
  - Beta-eudesmol
  - Guaiacol
  - Isoimperatorin
  - Isoquercitrin
  - P-cymene
  - Umbelliferone

- **Commercial Preparations**

  - Fresh or dried seeds
  - Tablets, various concentrations
  - Celery seed oil capsules
  - Alcohol or glycerine extract

Medicinal Uses/Indications

- Hypertension (celery seed contains both diuretic and directly hypotensive constituents)
- Arthritis/rheumatism (anti-inflammatory and analgesic constituents)
- Liver disorders (hepatoprotective and detoxifying constituents)
- Nervous restlessness (nervine and sedative constituents)
- Muscle spasms (spasmolytic, anti-inflammatory, and analgesic constituents)
- Gout and calculi (said to increase elimination of uric acid)
- Urinary tract infections (bactericidal and diuretic constituents)
- Digestive tonic and carminative
- Emmenogogue (uterine stimulant)
- Galactogogue
- May be useful cancer preventative (constituents that stimulate detoxifying enzymes; others with anti-tumor-promoting properties)
- Used as aphrodisiac in traditional medicine
- Anti-inflammatory

- **Pharmacology**

Arthritis and muscle spasm: Alpha-linoleic acid and umbelliferone have been shown to have anti-inflammatory activity. Umbelliferone is also an anti-prostaglandin, which may contribute to celery seed's effects on inflammation and arthritis. P-cymene is analgesic and antirheumatologic. Apiol, limonene, and umbelliferone are all antispasmodic. The high levels of calcium in celery seed may also aid in relaxing muscle spasm.

Urinary tract infections: Celery seed contains a number of consituents that have anti-bacterial properties. It also is a diuretic, which increases urine output to clear bacteria from the urinary tract. P-cymene, guaiacol, limonene, terpinen-4-ol, and umbelliferone are all bactericidal. Isoquercitrin and terpinen-4-ol have both bactericidal and diuretic properties. Apiol is also a diuretic.

Lowering of blood pressure: Alpha-linolenic acid has hypotensive properties; apiol and terpinen-4-ol act as diuretics; and isoquercitin has both hypotensive and diuretic activities. Celery seed also contains high levels of calcium, which may play a significant role in reducing blood pressure.

Liver disorders: In studies on rats, liver damage induced by hepatotoxins is inhibited by extracts of celery seed. Beta-eudesmol has hepatoprotective properties.

Uterine disorders: Apiol is a uterotonic and an emmenagogue (promotes menstruation). It also acts as an abortifacient, thereby contraindicating celery seed for use in pregnancy.

Anxiety and stress relief: Limonene has sedative properties. In addition, celery seeds contain high levels of calcium, which also tend to have a relaxing effect.

Anti-tumor and anti-oxidant properties: The phthalides, bitter liminoids, and sedanolide in celery seed stimulate the activity of the detoxifying enzyme glutathione S-transferase (GST). Compounds with this activity are potent anti-tumor agents. A number of other compounds found in celery seed also have anti-carcinogenic activity, including alpha-linoleic acid, isoimperatorin, isoquercitrin, limonene, and umbelliferone. In addition, alpha-linolenic acid has anti-metastatic lymphocytogenic, and immunostimulant properties.

Dosage Ranges and Duration of Administration

- The dosages found in different preparations on the market vary. Recommended dosage is to take the equivalent of 1 to 3 g dried seed tid.
- Tablets: various concentrations available. Take 1 to 3 g tid
- Celery seed oil capsules: one to two capsules tid
- Celery seed extract: 1/4 to 1/2 tsp. tid with 8 oz. juice or water
- Prepare a tea by pouring boiling water over 1 tsp. of freshly crushed seeds, 1 to 3 g dried seed tid. Let steep for 10 to 20 minutes before drinking.

Cautions

- **Adverse Effects/Toxicology**
  None reported

- **Warnings/Contraindications/Precautions**
  Do not use in pregnancy.
  Do not use seed sold for horticultural use. They are usually treated with fungicide.
  Do not use with active kidney inflammation. Phototoxic warnings as with St. John's wort are warranted here (i.e., not with UV therapy or with tanning booths).

Interactions

None reported

Regulatory and Compendial Status

N/A

References

Appel LJ, Moore TJ et al. A clinical trial of the effects of dietary patterns on blood pressure. *N Engl J Med.* 1997;336:1117–1124. Abstract.

Atta AH, et al. Anti-nociceptive and anti-inflammatory effects of some Jordanian medicinal plant extracts. *J Ethnopharmacol.* 1998;60:117–124.

Balch J, Balch P. *Prescription for Nutritional Healing: A-to-Z Guide to Drug-Free Remedies Using Vitamins, Minerals, Herbs, & Food Supplements.* New York, NY: Avery Publishing Group; 1990.

Banerjee S, Sharma R, Kale RK, Rao AR. Influence of certain essential oils on carcinogen-metabolizing enzymes and acid-soluble sulfhydryls in mouse liver. *Nutr Cancer.* 1994;21:263–269. Abstract.

Duke JA. *Handbook of Phytochemical Constituents of GRAS Herbs and Other Economic Plants.* Boca Raton, Fla: CRC Press; 1992.

Ko FN, et al. Vasodilatory action mechanisms of apigenin isolated from *Apium graveolens* in rat thoracic aorta. Biochim Biophys Acta. November 14; 1991;1115:69–74.

Lewis DA, et al. The anti-inflammatory activity of celery *Apium graveolens* L. *Int J Crude Drug Res.* 1985;23.

Mills SY. *Dictionary of Modern Herbalism: A Comprehensive Guide to Practical Herbal Therapy.* Rochester, Vt: Healing Arts Press; 1988.

Singh A, Handa SS. Hepatoprotective activity of Apium graveolens and Hygrophila auriculata against paracetamol and thioacetamide intoxication in rats. *J Ethnopharmacol.* 1995;49:119–126.

Steinmetz KA, Potter JD. Vegetables, fruit, and cancer. II. Mechanisms. *Cancer Causes Control.* 1991;2:427–442. Abstract.

Tsi D, et al. Effects of aqueous celery *(Apium graveolens)* extract on lipid parameters of rats fed a high fat diet. *Planta Med.* 1995;61:18–21.

Zheng GQ, et al. Chemoprevention of benzo [a] pyrene-induced forestomach cancer in mice by natural phthalides from celery seed oil. *Nutr Cancer.* 1993;19:77–86.

Zheng GQ, Kenney PM, Zhang J, Lam LK. Chemoprevention of benzo[a]pyrene-induced forestomach cancer in mice by natural phthalides from celery seed oil. *Nutr Cancer.* 1993;19:77–86.

© *Copyright Integrative Medicine Communications*

Chamomile, German

Names

- **English**
  Chamomile, German

- **Botanical**
  Matricaria recutita

- **Plant Family**
  Asteraceae

- **Pharmacopeial**
  Matricariae flos

Overview

German chamomile is used to relieve both external and internal inflammation. Externally, it reduces swelling caused by abrasions, exposure to chemicals or radiation, fungal invasion, or subdermal spasm or infection, and targets skin, mucous membranes, gums, and ano-genital areas. Inhaled, chamomile reduces spasm and inflammation of the respiratory tract. Used internally, it relieves colic and ulcers. It has been recommended for for carpal tunnel syndrome, insect bites, insomnia, gingivitis, and heartburn.

Beginning with the ancient Egyptians, Romans, and Greeks, who used chamomile flowers to relieve sun stroke, fevers, and colic, chamomile has held a prominent place in history. It is regarded by modern Europeans with a reverence similar to that given to ginseng by Asians. Germans describe chamomile as "alles zutraut," meaning that it is capable of anything. Most important, however, is that clinical studies support chamomile's broad range of use.

German chamomile is one of two chamomile species used medicinally. The hollow receptacle that lies beneath the flowers of *M. retutica* differentiates this species from Roman, or English, chamomile *(Chamaemelum nobile)*, which has a solid receptacle. Both chamomiles produce similar bioactive constituents and are used for similar ailments. They also share non-medicinal uses: chamomile extracts are added to hair dyes and shampoos to highlight hair or improve blonde tones, and chamomile oils add apple scents to soaps and perfumes.

Macro Description

Leaves, alternate, with thread-like divisions, grow from a light green, smooth, striated stem. From spring through summer, 10 to 20 cream-colored or silver-white petals bloom around a swollen, yellow central disk, or receptacle. Diameter of flower heads is 1/2 to 5/8 of an inch. The plant can grow to 2 or 3 feet but is often found low to the ground in native Europe, Africa, and Asia, and in North and South America where it has been naturalized.

Part Used/Pharmaceutical Designations

- Flower

- **Constituents/Composition**
  0.25% to 1% volatile oils including alpha-bisabolol, chamazulene; 2.4% flavonoids including apigenin; 5% to 10% pectin-like mucilage; also contains coumarins (umbelliferone, methyl ether heniarin), polysaccharide, anthemic acid, tricontane. Chamazulene, present in chamomile volatile oil, is blue, and is formed from its precursor, matricin, upon steam distillation of the oil.

- **Commercial Preparations**
  Crude dried flowers are available to buy in bulk. Chamomile tea is readily available, also aqueous or alcohol extracts and topical ointments. Because of its popular use with children, chamomile is also one of the most available herbs in glycerite form.

Medicinal Uses/Indications

- Traditional: anti-inflammatory, diuretic, vulnerary, antimicrobial, mildly sedative, carminative, aromatic, diaphoretic, and digestive tonic; actions, according to the German Commission E monograph, include antipholigistic, musculotropic, antispasmodic, deodorant, antibacterial, bacteriostatic

- Conditions: peptic ulcers, colic, childhood sleeplessness, hemorrhoids, spasmodic cough, excess gas, abrasions of the skin; skin irritation due to chemicals, radiation, fungi, subdermal spasm, infection; for respiratory tract irritation, insomnia, gingivitis or other oral cavity inflammation and pain

- Clinical Applications: inflammatory conditions of the skin, gastrointestinal, ano-genital, and respiratory tracts, including colic, ulcers, excess gas, heartburn, irritation from chest colds, slow-healing wounds, abcesses, fistulae, oral cavity/gum inflammation, skin inflammation due to X ray or other radiation (as for cancer patients), psoriasis, eczema, vaginal inflammations, and children's skin conditions such as impetigo, hives, chicken pox, infant acne, heat rash, diaper rash

- **Pharmacology**
  Whole extract and individual constituents have been studied for topical and internal antispasmodic, anti-inflammatory, and carminative effects. Chamazulene, alpha-bisabolol, and apigenin have the highest anti-inflammatory actions against pro-inflammatory agents used on laboratory rats. Matricin, the precursor of chamazulene, demonstrates anti-inflammatory activity superior to chamazulene. Chamazulene (azulene) has been reported to inhibit histamine release, alpha-bisabolol and cis-spiroether, another component of the volatile oil, blocked carrageenan-induced rat paw edema and demonstrated muscle relaxant actions.
  Alpha-bisabolol prevented the formation of indomethacin, stress, or alcohol-induced ulcers in laboratory animals.
  In vitro tests show that chamomile oil is actively antibacterial and fungicidal at concentrations of at least 25 mg/ml, as is bisabolol at concentrations of at least 1 mg/ml. Whole extracts and isolated flavonoid and bisabolol constituents also inhibit spasm in guinea pig intestine: 10 mg apigenin reduced spasm comparably to 1 mg papaverine. Volatile oil increases bile secretion in cats and dogs.
  Human studies demonstrate therapeutic efficiency for European propriety chamomile formulas used in weeping skin disorders, bedsores, contact dermatitis, eczema, and post-irradiation dermatitis. Chamomile was also antispasmodic and anti-inflammatory in both human duodenum and stomach; oral extracts promoted deep sleep in 10 out of 12 patients having cardiac catheterization; and topical ointments soothed and enhanced healing in patients using chamomile as adjunctive therapy for skin infections of the leg.

Dosage Ranges and Duration of Administration

- To relieve spasms or inflammations of the gastrointestinal tract: tea, 2 to 3 g herb steeped in hot water, tid or qid between meals; 1:5 tincture (5 ml tid), glycerite 1 to 2 ml tid for children
- To use as a gargle, prepare tea as above, cool, and gargle
- To use for respiratory tract inflammation, pour a few drops of essential oil into steaming water and inhale; or prepare tea and inhale steam
- For bath, to sooth inflammations of the skin, use 1/4 lb. dried flowers per bath made into a tea by slow cooking; or use essential oils in tub, instructing patient to enter tub only after sufficient water is mixed with oils.
- Douches, for vaginal inflammation, use 3% to 10% infusion
- Poultices for external application to skin inflammation, use 3% to 10% infusion
- For psoriasis, eczema, or dry, flaky skin, use creams with 3% to 10% crude drug content

Cautions

- **Adverse Effects/Toxicology**
  The American Herbal Products Association (AHPA) gives chamomile a class 1 safety rating: safe with appropriate use. The AHPA also notes that highly concentrated tea is reportedly emetic (flower heads contain anthemic acid).

- **Warnings/Contraindications/Precautions**
  Persons allergic to members of the aster family (ragweed) may have an allergic reaction to chamomile; two cases of anaphylactic reactions have been reported, and in both cases there was a pre-determined allergy to ragweed.
  According to the AHPA, in Germany chamomile labels are required to warn against using infusions near the eyes.
  Avoid excessive use during pregnancy and lactation.

Interactions

No interactions with other herbs or drugs are currently known, but because chamomile contains coumarins, it may interfere with anticoagulant therapy.

Regulatory and Compendial Status

In the United States, German chamomile is a dietary supplement and GRAS in the food industry; in England, German chamomile is a licensed product; and the Commission E approves of topical and internal use for inflammatory conditions in Germany.

References

Achterrath-Tuckermann U, et al. Pharmacological investigations with compounds of chamomile. V. Investigations on the spasmolytic effect of compounds of chamomile and Kamillosan on the isolated guinea pig ileum. *Planta Med.* 1980;39:38–50.

Blumenthal M, ed. *The Complete German Commission E Monographs.* Boston, Mass: Integrative Medicine Communications; 1998.

de la Motte S, Bose-O'Reilly S, Heinisch M, Harrison F. Doppelblind-vergleich zwischen einem apfelpektin/kamillenextrakt-prparat und plazebo bei kindern mit diarrhoe. *Arzneimittelforschung.* 1997;47:1247–1249.

Duke JA. *The Green Pharmacy.* Emmaus, Pa: Rodale Press; 1997.

Foster S. *Herbal Renaissance: Growing, Using and Understanding Herbs in the Modern World.* Salt Lake City, Utah: Gibbs-Smith; 1993.

Glowania HJ, Raulin C, Swoboda M. Effect of chamomile on wound healing - a clinical double-blind study. *Z Hautkr.* 1987; 62:1262, 1267–1271.

Kowalchik C, Hylton W, eds. *Rodale's Illustrated Encyclopedia of Herbs.* Emmaus, Pa: Rodale Press; 1998.

McGuffin M, Hobbs C, Upton R, Goldberg A. *American Herbal Products Associations's Botanical Safety Handbook.* Boca Raton, Fla: CRC Press; 1996.

Newall CA, Anderson LA, Phillipson JD. *Herbal Medicines: A Guide for Health Care Professionals.* London, England: The Pharmaceutical Press; 1996.

Salamon I. Chamomile: A medicinal plant. *Herb, Spice, and Medicinal Plant Digest.* 1992;10:1–4.

Schultz V, Hansel R, Tyler V. *Rational Phytotherapy: A Physician's Guide to Herbal Medicine.* Heidelberg: Springer; 1998.

Viola H, et al. Apigenin, a component of *Matricaria recutita* flowers, is a central benzodiazepine receptors-ligand with anxiolytic effects. *Planta Med.* 1995;61:213–216.

© Copyright Integrative Medicine Communications

Chamomile, Roman

Names

- **English**
  Roman chamomile

- **Botanical**
  Chamaemelum nobile

- **Plant Family**
  Asteraceae

- **Pharmacopeial**
  Chamomillae romanae flos

Overview

Roman, or English, chamomile reportedly reduces intestinal gas, calms muscle spasms, quells nausea and vomiting, induces a mild sedation, and has anti-inflammatory effects on skin and mucous membranes. Because of the similarity of its volatile oils, Roman chamomile acts similarly, if not identical to, German chamomile *(Matricaria recutita)*. It is used less often, however, because there exists less scientific documentation of its therapeutic effects. The origin of its many applications is largely empirical. Nevertheless, its high demand exceeds crop yields in native northern European countries, and chamomile is now exported from Argentina and Egypt.

At the dawn of the 20th century, chamomile was used as a folk medicine to restore tranquility and calm. Although more apt to be regarded in the United States as a pleasant-tasting tea with a nice aroma, chamomile is used medicinally today in Europe. There it is used not only as a mild sedative, but also as a tonic to speed recovery from numerous ailments. In particular, indications for use are indigestion caused by nervousness or mental stress accompanied by flatulence.

Roman chamomile differs from German chamomile in that the receptacle below the flower head is solid instead of hollow, and its leaf segments are thicker. The plant itself is lower to the ground. Double or semi-double flower heads are used in the commercial preparation of volatile oil. Both chamomiles share cosmetic, beverage, and food use; chamomile oils are added to hair dyes, ointments, shampoos, soaps, perfumes, liqueurs, and baked goods.

Macro Description

Perennial herb with a creeping rhizome. Grows low to the ground but sometimes reaches up to one foot in height. Stems are hairy, and either drooping or erect. Grayish-green leaves are alternate, segmented. Flower heads emit an apple-like fragrance. Disk flowers yellow, ray flowers white, and the cone-shaped receptacle is solid. Roman chamomile is native to northwestern Europe and Northern Ireland but has been cultivated throughout Europe, the United States, and parts of South America.

Part Used/Pharmaceutical Designations

- Flower

- **Constituents/Composition**
  0.4% to 1.75% volatile oil containing angelic and tiglic acid esters; 1,8-cineole, farnesol, nerolidol, sesquiterpenes chamazulene, alpha-bisabolol; amyl/isobutlyl alcohols; flavonoids (apigenin, luteolin, quercetin, and their glycosides); coumarins, anthemic acid, phenolic/fatty acids; phytosterol. Chamazulene is formed from matricin upon steam distillation. Volatile oil is blue.

- **Commercial Preparations**
  Crude dried flowers are available to buy in bulk; also, tea, tincture; Roman chamomile may be an additive in topical ointments and cosmetics.

Medicinal Uses/Indications

- Traditional: tonic, stomachic, diaphoretic, soporific, antispasmodic, and folk remedy for colic
- Conditions: ulcer, gastritis, slow-healing wounds, heartburn
- Clinical Applications: Roman chamomile is used alone or as a component of a number of European treatments for heartburn, anorexia, post-prandial bloating and fullness, nausea, newborn colic, spastic constipation, menstrual disorders, frontal sinus catarrh, hay fever, nasal and pharngeal mucositis, ear inflammation, wounds, burns, rashes, bedsores, hemorrhoids, Romeheld's syndrome, and diseases of the liver, and gallbladder. Due to lack of documentation, these uses are not approved by the German Commission E.

- **Pharmacology**
  In experiments with rats, Roman chamomile has been shown to reduce carrageenan-induced paw edema, a standard test for anti-inflammatory activity. Rat tests also demonstrate Roman chamomile-induced sedative and antidiuretic effects. Antitumor and cytotoxic activity have been demonstrated in vitro for various chamomile constituents. Farnesol is sedative and spasmolytic in vitro; and apigenin is associated with reductions in inflammation, spasm, and infection. However, Roman chamomile has not been tested as extensively as German chamomile, and it occurs as an unapproved botanical in the German Commission E monographs because of the lack of human data.

  The volatile oil of Roman chamomile contains the same active constituents as German chamomile, and Commission E notwithstanding it has been assumed to have similar pharmacological actions.

  Chamomiles are used in Europe in dermatology, pulmology, pediatrics, gynecology, gastroenterology, and otolaryngology. Their actions span a broad range of therapeutics, blocking convulsion, microbes, sepsis, inflammation, spasms, and viruses. Tests on humans demonstrate that German chamomile reduces inflammations in mucous membranes and on the skin that may be due to cuts, burns, yeasts, or other fungal growths. When it is inhaled, the volatile oil quells respiratory inflammations associated with colds. Investigations demonstrate that these actions are stimulated by volatile oil constituents chamazulene and alpha-bisabolol, and flavonoids and coumarins, also found in Roman chamomile.

Dosage Ranges and Duration of Administration

To reduce intestinal colic, flatulence, digestive disturbance, lack of appetite, painful menstruation, gingivitis, or oral inflammation, choose from the following.

- Dried flowers, as tea, 1 to 4 g tid
- 70% alcohol extract, 1 to 4 ml tid

For hemorrhoids/skin inflammation, add a few teabags or chamomile tincture to bathwater. Ointments should contain 3% to 10% crude drug.

Cautions

- **Adverse Effects/Toxicology**
  Roman chamomile has a class 2b safety rating from The American Herbal Products Association (AHPA). Class 2b indicates that the AHPA advises against use during pregnancy, and lists it as a potential abortifacient due to its action on uterine smooth muscle and tendency to induce menstruation when taken at high doses. Normal dietary intake of Roman chamomile in tea is not associated with these actions. Roman chamomile in high doses may also stimulate emesis, due to anthemic acid in the flower heads.

  One case of anaphylaxis reportedly resulted from Roman chamomile tea ingestion in patients with ragweed allergy.

- **Warnings/Contraindications/Precautions**
  Avoid use in patients with known allergies to the aster family (ragweed). In laboratory tests, cross reactions were noted with German chamomile, yarrow, lettuce, and chrysanthemum. Allergic rhinitis may develop in patients with atopic reactions to mugwort.

  Do not use during pregnancy or lactation.

Interactions

No interactions with other herbs or drugs are currently known, but chamomile contains coumarins, which may interfere with anticoagulant therapy.

Regulatory and Compendial Status

Roman chamomile is on the General Sales List in England. The German Commission E does not approve of its medicinal use due to lack of demonstrated efficacy, but use of flower head as tea is permitted.

References

Achterrath-Tuckermann U, et al. Pharmacologisch untersuchungen von kamillen-inhaltestoffen. *Planta Med.* 1980;39:38–50.

Berry M. The chamomiles. *Pharm J.* 1995;254:191–193.

Blumenthal M, ed. *The Complete German Commission E Monographs.* Boston, Mass: Integrative Medicine Communications; 1998.

Bradley PR. *British Herbal Compendium.* Dorset, England: British Herbal Medicine Association; 1992:1.

DeSmet PAGM, Keller K, Hansel R, Chandler RF. *Adverse Effects of Herbal Drugs.* New York, NY: Springer-Verlag; 1992:2.

Evans WC. *Trease and Evans' Pharmacognosy.* 13th ed. London, England: Bailliere Tindall; 1989.

Foster S. *Herbal Renaissance: Growing, Using and Understanding Herbs in the Modern World.* Salt Lake City, Utah: Gibbs-Smith; 1993.

Harborne J, Baxter H. *Phytochemical Dictionary: A Handbook of Bioactive Compounds from Plants.* Washington, DC: Taylor and Francis; 1993.

Harris B, Lewis R. Chamomile part 1. *Int J Alt Comp Med.* September 1994;12.

Hausen BM, et al. The sensitizing capacity of Compositae plants. *Planta Med.* 1984;50.

Leung A, Foster S. *Encyclopedia of Common Natural Ingredients Used in Food, Drugs, and Cosmetics.* 2nd ed. New York, NY: Wiley & Sons; 1996.

McGuffin M, Hobbs C, Upton R, Goldberg A. *American Herbal Products Associations's Botanical Safety Handbook.* Boca Raton, Fla: CRC Press; 1996.

Newall CA, Anderson LA, Phillipson JD. *Herbal Medicines: A Guide for Health Care Professionals.* London, England: The Pharmaceutical Press; 1996:72–73.

Opdyke DLJ. Chamomile oil roman. *Food Cosmet Toxicol.* 1974;12:853.

Weiss RF. *Herbal Medicines.* Beaconsfield, England: Beaconsfield Publishers, Ltd; 1988.

© *Copyright Integrative Medicine Communications*

Comfrey

Names

- **English**
  Comfrey leaf/Comfrey root

- **Botanical**
  Symphytum officinale

- **Plant Family**
  Boraginazeae

- **Pharmacopeial**
  Symphyti folium/Symphyti radix

Overview

Comfrey is a herbaceous perennial native to Europe and temperate Asia. It is now naturalized in the United States. Also known as knitbone, comfrey has traditionally been used to treat superficial wounds as well as the inflammation of sprains and broken bones.

Allantoin, a key constituent found in the roots and leaves, is a cell proliferant that promotes wound healing and tissue regeneration. Comfrey leaf contains rosmarinic acid, which decreases inflammation and microvascular pulmonary injury. The mucilages in comfrey are responsible for its efficacy as a local demulcent (a slippery medicine for inflamed surfaces).

Although many traditional herbalists consider comfrey a beneficial herb, several pharmacological studies show that it is potentially quite toxic. Comfrey preparations, especially those taken internally, have been associated with veno-occlusive disease and even death. Many comfrey species contain poisonous pyrrolizidine alkaloids, compounds known to be highly toxic to the liver. Echimidine is one of the most toxic pyrrolizidine alkaloids. Dangerously high levels of this alkaloid have been found in both prickley comfrey *(Symphytum asperum)* and Russian comfrey *(S. uplandicum)*. Although common comfrey *(S. officinale)* does not usually contain echimidine, other harmful pyrrolizidine alkaloids have been isolated from it. According to some research, small quantities of echimidine have been detected in about 25% of samples of common comfrey. Products made from the root should be used with extreme caution since the quantity of pyrrolizidine alkaloids in comfrey root is nearly ten times that in the leaves.

While *S. officinale* is the preferred source of comfrey herbal products, some comfrey preparations sold in the United States and Europe may unknowingly be made from Russian and prickley comfrey. Collectors who harvest raw plant material are not always able to identify different species of comfrey. Consequently, there are mislabeled comfrey products on the market that do not actually come from *S. officinale,* but instead come from other *Symphytum* species containing high echimidine levels. For this reason, special care must be taken in determining the source and botanical authenticity of commercial comfrey products.

Macro Description

Fond of moist soils, comfrey has an erect and stiff-haired stem, and it grows to a height of 20 to 120 cm. Its flowers are dull purple, violet, or whitish, and densely arranged in clusters. The wrinkly and hairy leaves are oblong, and often differ in appearance depending upon their position on the stem: the lower leaves are broad at the base and tapered at the ends while the upper leaves are broad throughout and narrowed only at the ends. The slimy roots show a horn-like appearance when dried. The root has a black exterior and fleshy whitish interior filled with a glutinous juice.

Part Used/Pharmaceutical Designations

- Leaves
- Roots (rhizome)
- Aerial parts

- **Constituents/Composition**
  Pyrrolizidine-type alkaloids (0.3%), including symphytine, symlandine, echimidine, intermidine, lycopsamine, myoscorpine, acetyllycopsamine, acetylintermidine, lasiocarpine, heliosupine, viridiflorine, echiumine; carbohydrates (gum, mucilage); pyrocatechol-type tannins (2.4%); triterpenes (phytosterols, steroidal saponins, isobauerenol); allantoin (0.75 to 2.55%), caffeic acid, carotene (0.63%), chlorogenic acid, choline, lithospermic acid, rosmarinic acid, silicic acid.

- **Commercial Preparations**
  Comfrey ointments (containing 5% to 20% of the drug), creams, mucilaginous decoctions, poultices, and liniments are made from the fresh or dried aerial parts, fresh or dried leaf, and/or root of comfrey species and are used for external application. Experts advise using only products made from the mature leaves of *S. officinale*. Root preparations are available but are not recommended for either internal or external use. PA-free comfrey preparations are also available.

Medicinal Uses/Indications

Traditional herbal actions: demulcent; internal and external vulnerary (wound healer), relaxing expectorant, astringent, emollient, pectoral tonic.

Comfrey preparations are used externally (only on intact skin) for bruising, pulled muscles and ligaments, sprains, and blunt injuries. The root has anti-inflammatory, callus-promoting, and antimitotic action.

Clinical applications: Comfrey is a stimulant to fibroblast, osteoblast, and chrondroblast activity, and is thus used for fractures, sprains, and strains. The pyrrolizidine alkaloid-free form is used internally for ulceration or erosion of the gut wall and congestive bronchial conditions.

- **Pharmacology**
  In in vivo studies, unsaturated pyrrolizidine alkaloids isolated from comfrey have been shown to have hepatotoxic, carcinogenic, and mutagenic effects. In experiments in animals, comfrey extract given orally to rats had wound healing and analgesic properties and stimulated the actions of the drug-metabolizing enzyme, aminopyrine N-demethylase in the liver. In in vitro research, comfrey extract increased uterine tone.

  Rosmarinic acid isolated from comfrey is responsible for in vitro anti-inflammatory effects. In other studies, pyrrolic esters found in comfrey exhibited weak antimuscarinic effects in clinical trials. Sarracine and platyphylline are nonhepatotoxic pyrrolizidine alkaloids used clinically to treat gastrointestinal hypermotility and peptic ulcers in human patients.

Dosage Ranges and Duration of Administration

Herb and leaf ointments—root extracts and semi-solid products for external use: 5% to 20% dried drug or equivalent preparation. Daily dosage should not exceed 100 mcg of pyrrolizidine alkaloids with 1,2-unsaturated necine structure, including their N-oxides, for more than four to six weeks per year. Comfrey is also available as a 1:5 tincture of root and leaves (PA-free tincture, 1 to 2 ml tid). Capsules are not currently available due to concerns about PA content.

Cautions

- **Adverse Effects/Toxicology**
  Comfrey is basically safe if taken within recommended therapeutic dosages and if used only as external preparations on unbroken skin. However, internal consumption of comfrey over prolonged periods of time may cause hepatic veno-occlusive disease. Oral intake of comfrey is also associated with several cases of atropine poisoning. However, reported cases of atropine toxicity may have been due to deadly nightshade (belladonna leaf) contaminants in raw plant material used to manufacture comfrey products. Contamination can occur because comfrey and belladonna leaves resemble each other.

- **Warnings/Contraindications/Precautions**
  Topical comfrey preparations should never be used on broken skin. Pregnant and lactating women should not use comfrey products under any circumstances.

Interactions

No interactions have been reported between comfrey and other drugs.

Regulatory and Compendial Status

Comfrey products are sold in the United Kingdom, France, and Germany as nonprescription drugs. The U.S. FDA classifies common comfrey as a dietary supplement.

References

Behninger C, et al. Studies on the effect of an alkaloid extract of *Symphytum officinale* on human lymphocyte cultures. *Planta Med.* 1989;55:518–522.

Blumenthal M, ed. *The Complete German Commission E Monograph; Therapeutic Guide to Herbal Medicines.* Boston. Mass: Integrative Medicine Communications; 1998:115–116.

Bradley P. ed. *British Herbal Compendium. Vol. I.* Dorset, England: British Herbal Medicine Association; 1992:66–68.

Dorland's Illustrated Medical Dictionary. 25th ed. Philadelphia, Pa: WB Saunders; 1974

Furmanowa M, et al. Mutagenic effects of aqueous extracts of *Symphytum officinale* L. and of its alkaloidal fractions. *J Appl Toxico.* 1983; Jun;3(3):127–30.

Goldman RS, et al. Wound healing and analgesic effect of crude extracts of *Symphytum officinale. Fitoterapi.* 1985;(6):323–329.

Gruenwald J, Brendler T, Jaenicke C, eds. *PDR for Herbal Medicines.* Montvale, NJ: Medical Economics Co; 1998:1163–1166.

Heinerman J. *Heinerman's Encyclopedia of Fruits, Vegetables and Herbs.* Englewood Cliffs, NJ: Prentice Hall; 1988:112–113.

Newall CA, Anderson LA, Phillipson JD. eds. *Herbal Medicines: A Guide for Health-care Professionals.* London: Pharmaceutical Press; 1996:87–89.

Olinescu A, et al. Action of some proteic and carbohydrate components of *Symphytum officinale* upon normal and neoplastic cells. *Roum Arch Microbiol Immunol.* 1993; 52:73–80.

Ridker PM, et al. Hepatic venocclusive disease associated with the consumption of pyrrolizidine-containing dietary supplements. *Gastroenterology.* 1985;(88):1050–1054.

Schulz V, Hnsel R, Tyler VE. *Rational Phytotherapy: A Physician's Guide to Herbal Medicine.* 3rd ed. Berlin: Springer; 1998:262.

Shealy C. *The Illustrated Encyclopedia of Healing Remedies.* Dorset, UK: Element Books; 1998:132.

Tyler VE. *Herbs of Choice: The Therapeutic Use of Phytomedicinals.* Binghamton, NY: Pharmaceutical Products Press; 1994:158–169.

Tyler VE. *The Honest Herbal: A Sensible Guide to the Use of Herbs and Related Remedies.* 3rd Ed. Binghamton, NY: Pharmaceutical Products Press; 1993:97–100.

© Copyright Integrative Medicine Communications

Dandelion

Names

- **English**
  Dandelion Herb/Dandelion Root With Herb

- **Botanical**
  Taraxacum officinale

- **Plant Family**
  Asteraceae

- **Pharmacopeial**
  Taraxaci herba/Taraxaci radix cum herba

Overview

Indigenous to Europe, dandelion is now widespread throughout North America. Hundreds of subspecies of *Taraxacum officinale* with distinctive appearances are found in the temperate regions of Europe and Asia as well. Dandelion is a common weed, but it is heralded for both its culinary and medicinal value. It is consumed mainly as a food, and its leaves contain the highest vitamin A content of all greens. This plant is also a source of wine, beer, and coffee substitutes.

In traditional medicine, dandelion roots and leaves are used largely in treatments for hepatic disorders. In Europe, herbalists incorporate it into remedies for liver congestion, fever, skin ailments, eye problems, diarrhea, fluid retention, and heartburn. The leaves produce a transient diuretic effect while the roots act as an appetite stimulant and digestive aid. Chinese medicinal practitioners traditionally used dandelion to treat digestive problems, appendicitis, and breast cancer. Today, herbal practitioners still tout dandelion leaves as an effective diuretic and weight-loss agent.

Dandelion is generally considered nontoxic and devoid of adverse side effects. Pharmacological studies confirm that dandelion stimulates diuresis, and acts on the liver and digestive processes. Taraxacin, an undefined bitter principle in dandelion, may be responsible for its therapeutic effects on digestion. However, there is only limited scientific evidence supporting the efficacy of dandelion for its varied traditional uses. Even though numerous active principles have been isolated from the rhizomes and roots, only a few structure-activity relationships have been established.

Macro Description

Dandelion is a hardy, variable perennial that can grow to a height of nearly 12 inches. Its short rhizome divides at the crown into a tapered, multi-headed taproot. It has a distinctive basal rosette of deeply notched, toothy, spatula-like leaves that are shiny and hairless. Each rosette is capped by a head of composite bright yellow flowers. The grooved leaves funnel the flow of rainfall into the tapered root.

Dandelion flowers are light-sensitive, characteristically opening in the morning and closing in the evening and during gloomy weather. The roots are fleshy and brittle, with a dark brown exterior, and filled with a white milky latex that is bitter and slightly odorous.

Part Used/Pharmaceutical Designations

- leaves
- roots

- **Constituents/Composition**
  Acids (e.g., caffeic acid, *p*-hydroxyphenylacetic acid, chlorogenic acid, linoleic acid, linolenic acid, oleic acid, palmitic acid), resin (undefined bitter complex, taraxacin), terpenoids (sesquiterpene lactones, or bitter substances: e.g., taraxinacetyl-1'-O-glucosides, 11,13-dihydrotaraxinacetyl-1'-O-glucosides, taraxacolide-1'-O-glucosides, taraxinic acid), flavonoids, vitamin A (14,000 IU/100 g leaf), carotenoids, choline, mucilage, inulin, pectin, phytosterols, sugars, potassium.

- **Commercial Preparations**
  Commercial preparations of dandelion are available as liquids and solids for oral use. Root preparations are made from dandelion root harvested in autumn, and the roots are then air-dried. Both dried leaves and dried aerial parts are collected before the flowering season. Root products are preferably prepared from large, fleshy, and well-formed roots on plants that are two years old. Dandelion products when stored should be protected from light and moisture.

Medicinal Uses/Indications

Traditional uses: mild diuretic and weight loss aid (leaf preparations); laxative, cholagogue (stimulates flow of bile to duodenum), muscular rheumatism and other rheumatic ailments, cholecystitis (gallbladder inflammation), gallstones, jaundice, dyspepsia with constipation, oliguria (diminished urination), poor circulation, liver and gallbladder disorders, hemorrhoids, congestion in the portal system, gout, skin ailments

Conditions: dyspepsia, infections of urinary tract, kidney stone and gravel formation, liver and gallbladder complaints, loss of appetite, disturbances in bile flow, stimulation of diuresis, diabetes

Clinical applications: loss of appetite, dyspepsia, bile flow disorders, diuretic

- **Pharmacology**
  An aqueous extract of dandelion showed antitumor activity in vitro. Oral administration of dandelion extracts, particularly herb extracts, produced diuretic activity in rats and mice. Dried dandelion herb (2 g/kg, or 50 ml) exhibited a diuretic effect comparable to that of 80 mg/kg furosemide (Lasix) without the potentially adverse side effects of Lasix.

  An alcohol extract of dandelion was given to mice inoculated with Ehrlich ascites cancer cells, with the test animals receiving dandelion over a 10-day period. The extract significantly suppressed the growth of cancerous cells within one week after treatment. In other research, dandelion stimulated production of antibodies to active polypeptides in tumor-induced ascites fluid in mice.

  Dandelion and one of its constituents, inulin, showed hypoglycemic activity in normoglycemic but not in alloxan-treated hyperglycemic (diabetic) rabbits. The blood-sugar-lowering effect of dandelion may result from stimulation of pancreatic beta-cells, the mechanism responsible for the hypoglycemic activity of the sulfonylureas. In another investigation, a dandelion root extract produced moderate anti-inflammatory action against carrageenan rat paw edema.

Dosage Ranges and Duration of Administration

- Dried leaf infusion: 4 to 10 g tid
- Dried root (infusion or decoction): 2 to 8 g tid
- Herb: 4 to 10 g tid
- Leaf tincture (1:5) in 30% alcohol: 5 ml tid
- Powdered solid extract (4:1): 250 to 500 mg/day
- Root tincture (1:2) fresh root in 45% alcohol: 5 ml tid

Cautions

- **Adverse Effects/Toxicology**
  Dandelion is considered safe even in large quantities. Dandelion can be used for an unlimited duration.

  The toxicity of this plant is extremely low. It is reportedly free of adverse side effects when used both externally and internally. LD_{50} values (mice, I.P.) for the root and herb are 36.8 g/kg and 28.8 g/kg, respectively. Rabbits given dandelion extracts by mouth 3, 4, 5, and 6 g/kg body-weight for periods of up to one week showed neither visible signs of toxicity nor behavioral changes.

  However, the bitter substances in this plant can cause gastric hyperacidity in some individuals. Though rare, contact allergic reactions can occur in response to sesquiterpene lactones in the latex. Also, dandelion has a weak sensitizing capacity.

- **Warnings/Contraindications/Precautions**
  Susceptible individuals may develop contact allergic reactions to dandelion; however, ingestion does not appear to cause allergic responses. Pregnant and lactating women can use dandelion safely if their intake is limited to quantities used in foods.

  Dandelion may precipitate closure of the biliary ducts, gallbladder empyema (inflammation), and ileus. Individuals with biliary conditions and gallstones should first consult with a doctor before ingesting dandelion.

Interactions

Dandelion may augment the effects of other diuretic agents. It may interfere with the hypoglycemic action of other medications.

Regulatory and Compendial Status

In Britain, dandelion is included in the General Sale List (GSL). The Council of Europe classifies this herb as a natural source of food flavoring (category N2) approved as an additive to foodstuffs in small quantities. Dandelion is listed as an approved herb in *The Complete German Commission E Monographs*.

References

Akhtar M, Khan Q, Khaliq T. Effects of *Portulaca oleraceae* (kulfa) and *Taraxacum officinale* (dhudhal) in normoglycaemic and alloxan-treated hyperglycaemic rabbits. *J Pakistan Med Assoc*. 1985;35:207–201.

Baba K, Abe S, Mizuno D. Antitumor activity of hot water extract of dandelion, *Taraxacum officinale*-correlation between antitumor activity and timing of administration [in Japanese]. *Yakugaku Zasshi*. 1981;101(ISS 6):538–43.

Blumenthal M, ed. *The Complete German Commission E Monographs*. Boston, Mass: Integrative Medicine Communications; 1998:118–120.

Davies MG, Kersey PJ. Contact allergy to yarrow and dandelion. *Contact Dermatitis*. 1986;14 (ISS 4):256–7.

Dorland's Illustrated Medical Dictionary. 25th ed. Philadelphia, Pa: W.B. Saunders; 1974.

Grieve M. *A Modern Herbal*. Vol. I. New York, NY: Dover; 1971:249–255.

Gruenwald J, Brendler T, Jaenicke C. *PDR for Herbal Medicines*. Montvale, NJ: Medical Economics Company; 1998:1174–76.

Hobbs C. *Taraxacum officinale*: A monograph and literature review. In: *Eclectic Dispensatory*. Portland, Ore: Eclectic Medical Publications; 1989.

Mascolo N, et al. Biological screening of Italian medicinal plants for anti-inflammatory activity. *Phytotherapy Res* 1987:28–29.

Murray MT. *The Healing Power of Herbs*. 2nd ed. Rocklin, Calif: Prima Publishing; 1995: 86–91.

Newall C, Anderson L, Phillipson J. *Herbal Medicines: A Guide for Health-care Professionals*. London, England: Pharmaceutical Press; 1996:96–97.

Racz-Kotilla E, Racz G, Solomon A. The action of *Taraxacum officinale* extracts on the body weight and diuresis of laboratory animals. *Planta Med*. 1974;26: 212–217.

Tyler V. *The Honest Herbal: A Sensible Guide to the Use of Herbs and Related Remedies*. 3rd ed. New York, NY: Pharmaceutical Products Press; 1993:109–110.

Yamashita K, Kawai K, Itakura M. Effects of fructooligosaccharides on blood glucose and serum lipids in diabetic subjects. *Nutr Res*. 1984;4:491–496.

© *Copyright Integrative Medicine Communications*

Devil's Claw

Names

- **English**
  Devil's claw root

- **Botanical**
  Harpagophytum procumbens

- **Plant Family**
  Pedaliaceae

- **Pharmacopeial**
  Harpagophyti radix

Overview

Harpagophytum procumbens and a closely related plant, Harpagophytum zeyheri, are native to southern Africa and Madagascar. They are the only two species in *Harpagophytum*, a genus in the sesame family. Both species have comparable anti-inflammatory and pain-reducing activity, and both are used as a source of *Harpagophytum radix*.

According to traditional folklore, the Khoisan of the Kalahari used the dried root in remedies to treat pain, pregnancy complications, and skin disorders. Devil's claw has appetite stimulating and mildly analgesic pharmacological actions. Today, this bitter-tasting plant is sold in Europe and Canada as a digestive aid and appetite stimulant.

Devil's claw is collected from the savannas and outskirts of the Kalahari Desert in South Africa and Namibia. The drug is made from dried, secondary tubers. The root tubers are always sliced or pulverized before they are dried because they are nearly impossible to cut once they have dried.

Macro Description

Devil's claw is a leafy perennial with a branched root system and branched shoots. The fruit consists of large woody grapples that are pointed and barbed. The secondary tuber roots grow out of the main and lateral roots. The root tubers (also called peripheral tubers) can reach a size of 20 cm long and 3 cm thick. The crude drug is made from the dried, yellowish-gray to bright pink tubers.

Part Used/Pharmaceutical Designations

- Roots (rhizome)
- Dried secondary tubers

- **Constituents/Composition**
  Monoterpenes include mainly harpagoside (0.5% to 1.6%; extremely bitter iridoid glycoside), harpagide, procumbide; phenylethanol derivatives include acteoside (verbascoside), isoacetoside; oligossacharides; harpagoquinones; other compounds (carbohydrates, amino acids, flavonoids).

- **Commercial Preparations**
  Dried powder capsules and fluid extract preparations are made from dried secondary tubers.

Medicinal Uses/Indications

Traditional herbal actions: antirheumatic, analgesic, sedative, diuretic, antipyretic, anti-inflammatory; Newall painful arthroses, tendinitis, dyspepsia, liver and gallbladder problems, loss of appetite (anorexia); supportive treatment for degenerative musculoskelatal conditions (disorders of locomotive system)

Clinical applications: Rheumatic and joint disorders such as rheumatoid arthritis, osteo arthritis, and gout. Conditions involving inflammation of connective tissues such as fibromyalgia, fibrositis, tendinitis, adhesions due to scar tissue. Liver, kidney, and bladder disorders; allergies; arteriosclerosis; lumbago; gastrointestinal problems; menstrual symptoms; neuralgia; headache; heartburn; nicotine poisoning

- **Pharmacology**
  Several in vitro and in vivo investigations confirm that aqueous extracts of devil's claw and its primary active principle, harpagoside, have anti-inflammatory and anti-exudative effects. In one study, devil's claw exhibited anti-inflammatory effects comparable to those of the antiarthritic drug, phenylbutazone. Anti-inflammatory effects have been strongest in semi-chronic rather than in acute inflammatory animal models. In another investigation, however, devil's claw failed to show anti-inflammatory properties when compared to aspirin and indomethacin. Other studies have not unequivocally shown that devil's claw reduces inflammation in either animals or humans. Inconsistent findings on efficacy may be due to different modes of administering the drug. Gastric juices apparently inactivate some of the active constituents. Therapeutic effects may be difficult to demonstrate in animal models unless devil's root extracts are protected from gastric enzymes.

In an in vitro experiment, indomethacin and aspirin caused a 5% inhibition of prostaglandin synthetase activity, but devil's claw did not produce a significant reduction in enzyme activity. In vitro research also shows that harpagoside diminished the contractile response of smooth muscle in isolated muscle preparations. Harpagoside and other active principles presumably are able to alter the contractile response by disrupting calcium influx. In addition, devil's claw extracts have weak antifungal properties.

Devil's claw extracts are cardioactive and have protective activity against ventricular arrhythmias. However, the cardioactive effects are not entirely due to harpagoside. Instead, cardioprotecive properties are attributed to a synergy between hapagoside and other active constituents in the crude extract.

The biochemical action of devil's claw on arachidonic acid metabolism apparently differs from the mechanisms of action found in NSAIDs. The therapeutic effects are perhaps explained by in vivo conversion (via enzymatic hydrolysis) of either harpagoside or harpagide into harpagogenin.

In a double-blind, placebo-controlled clinical study, 89 patients with rheumatoid symptoms were given two g of powdered devil's claw daily for two months. The treatment group had significant improvements compared to the placebo group in sensitivity to pain and in flexibility measured by fingertip-floor distance.

Dosage Ranges and Duration of Administration

- Dried tuber: Take 0.1 to 0.25 g tid, encapsulated or as decoction.
- Fluid extract (1:1 in 25% alcohol): Take 0.1 to 0.25 ml tid.
- Tincture (1:5 in 25% alcohol): Take 0.5 to 1.0 ml tid.

Cautions

- **Adverse Effects/Toxicology**
  Most experts consider devil's claw nontoxic and safe.

- **Warnings/Contraindications/Precautions**
  No side effects have been reported for devil's claw root when it is administered in recommended therapeutic doses. However, this herb should not be used in excess because information on toxicology is limited. Cardioactivity makes it potentially risky for individuals with certain medical conditions because devil's claw stimulates gastric secretions. Individuals with gastric and/or duodenal ulcers, and/or gallstones should not take devil's claw without the advice of a physician or other qualified health care provider. Cinnamylic acid and terpene in devil's claw may trigger allergic effects. Despite a common misconception that devil's claw is an abortifacient, pharmacological research suggests that this plant does not induce abortion. However, digestive stimulants such as devil's claw should not be used in pregnancy because of the reflexive action on uterine muscle.

Interactions

None known

Regulatory and Compendial Status

The U.S. FDA classifies devil's claw as a dietary supplement. The plant is accepted in France for specified indications. It is approved by the German Commision E. Devil's claw is not included on the GSL in Britain.

References

Baghdikian B, Lanhers M, Fleurentin J, et al. An analytical study, anti-inflammatory and analgesic effects of *Harpagophytum procumbens and Harpagophytum zeyheri*. *Planta Med.* 1997;63:171–176.

Blumenthal M, ed. *The Complete German Commission E Monographs: Therapeutic Guide to Herbal Medicines*. Boston, Mass: Integrative Medicine Communications; 1998.

Bradley P, ed. *British Herbal Compendium*. Dorset, England: British Herbal Medicine Association; 1992;1:96–98.

British Herbal Pharmacopoeia 1996. 4th ed. Dorset, England: British Herbal Medicine Association; 1996.

Costa de Pasquale R, Busa G, Circosta C, et al. A drug used in traditional medicine: *Harpagophytum procumbens DC.* III. Effects on hyperkinetic ventricular arrhythmias by reperfusion. *J Ethnopharmacology.* 1985;(13):193–9.

Grahame R, Robinson B. Devil's claw (*Harpagophytum procumbens*): pharmacological and clinical studies. *Ann Rheum Dis.* 1981;40:632.

Guyader M. 1984. Les plantes antirhumatismales. Etude historique et pharmacologique, et etude clinique du nebulisat *d'Harpagophytum procumbens* DC chez 50 patients arthrosiques sivis en service hospitalier. Paris: Universite Pierre et Marie Curie.

Lanhers MC, Fleurentin J, Mortier F, Vinche A, Younos C. Anti-inflammatory and analgesic effects of an aqueous extract of *Harpagophytum procumbens. Planta Med.* 1992;58:117–123.

Mabberley DJ. *The Plant-Book: A Portable Dictionary of the Higher Plants.* Cambridge, England: Cambridge University Press; 1987.

McLeod D, et al. Investigations of *Harpagophytum procumbens* (Devil's Claw) in the treatment of experimental inflammation and arthritis in the rat. *Br J Pharmacol.* 1979;66:140P

Moussard C, Alber D, Toubin M, Thevenon N, Henry JC. A drug used in traditional medicine, *Harpagophytum procumbens:* no evidence for NSAID-like effect on whole blood eicosanoid production in human. *Prostaglandins Leukot Essent Fatty Acids.* 1992;46:283–286.

Newall C, Anderson L, Phillipson J. *Herbal Medicines: A Guide for Health-care Professionals.* London, England: Pharmaceutical Press; 1996.

Occhiuto F, Circosta C, Ragusa S, Ficarra P, Costa De Pasquale R. A drug used in traditional medicine: *Harpagophytum procumbens* DC. IV. Effects on some isolated muscle preparations. *J Ethnopharmacol.* 1985;13:201–208.

Schulz V, Hnsel R, Tyler VE. *Rational Phytotherapy: A Physician's Guide to Herbal Medicine.* 3rd ed. Berlin, Germany: Springer-Verlag; 1998.

Tyler VE. *The Honest Herbal: A Sensible Guide to the Use of Herbs and Related Remedies.* 3rd ed. Binghampton, NY: Pharmaceutical Products Press; 1993.

Whitehouse L, et al. Devil's Claw *(Harpagophytum procumbens):* no evidence for anti-inflammatory activity in the treatment of arthritic disease. *Can Med Assoc J.* 1983;129:249–251.

© *Copyright Integrative Medicine Communications*

Echinacea

Names

■ **English**
Echinacea Angustifolia herb-root/Echinacea Pallida herb-root/Echinacea Purpurea herb-root

■ **Botanical**
Echinacea angustifolia/Echinacea pallida/Echinacea purpurea

■ **Plant Family**
Asteraceae

■ **Pharmacopeial**
Echinacea angustofoliae herba-radix/Echinacea pallidae herba-radix/Echinacea purpureae herba-radix

Overview

Echinacea may reduce the symptoms and duration of colds, flu, chronic infections of the respiratory tract, or infections of the lower urinary tract. Topically, it may speed the healing of chronic or slow-healing wounds. Its nonspecific, immune-stimulant activity is currently under investigation, yet it is believed to particularly activate phagocytosis and stimulate fibroblasts.

The species is named for the sharp, spiny pales of its large conical seed head, which resemble the spines of an angry hedgehog (*echinos* is Greek for hedgehog). Of nine species, the three noted above are used medicinally.

An archeological dig in the region of the Lakota Sioux unearthed echinacea dating to the 1600s. Native Americans used echinacea for snakebites, oral lesions and pain, sepsis, sore throat, colic, and stomachaches. It was also historically used for scarlet fever, syphilis, malaria, blood poisoning, and diphtheria. Through the 1800s, it was the most widely used plant drug in the United States, dispensed by both eclectic physicians and more traditional doctors. It remained on the national list of official plant drugs in the United States until the 1940s, most likely taken off this list because the conditions it had been used for were then being treated with antibiotics.

Macro Description

Native to North America, echinacea consists of erect stems and alternate or opposite leaves that vary from appearing oval shaped, to oval-shaped ending in points, with varying degrees of teeth along the edges. Flowers grow singly on stem ends. Blooms are large, bear both ray and disk flowers, and have a characteristic cone-shaped receptacle. Roots grow either vertically or horizontally.

E. angustifolia has purplish-red ray flower with darker disk flowers; *E. purpurea* bears deep rose-purple ray flowers, and pales in the seed head may be tipped with orange. *E. pallida*'s flowers are pale rose, usually drooping.

Part Used/Pharmaceutical Designations

- Flower
- Seeds
- Leaves
- Roots
- Stems

■ **Constituents/Composition**
Polysaccharides, flavonoids, caffeic acid derivatives (echinoside, cichoric acid, chlorogenic acid, and isochlorogenic acids), essential oils, polyacetylenes, alkylamides, alkaloids

■ **Commercial Preparations**
Many dozens of preparations are available as urological, wound, and flu remedies, but preparations standardized to 1:2 tincture, with 50% alcohol, 3 to 5 ml qid, made from fresh root or fresh root and cone are preferred. Extracts, tinctures, tablets, capsules, ointments and stabilized fresh extracts are available. In Europe, intraperitoneal and intravenous forms are sometimes used.

Medicinal Uses/Indications

Traditional herbal actions: anti-microbial, immunostimulant, anti-infective, anti-inflammatory, alterative

Clinical applications: Furunculosis and boils, septicemia, nasopharyngeal inflammation, pyorrhea, tonsillitis, carbuncles, abscesses, viral, fungal, and bacterial illness, chronic respiratory infection, colds and flu. Used topically for wounds and dermal ulceration.

■ **Pharmacology**
Echinacea is an immune stimulant with anti-inflammatory, antiviral, and antibacterial effects. These effects are largely due to nonspecific immune system activation. Carbon clearance tests have measured significant echinacea-induced macrophage activation. Echinacea's polysaccharides are immunostimulatory; its polyacetylenes are anti-inflammatory.

Echinacea increases phagocytosis; activates T lymphocytes; stimulates tumor necrosis factor, properdin, and interferon; inhibits hyaluronidase; and stimulates the adrenal cortex.

One in vitro study showed that when mouse cells were injected with echinacea extracts and incubated, a 24-hour period of resistance to influenza, herpes, and vesicular viruses resulted, likely due to nonspecific T-cell activation.

In animal studies, Echinacea's polysaccharides induce tissue regeneration; polyacetylenes are anti-inflammatory when injected. Echinacea also exerts spasmolytic effects to acetylcholine-induced spasm.

A lipid-soluble alkene, Z-1,8-pentadecadiene exerts significant anticancer effects in vivo against Walker tumors in rats and P388 leukemia in mice.

In studies in humans, a respected double-blind trial using 100 patients and an initial 2-day dose of 30 ml of echinacea followed by 15 ml for 4 more days demonstrated that echinacea could reduce the duration of a cold from 10 days to 7. In a double-blind, placebo-controlled study of 180 patients, 450 mg doses of *E. purpurea* herb extract was as effective as placebo in providing flu relief, but patients receiving 900 mg doses reported significant relief. Prophylaxis was demonstrated in a double-blind, placebo-controlled study: of 108 cold-prone patients, those receiving 4 ml of a proprietary echinacea formula bid significantly reduced cold recurrence. Fifteen drops of *E. purpurea* tid reduced rheumatoid inflammation up to 21.8% in an uncontrolled study; effects were almost half those exerted by cortisone and prednisone and did not cause additional adverse effects.

As part of a proprietary microbicide, *E. purpurea* demonstrated possible applications against both acyclovir-resistant and acyclovir-susceptible herpes simplex virus. In a recent double-blind, placebo-controlled crossover trial, *E. angustifolia* significantly enhanced natural-killer-cell activity against HIV transinfected cells. Echinacea's therapeutic potential in these diseases deserves further study.

Dosage Ranges and Duration of Administration

For immune stimulation during viral or bacterial infection, choose equivalent form of the following and take three times daily.

- 1 to 2 g dried root, as tea
- 2 to 3 ml of 22% ethanol extract standardized to contain 2.4% beta-1,2-fructofuranosides
- 200 mg of powdered extract containing 6.5:1, or 3.5%, echinacoside
- Fluid extract (1:1): .5 ml to 1 ml tid
- Tincture (1:5): 1 to 3 ml tid
- Stabilized fresh extract: .75 ml tid

Commission E advises to discontinue use of internal *E. purpurea* and *E. pallida* after eight weeks, and parenteral *E. purpurea* after three weeks.

Cautions

■ **Adverse Effects/Toxicology**
The American Herbal Products Association safety rating is class 1 (safe with appropriate use).

Echinacea is a member of the *Compositae* family and as such may rarely cause allergic reaction.

■ **Warnings/Contraindications/Precautions**
Isobutylamides, found only in *angustifolia* roots and *purpurea* seed heads, are responsible for the characteristic numbing and burning sensations when echinacea herb and root extracts are placed on the tongue. Sensation dissipates quickly.

Rare reports of dermatitis. Not recommended for use in systemic diseases (tuberculosis, leukoses, diabetes, collagenosis, multiple sclerosis, AIDS, HIV infection, other autoimmune diseases) or during immunosuppressant therapy. Safety during pregancy has not been studied.

Interactions

Do not use with immunosuppressant therapy.

Regulatory and Compendial Status

Dietary supplement in the United States. *E. pallida* root approved by Germany's Commission E for relief during flu-like infections; *E. purpurea* approved topically for chronic ulcers and slow healing wounds, internally for flu-like infections. On the General Sales List in England.

References

Berman S. Dramatic increase in immune-mediated HIV killing activity induced by *Echinacea angustifolia*. *Int Conf AIDS* 12 (582). Abstract 32309.

Blumenthal M, ed. *The Complete German Commission E Monographs: Therapeutic Guide to Herbal Medicine*. Boston, Mass: Integrative Medicine Communications; 1998.

Brünig B, Dorn M, Knick E. *Echinacea purpurea radix* for strengthening the immune response in flu-like infections. *Z Phytotherapie*. 1992;13:7–13.

Dorn M, Knick E, Lewith G. Placebo-controlled, double-blind study of *Echinacea pallidae radix* in upper respiratory tract infections. *Complementary Therapies in Medicine*.1997;5:40–42.

Hobbs C. Echinacea: a literature review. *Herbalgram* 1994;30:33–47.

Hoheisel O, Sandberg M, Bertram S, Bulitta M, Schfer M. Echinagard treatment shortens the course of the common cold: a double-blind, placebo-controlled clinical trial. *European Journal of Clinical Research*. 1997;9:261–269.

Hyman R, Pankhurst R. *Plants and Their Names: A Concise Dictionary*. New York, NY: Oxford University Press; 1995.

McGuffin M, Hobbs C, Upton R, Goldberg A, eds. *American Herbal Products Association's Botanical Safety Handbook*. Boca Raton, Fla: CRC Press; 1996.

Melchart D, Walther E, Linde K, Brandmaier R, Lersch C. Echinacea root extracts for the prevention of upper respiratory tract infections: a double-blind, placebo-controlled randomized trial. *Arch Fam Med*. 1998;7:541–545.

Melchart D, Linde IK, Worku F, Sarkady L, Holzmann M, Jurcic K, et al. Results of Five Randomized Studies on the Immunomodulatory Activity of Preparations of Echinacea. *J Alt Comp Med*. 1995;1(2):145–160.

Murray MT. *The Healing Power of Herbs: The Enlightened Person's Guide to the Wonders of Medicinal Plants*. Rocklin, Calif: Prima Publishing; 1995.

Newall CA, Anderson LA, Phillipson JD. *Herbal Medicines: A Guide for Health-Care Professionals*. London: The Pharmaceutical Press; 1996.

Schulz V, Hñsel R, Tyler VE. *Rational Phytotherapy: A Physicians' Guide to Herbal Medicine*. 3rd ed. Berlin: Springer; 1998.

Snow JM. Echinacea. *Protocol J Botanical Medicine*. 1997;2:18–24.

Thompson KD. Antiviral activity of Viracea against acyclovir susceptible and acyclovir resistant strains of herpes simplex virus. *Antiviral Res*. 1998;39:55–61.

Tyler VE. *Herbs of Choice: The Therapeutic Use of Phytomedicinals*. Binghamton, NY: Pharmaceutical Products Press; 1994.

Verhoef MJ, Hagen N, Pelletier G, Forsyth P. Alternative therapy use in neurologic disease: use in brain tumor patients. *Neurology* 1999;52:617–622.

© *Copyright Integrative Medicine Communications*

Eucalyptus

Names

■ **English**
Eucalyptus leaf/Eucalyptus oil

■ **Botanical**
Eucalyptus globulus/Eucalyptus fructicetorum/Eucalyptus polybractea/Eucalyptus smithii

■ **Plant Family**
Myrtaceae

■ **Pharmacopeial**
Eucalypti folium/Eucalypti aetheroleum

Overview

Eucalyptus leaf is antibacterial, antiseptic, and astringent. It was most likely first used by the Aborigines of Australia, who applied it as a poultice for wounds, abscesses, and fungal infections of the skin. They also drank eucalyptus leaf tea to reduce fevers. In 19th century England, eucalyptus oil was used in hospitals to clean urinary catheters. Today, herbalists use fresh leaves as a topical antiseptic for wounds and recommend eucalyptus gargles for sore throats, as well as inhalation of the essential oil vapors for the treatment of croup, bronchitis, asthma, nasal congestion, and flu. The oil is antiviral and expectorant; eucalyptus oil-based chest rubs and vapor inhalations relieve respiratory ailments.

Eucalyptus is added to perfumes, soaps, foods, and beverages. It's also found in wax candles and topical sprays to repel insects. Recent research suggests that washing bedclothes with eucalyptus oil may decrease asthmatic patients' exposure to dust mites. Its effects on insect habitats gave it the nickname Australian fevertree: eucalyptus trees dried marshes in which it was planted, so that malaria-bearing mosquitos could not proliferate. It also kills cockroaches. Eucalyptus oil is highly toxic to humans and should be used with care.

Macro Description

There are over 500 species of eucalyptus plants, ranging in height from five-foot shrubs to 480-foot trees. Of these, blue gum is the most common. Reaching up to 230 feet in height, it has smooth, blue-gray bark that peels in shreds, revealing a cream-colored trunk beneath.

Young leaves are opposite and broad; mature 4- to 12-inch leaves are alternate, swordlike, thick, dark green, and shiny. Clusters of flowers grow near axils, bear no petals but white flower stamens, and give way to seeded fruits. The roots, which collect water, quench thirst. When one end of a root is blown into, water drips out the other end and can be collected in a vessel. Eucalyptus is native to Australia and cultivated in Europe, the U.S., China, Africa, and South America. The leaves and branch tips are the source of crude extracts and steam-distilled oil.

Part Used/Pharmaceutical Designations

- Leaves
- Branch tips

■ **Constituents/Composition**
Fresh and dried leaves and branch tips yield yellow, sometimes colorless, volatile oil which consists primarily of cineole (70% to 85%; formerly called eucalyptol); also, monoterpenes (borneol, terpenines, a-terpineol, citronellal, geraniol, iso-fenchone, limonene, linalool, myrcene, a-phellandrene, a- and b-pinene, camphene, trans-pinocarveol, piperitone); sesquiterpenes (aromadendrene, cadinene, caryophyllene, a-copaene, a-,b-, and gamma-eudesmol, globulol); alkanes; flavonoids (eucalyptin). Leaf contains tannins, flavonoids (procyanidin b-2,3'-O-galloyl, prodelphinidin b-2,3'-O-galloyl, prodelphinidin, quercetin, hyperoside, rutin).

■ **Commercial Preparations**
Liquid essential oil (dilute with water, oil, or rubbing acohol before using), topical creams containing essential oil. To be used commercially, eucalyptus oil must have a high percentage of cineole (not less than 70%). Concentrations of phellandrene and aldehydes must be low. Crude leaf and aqueous extracts from leaf material are also available.

Commercial cough drops, syrups, vaporizer fluid, liniments, toothpaste, and mouthwash may contain eucalyptus oil or 1.8-cineole; both are also used in dentistry. Used in perfume, no more than 1.0% oil is allowed in products; 0.002% is the allowable limit for 1.8-cineole content in foods.

Medicinal Uses/Indications

Traditional actions: oil—antiseptic, expectorant, antiviral, febrifuge; leaves—decongestant, astringent, stimulant. Eucalyptus was historically used for pulmonary tuberculosis, bacterial dysentery, and aching joints, but it is no longer used clinically for these conditions.

Eucalyptus leaves are currently used internally for bronchial and throat inflammation, excess mucus, congestive chest conditions, to combat colds and influenza. Eucalyptus oil is used externally for chest congestion, aches and pains, ringworm, tinnea, and as a deoderant.

Clinical applications: The German Commission E approves internal use of leaf extracts and steam inhalation of essential oil for catarrh of the upper respiratory tract, and dilute essential oil topical applications to relieve rheumatic discomfort.

■ **Pharmacology**
Essential oil is antibacterial against *Escherichia coli, Staphylococcus spp., Pseudomonas, Enterobacter species, Hemophilus influenzae, Proteus mirabilis,* and *Klebsiella* species in agar plate tests. It is antifungal to *Aspergillus aeguptiacus* and *Trichoderma viride.* Gram-positive bacteria are apparently the most sensitive to eucalyptus preparations. Oral doses and external application are expectorant.

Crude leaf extract lowers high blood sugar levels in rabbits. The flavonoids quercetin and hyperoside demonstrate in vitro anti-influenza (Type A) activity.

In humans, a combination formula including eucalyptus oil has been used to successfully treat suppurative otitis. Topical application inhibits prostaglandin synthesis, and stimulates mild hyperemic, expectorant, and secretolytic effects. Leaf extracts stimulate the same effects.

Dosage Ranges and Duration of Administration

- Eucalyptus leaf as infusion: 1 to 2 g per cup tid
- Eucalyptus leaf tincture (for catarrh): $1/2$ to 1 ml/day
- Oil for topical application (sore joints or chest rub for catarrh): 30 ml oil to 500 ml lukewarm water.
- Eucalyptol (catarrh): 0.05 to 0.2 ml (1 to 2 drops per cup boiling water) daily
- Eucalyptus oil (for topical application): add $1/2$ to 1 ml (15 to 30 drops) of oil to $1/2$ cup of carrier oil (sesame, olive, etc.). For inhalation, add 5 to 10 drops of oil to 2 cups boiling water; place towel over head and inhale steam.

Cautions

■ **Adverse Effects/Toxicology**
When used externally, eucalyptus oil is non-toxic, non-sensitizing, and does not promote phototoxicity. Internally, eucalyptus oil is toxic and must be diluted. Ingestion of 3.4 ml oil has resulted in death.

The American Herbal Products Association gives eucalyptus leaf a class 2d safety rating, specifying gastric and bile duct inflammatory disease as contraindications, and cautioning against use on the faces of children under age 2. Tannins (comprising 11% of leaf extract constituents) in the leaves may cause gastrointestinal distress or kidney and liver damage if leaf preparations are ingested in large amounts.

Symptoms of poisoning include epigastric burning, miosis, cyanosis, and convulsions. Charcoal lavage, diazepam, atropine, electrolyte replenishment, sodium bicarbonate, intubation, or oxygen respiration may be required as treatments. Non-fatal doses of leaf extracts or essential oil caused nausea, vomiting, diarrhea.

■ **Warnings/Contraindications/Precautions**
Eucalyptus oil should not be ingested; should be in diluted form when used topically. Do not use while pregnant or breastfeeding. Not for use in patients with inflammatory disease of gastrointestinal tract or bile ducts, or severe liver disease. Eucalyptus oil should not be applied to the face of infants or young children, and especially not near the nose or mouth; glottal spasm, bronchial spasm, or asphyxiation may result.

Interactions

Eucalyptus extract and oil may interfere with hypoglycemic therapy.

Regulatory and Compendial Status

Approved for food use in appropriate quantities in the U.S., and also as a dietary supplement. Licensed through the General Sales List in England. Approved for the treatment of respiratory catarrh and rheumatic complaints by the German Commission E.

References

Belzner S. [Eucalyptus oil dressings in urinary retention] Eukalyptusol-kompresse bei harnverhalten. *Pflege Aktuell.* 1997;51:386–387.

Benouda A, Hassar M, Menjilali B. In vitro antibacterial properties of essential oils, tested against hospital pathogenic bacteria. *Fitoterapia.* 1988;59:115–119.

Blumenthal M, ed. *The Complete German Commission E Monographs.* Boston, Mass: Integrative Medicine Communications; 1998.

Bremness L. *Herbs.* New York, NY: DK Publishing; 1994.

Burrow A, Eccles R, Jones AS. The effects of camphor, eucalyptus and menthol vapour on nasal resistance to airflow and nasal sensation. *Acta Otolaryngol (Stockh).* 1983;96(1-2):157–161.

Castleman M. *The Healing Herbs.* Emmaus, Pa: Rodale Press; 1991.

El-keltawi NEM, Megalla SE, Ross SA. Antimicrobial activity of some Egyptian aromatic plants. *Herba Pol.* 1980;26:245–250.

Evans WC. *Trease and Evans' Pharmacognosy.* 13th ed. London, England: Bailliere Tindall; 1989.

Gruenwald J, Brendler T et al, eds. *PDR for Herbal Medicines.* Montvale, NJ: Medical Economics Company Inc; 1998.

Kumar A, et al. Antibacterial properties of some *Eucalyptus* oils. *Fitoterapia.* 1988;59:141–144.

Leung A, Foster S. *Encyclopedia of Common Natural Ingredients Used in Food, Drugs, and Cosmetics.* 2nd ed. New York, NY: Wiley & Sons; 1996.

McGuffin M, Hobbs C, Upton R, Goldberg A. *American Herbal Products Associations's Botanical Safety Handbook.* Boca Raton, Fla: CRC Press; 1996.

Newall CA, Anderson LA, Phillipson JD. *Herbal Medicines: A Guide for Health Care Professionals.* London, England: The Pharmaceutical Press; 1996:72–73.

Nichimura H, Calvin M. Essential oil of Eucalyptus globulus in California. *J Agr Food Chem.* 1979;27:432–435.

Osawa K, et al. Macrocarpals H, I, and J from the Leaves of *Eucalyptus globulus. J Nat Prod.* 1996;59:823–827.

Tovey ER, McDonald LG. Clinical aspects of allergic disease: A simple washing procedure with eucalyptus oil for controlling house dust mites and their allergens in clothing and bedding. *J Allergy Clin Immunol.* 1997;100:464–467.

Whitman BW, Ghazizadeh H. Eucalyptus oil: therapeutic and toxic aspects of pharmacology in humans and animals [letter; comment]. *J Paediatr Child Health.* 1994;30(2):190–191.

© *Copyright Integrative Medicine Communications*

Evening Primrose

Names

- **English**
  Evening primrose

- **Botanical**
  Oenothera biennis

- **Plant Family**
  Onagraceae

Overview

Currently, evening primrose seed oil (EPO) is used to treat atopic dermatitis and cyclical/non-cyclical mastalgia. It is also considered to be potentially useful for the treatment of premenstrual syndrome and many other inflammatory conditions. The plant that the seed oil comes from, evening primrose, has served as both food and medicine at previous times in history. Native Americans ate the boiled, nutty-flavored root, and used leaf poultices from the plant for bruises and hemorrhoids. European settlers took the root back to England and Germany, where it was introduced as food and became known as German rampion. The plant was also a Shaker medicine, sold commercially.

Recent investigation of dietary fatty acids and their roles in health stimulated interest in evening primrose. EPO contains the essential fatty acids linoleic acid (LA) and gamma-linolenic acid (GLA). GLA, an omega-6 series fatty acid, normally forms in the body during the desaturation of LA. Both GLA and its break-down product, dihomogamma-linolenic acid (DGLA), are involved with the formation of prostaglandins E1 (PGE1) and E2 (PGE2). PGE1 are vasodilatory, immune-modulating, and anti-inflammatory prostaglandins. They also inhibit platelet aggregation and phospholipase A2, block cholesterol synthesis, and lower blood pressure. PGE2 prostaglandins, on the other hand, tend toward the opposite of these actions.

EPO ingestion, and subsequent GLA and DGLA formation, may result in reductions to PGE2 stimulation by arachadonic acid. Tests demonstrate that DGLA-stimulated PGE1 reduces PGE2. EPO delivers GLA, bypasses conversion, and favors PGE1 formation over PGE2. The many potential uses of EPO include atopic eczema, diabetes, cardiovascular disease, high cholesterol, chronic fatigue syndrome, and cancer. Patients with some of these illnesses have demonstrated a slower LA-GLA conversion rate, as well as, in some cases, deficient levels of LA due to poor diet.

Macro Description

Biennial plant native to North America, evening primrose grows a rosette of leaves in the first year, and creamy yellow or bright yellow flowers in the second. Flowers bloom after sunset, June through September, or on overcast days. Stems are branched, with alternate, lanceolate leaves; flowers contain a predominant X-shaped stamen and seeds. This monograph focuses on the seed from which the oil is extracted.

Part Used/Pharmaceutical Designations

- Flower
- Leaves
- Roots
- Seed oil

- **Constituents/Composition**
  Seed oil contains up to 25% fatty oil, which is extracted with hexane (except in the case of products labeled "hexane free") to produce a 60% to 80% linoleic acid/8% to 14% gamma-linolenic acid product.

- **Commercial Preparations**
  Standardized preparations (8% gamma-linolenic acid), in capsules or as oil.

Medicinal Uses/Indications

Traditional actions of the leaf, flower, and root bark include vulnerary, stomachic, demulcent, and anti-inflammatory. Oil is used topically for infantile eczema. Conditions for which it is used clinically today include bruises, wounds, obesity, hemorrhoids, infantile eruptions.

In clinical applications, there are two categories of potential indications.

- Conditions associated with essential fatty acid deficiency or imbalance: acne, arthritis, rheumatoid arthritis, asthma, chronic fatigue syndrome, platelet aggregation and high blood pressure relative to congestive heart failure, diabetic neuropathy, developmental disorders, diabetes, dry scaly skin, eczema, fibrocystic breast disease, inflammation, intermittent claudication, hypercholesterolemia, mastalgia, metabolic disorders, migraine, multiple sclerosis, premenstrual syndrome, psoriases, psychological disorders, Raynaud's syndrome, Sjogren's syndrome
- Conditions associated with difficulty or inability to convert cis-linoleic acid to prostaglandin E1: aging-related disorders, alcoholism, cancer, poor nutrition, radiation damage

- **Pharmacology**
  Anti-inflammatory and relaxed smooth muscle response may result from alterations in prostaglandin biosynthesis. Effects of EPO vary and indicate a need for future research.

  Placebo-controlled studies show positive effects for EPO in: rheumatoid arthritis patients (resulting in a lesser need for NSAIDs in 60% of RA patients despite the lack of changes in biochemical indicators); Sjogren's syndrome (mild increase in tear flow); irritable bowel syndrome (symptom improvement); chronic fatigue syndrome (symptom improvement); kidney transplant graft survival rate; endometriosis (90% symptom reduction in EPO group, versus 10% symptom reduction in placebo group); schizophrenic symptoms (EPO/zinc/B_6/C/niacin combination, also improved tardive dyskenesia, memory loss); alcohol withdrawal; Alzheimer's disease.

  Two large double-blind, placebo-controlled trials showed no effect of EPO on atopic dermatitis. Smaller studies, with severe cases, showed positive results.

  Most studies support EPO in the treatment of non-cyclic breast pain and inflammation. A daily dosage of 3 g EPO had an equal effect to bromocriptine. Neither EPO nor bromocriptine were as effective as danazol, but the EPO recipients had significantly fewer side effects (4%) than did the pharmaceutical recipients (danazol: 30%; bromocriptine: 35%).

  Both positive results and no results have been demonstrated in studies on the effects of EPO on premenstrual syndrome, and studies on EPO in multiple sclerosis also yield conflicting results; patients in early or less severe stages of the disease showed the greatest benefit.

  Effects of EPO and GLA on human cancers are currently under study.

Dosage Ranges and Duration of Administration

Products are standardized to contain 8% gamma-linolenic acid. A three-month treatment period may be necessary in order to achieve a clinical response. The recommended doses are as follows.

- Atopic dermatitis: 6 to 8 g (adult); 2 to 4 g (child)
- Cyclical and non-cyclical mastalgia: 3 to 4 g daily
- Premenstrual syndrome: 3 g daily

Cautions

- **Adverse Effects/Toxicology**
  American Herbal Products Association (AHPA) safety rating: class 1 (safe with appropriate use). Reported side effects are rare and mild, and include nausea, stomach pain, headache. Soft stool and abdominal pain indicate excess dosage.

- **Warnings/Contraindications/Precautions**
  EPO may trigger latent temporal lobe epilepsy. Schitzophrenics receiving phenothiazines are at greatest risk; occurrence not yet observed in non-phenothiazine therapy.

  Breast milk contains LA and GLA; EPO safety while breastfeeding is inferred. During pregnancy, use with caution as for any herbal preparation or dietary supplement.

Interactions

Increases risk of temporal lobe epilepsy when used in combination with epileptogenic drugs for schizophrenia.

Regulatory and Compendial Status

In the Unites States, EPO is a dietary supplement. In England, a proprietary evening primrose oil is licensed for use in atopic eczema and mastalgia.

Germany has approved evening primrose as a food, but the oil is not included in the Commission E monographs.

References

Belch JJR, Ansell D, Madhok R, O'Dowd A, Sturrock RD. Effects of altering dietary essential fatty acids on requirements for NSAIDs in patients with rheumatoid arthritis. *Ann Rheum Dis.* 1988;47:96–104.

Blumenthal M, Riggins C. *Popular Herbs in the U.S. Market: Therapeutic Monographs.* Austin, Tex: The American Botanical Council; 1997.

Brehler R, Hildebrand A, Luger TA. Clinical reviews: recent developments in the treatment of atopic eczema. *J Am Acad Dermatol.* 1997;36: 989–990.

Foster S. *Herbal Renaissance: Growing, Using and Understanding Herbs in the Modern World.* Salt Lake City, Utah: Gibbs-Smith; 1993.

Fugh-Berman A. Complementary and Alternative Therapies in Primary Care: Clinical trials of herbs. *Primary Care: Clinics in Office Practice.* 1997;24: 889–903.

Graham-Brown R. Psychodermatology: Managing adults with atopic dermatitis. *Dermatologic Clinics.* 1996;14: 536.

Greenfield S.M. et al. A randomized controlled study of evening primrose oil and fish oil in ulcerative colitis. *Aliment Pharmacol Ther.* 1993;7:159–166.

Horrobin DF. Interactions between n-3 and n-6 essential fatty acids (EFAs) in the regulation of cardiovascular disorders and inflammation. *Prostaglandins Leukot Essent Fatty Acids.* 1991;44:127–131.

Horrobin DF. The relationship between schizophrenia and essential fatty acid and eicosanoid metabolism. *Prostaglandins Leukot Essent Fatty Acids.* 1992;46:71–77.

Jamal GA, Carmichael H. The effect of y-linolenic acid on human diabetic peripheral neuropathy: A double-blind placebo-controlled trial. *Diabetic Med.* 1990;7(4):319–323.

Khoo S.K., C. Munro, D. Battistutta. Evening primrose oil and treatment of premenstrual syndrome. *Med J Aust.* 1990;153(4):189–192.

Leung A, Foster S. *Encyclopedia of Common Natural Ingredients Used in Food, Drugs, and Cosmetics.* 2nd ed. New York, NY: Wiley & Sons; 1996.

McGuffin M, Hobbs C, Upton R, Goldberg A. *American Herbal Products Associations' Botanical Safety Handbook.* Boca Raton, Fla: CRC Press; 1996.

Murray M. *The Encyclopedia of Nutritional Supplements.* Rocklin, Calif: Prima Publishing; 1996.

Newall CA, Anderson LA, Phillipson JD. *Herbal Medicines: A Guide for Health Care Professionals.* London, England: The Pharmaceutical Press; 1996.

Scarff DH, Lloyd DH. Double-blind, placebo-controlled crossover study of evening primrose oil in the treatment of canine atopy. *Veterinary.* 1992.

Schultz V, Hansel R, Tyler V. *Rational Phytotherapy: A Physician's Guide to Herbal Medicine.* Heidelberg: Springer-Verlag; 1998.

Stewart JCM, et al. Treatment of severe and moderately severe atopic dermatitis with evening primrose oil (Epogam): a multi-center study. *J Nut Med.* 1991;2:9–16.

© Copyright Integrative Medicine Communications

Feverfew

Names

- **English**
  Feverfew

- **Botanical**
  Tanacetum parthenium/Chrysanthemum parthenium

- **Plant Family**
  Compositae

- **Pharmacopeial**
  Tanaceti parthenii herba

Overview

A wealth of scientific evidence shows that feverfew is an effective treatment and prophylactic for migraine headaches. Used for centuries in European folk medicine, feverfew was traditionally utilized for headache, arthritis, and fever. The word feverfew is a corruption of the Latin febrifuge, which literally means fever-reducing.

In a survey conducted in Britain in the 1980s, 70% of migraine sufferers who ate two to three fresh feverfew leaves daily experienced considerable relief from their headaches. A clinical study later revealed that feverfew significantly reduced the symptoms of migraine when compared with placebo. Feverfew also lessened accompanying symptoms of nausea and vomiting. In 1997, this medicinal herb ranked #19 on a list of the top herbs sold at health food stores in the United States.

Feverfew's anti-migraine activity comes from parthenolide, a sesquiterpene lactone. Parthenolide is a spasmolytic that makes smooth muscle in the walls of cerebral blood vessels less reactive to vasoconstrictors. Parthenolide helps prevent migraines and lessen the severity of existing migraines by acting as an antagonist to vasoconstrictors such as serotonin, prostaglandins, and norepinephrine.

Parthenolide and standardized extracts of feverfew containing parthenolide block the release of serotonin from blood vessels and prevent platelets from over-aggregating. Parthenolide also inhibits the actions of compounds released from cells that cause inflammation.

Macro Description

Native to southeastern Europe, feverfew is now widespread throughout Europe, North America and Australia. It is a short, herbaceous, composite perennial. It is a member of the daisy family, and it blooms between July and October. This aromatic plant gives off a strong and bitter odor. Its yellow-green leaves are alternate and bipinnatifid. The small, daisy-like yellow flowers are arranged in a dense corymb.

Part Used/Pharmaceutical Designations

- Leaves (dried leaves)
- Dried aerial parts

- **Constituents/Composition**
  Flavonoids, polyenes, volatile oil (camphor, borneol, terpenes, various esters); sesquiterpene lactones (85% is parthenolide) (0.1% to 0.9% of plant); sesquiterpenes, monoterpenes, spiroketal enol ether polyenes.

- **Commercial Preparations**
  Parthenolide content varies tremendously and depends on geographical origin. Nearly 50% of feverfew products from Canada lacked parthenolide. And no parthenolide could be detected in samples from Mexico and Eastern Serbia. It is for this reason that feverfew preparations should be standardized for at least 0.2% parthenolide.

Medicinal Uses/Indications

Traditional actions: relaxant, anti-inflammatory, vasodilator, digestive bitter, emmenagogue. Historically, feverfew was used for intestinal parasites, anemia, insect bites, irregular menses, stomachaches, and as an abortifacient, although it is rarely used this way now.

Clinical applications of feverfew include preventing and treating migraine, initial inflammatory stages of arthritis, rheumatic diseases, allergies, congestive dysmenorrhea, vertigo, and tinnitus.

Conditions: migraine, arthritis, rheumatic diseases, allergies.

- **Pharmacology**
  In vitro and in vivo studies show that feverfew has anti-inflammatory activity and prophylactic action against migraines. The underlying cause of migraine headaches presumably involves two primary mechanisms: (1) over-aggregation of platelets; and (2) release of serotonin and inflammatory compounds from platelets. In vivo and in vitro studies show unequivocally that parthenolide disrupts both mechanisms.

Parthenolide apparently neutralizes sulfhydryl groups on enzymes crucial for platelet aggregation. And it probably achieves its prophylactic effects by suppressing the release of serotonin from platelets. In in vivo studies, extracts of feverfew blocked the synthesis of prostaglandin, thromboxane, and leukotriene.

In vitro findings indicate that feverfew may be beneficial for arthritis. The anti-arthritic effects may be due to the ability of feverfew to destroy peripheral blood mononuclear cells in the synovium.

The first human clinical study of feverfew involved a small sample of only 17 patients, but the results were dramatic. All patients enrolled in this study had taken feverfew for several years. Nine patients were given a placebo and eight were given 50 mg of feverfew daily. During the six-month study period, the patients remaining on feverfew experienced continued relief. Migraines increased almost threefold in the patients taking placebo. However, the increase in symptoms in the placebo group may have actually been part of a feverfew-withdrawal syndrome.

In a double-blind, placebo-controlled, crossover study of 72 migraine sufferers, the treatment group received 70 to 114 mg of feverfew. They had a 24% reduction in the number of migraines when compared with the placebo group. The treatment group had fewer symptoms, although the length of each individual migraine episode did not change.

In another investigation, feverfew showed no clear-cut clinical benefits for rheumatoid arthritis. However, a low dosage of powdered leaf product was used and the parthenolide content was not determined in this trial. Because of the limitations of this study, the efficacy of feverfew for arthritis is inconclusive.

Dosage Ranges and Duration of Administration

Recommended dosage:

- Treatment and prevention of migraine: standardized feverfew extract (minimum 0.25 mcg parthenolide) bid
- Acute migraine attack: 1 to 2 g parthenolide daily
- For other conditions: 1 to 2 ml bid of 1:1 fluid extract; 2 to 4 ml bid of 1:5 tincture

Cautions

- **Adverse Effects/Toxicology**
  There are no long-term studies on feverfew toxicology. Minor side effects of nervousness and mild gastrointestinal irritation have been reported with use of standardized feverfew tablets. Adverse side effects of abdominal pain, indigestion, flatulence, diarrhea, nausea, and vomiting have also been observed. Mouth ulcerations, loss of taste, and swelling of the lips, tongue, and mouth occur in about 10% of individuals who chew the leaves.

In vivo studies revealed little evidence of negative reactions to feverfew in daily doses 100 times the dose given to humans. A histological examination of human lymphocytes showed that feverfew does not cause chromosomal abnormalities.

- **Warnings/Contraindications/Precautions**
  Feverfew is indicated for migraine sufferers who do not respond to conventional treatment. Because this herb can alter the menstrual cycle, menstruating women should use it with caution. Pregnant and lactating women and children under 2 years of age should not take feverfew.

Interactions

In vivo and in vitro findings suggest that feverfew may interact with antithrombotic drugs such as aspirin and warfarin. Individuals taking these medications should use feverfew only under the supervision of a qualified health care provider.

Regulatory and Compendial Status

The U.S. FDA classifies feverfew as a dietary supplement. Feverfew is used as a nonprescription drug for migraine headache in Britain and Germany.

References

Blumenthal M, ed. *The Complete German Commission E Monographs. Therapeutic Guide to Herbal Medicines.* Boston, Mass: Integrative Medicine Communications; 1998:12.

Bradley P, ed. *British Herbal Compendium.* Dorset, England: British Herbal Medicine Association; 1992:1:96–98

Brown D. *Herbal Prescriptions for Better Health.* Rocklin, Calif: Prima Publishing; 1996:91–95

De Weerdt CJ, Bootsma HPR, Hendriks H. Herbal Medicines in migraine prevention. Randomized double-blind placebo controlled crossover trial of a feverfew preparation. *Phytomedicine.* 1996;3:225–230.

Grieve M. *A Modern Herbal.* New York, NY: Dover; 1971:1:309–310.

Gruenwald J, Brendler T, Jaenicke C et al, eds. *PDR for Herbal Medicines.* Montvale, NJ: Medical Economics Company; 1998:1171–1173.

Heptinstall S, Groenewegen W, Spangenberg P, Lsche W. Inhibition of platelet behavior by feverfew: a mechanism of action involving sulfhydryl groups. *Folia Haematol Int Mag Klin Morphol Blutforsch.* 1988;43:447–449.

Johnson ES, Kadam NP, Hylands DM, Hylands PJ. Efficacy of feverfew as prophylactic treatment of migraine. *Br Med J.* 1985;291:569–573.

Johnson ES. Patients who chew chrysanthemum leaves. *MIMS Magazine* May 15, 1983: 32–35.

Murphy JJ, Heptinstall S, Mitchell JR. Randomised double-blind placebo-controlled trial of feverfew in migraine prevention. *Lancet.* 1988;2:189–192.

Murray MT. *The Healing Power of Herbs: The Enlightened Person's Guide to the Wonders of Medicinal Plants.* 2nd ed. Rocklin, Calif: Prima Publishing; 1995.

Newall CA, Anderson LA, Phillipson JD. *Herbal Medicines: A Guide for Health-care Professionals.* London, England: Pharmaceutical Press; 1996:119–120.

Palevitch D, Earon G, Carasso R. Feverfew *(Tanacetum parthenium)* as a prophylactic treatment for migraine: a double-blind controlled study. *Phytotherapy Res.* 1997;11: 508–511.

Pattrick M, Heptinstall S, Doherty M. Feverfew in rheumatoid arthritis: a double-blind, placebo controlled study. *Ann Rheum Dis.* 1989;48:547–549.

Tyler VE. *Herbs of Choice: The Therapeutic Use of Phytomedicinals.* Binghamton, NY: Pharmaceutical Products Press; 1994:126–134.

Tyler VE. *The Honest Herbal: A Sensible Guide to the Use of Herbs and Related Remedies.* 3rd ed. Binghampton, NY: Pharmaceutical Products Press; 1993.

© *Copyright Integrative Medicine Communications*

Flaxseed

Names

- **English**
  Flaxseed

- **Botanical**
  Linum usitatissimum

- **PlantFamily**
  Linaceae

- **Pharmacopeial**
  Lini semen

Overview

Used by the ancient Egyptians, flax was originally grown in the Mediterranean and Western Europe for industrial, nutritional, and medicinal uses. It is now found as both a cultivated and semi-wild plant throughout temperate and tropical regions.

Flax is a rich source of dietary fiber that can lower cholesterol levels. The oil in flaxseed (linseed) is medicinally important for cardiovascular conditions and cancer prevention. Linseed oil contains both omega-3 fatty acids and omega-6 fatty acids as well as plant nutrients such as phytoestrogens. Linoleic and alpha-linolenic acid are essential fatty acids that the body requires for normal cellular function.

Alpha-linolenic acid (ALA) is an omega-3 oil while linoleic acid is an omega-6 oil. Flaxseed oil is nature's richest storehouse of omega-3 fatty acids. The content of omega-3 oils in flaxseed is more than double the quantity in fish oils. Experts think that the high amount of unsaturated fatty acids in flaxseed oil significantly reduces the risk for arteriosclerosis.

Macro Description

Flax is an annual plant that grows up to five feet in height. It flourishes in deep moist soils rich in sand, silt, and clay. Ideally, flax should be quickly grown and harvested. Its gray-green leaves and delicate cordial blue (or sometimes white) flowers make it easily recognizable. The plant flowers only in the morning. The spherical, pea-size fruit contain flat, shiny, brown seeds filled with linseed oil. Mucilage is obtained from the husks of the seeds. Both the oil and mucilage of linseed are used for a variety of health conditions. The fruits are threshed to loosen the seeds, and the seeds do not actually ripen until after the plant has been harvested.

Part Used/Pharmaceutical Designations

- Flowers (fresh flowering plant)
- Seeds (flaxseed oil)

- **Constituents/Composition**
  Mucilages (3% to 10%); cyanogenic glycosides 0.05% to 0.1% (linustatin and neolinustin); fatty oil (30% to 45%), includes linolenic acid (40% to 70%), linoleic acid (10% to 25%), oleic acid (13% to 30%); mono- and triglycerides, free sterols, sterol esters, hydrocarbons: proteins (25%), ballast (25%), lignans, phenylpropane derivatives.

- **Commercial Preparations**
  Flaxseed is available as whole, bruised, or milled seeds. Linseed oil can be purchased in liquid form (to use in preparing food) or as soft gels for dietary supplementation. For optimal benefits, flaxseed oil should be added to foods (such as salad dressings) but not cooked or heated.

Medicinal Uses/Indications

Traditional Actions: whole seed, crushed seed, seed oil: bulking laxative, anti-inflammatory, demulcent, antitussive, emollient, vulnerary and expectorant. Was also historically used from gonorrhea, dysentary and diarrhea, although herbalists no longer use it for these conditions.

Internal conditions: whole or cracked seed preparations for chronic constipation, colon problems due to laxative abuse, irritable colon, diverticulitis, mucilage for gastritis and enteritis. Decoction used for cough and bronchial irritation, bladder or urinary tract inflammation.

External conditions: poultice for burns and scalds, local skin irritation, drawing poultices for local infections, pimples, boils, etc.

Clinical applications: elevated cholesterol and triglycerides; preventative for cardiovascular disease and cancer

- **Pharmacology**
  Epidemiological studies suggest that omega-3 oils significantly reduce the risk of heart disease. Omega-3 fatty acids lower LDL cholesterol and triglyceride levels. They also block platelet over-aggregation, reduce blood pressure in persons with hypertension, and lower fibrinogen levels. Consequently, omega-3 oils are clinically beneficial for hypercholesterolemia, angina, hypertension, psoriasis, eczema, cancer, and autoimmune disorders such as rheumatoid arthritis and multiple sclerosis.

  ALA, the main fatty acid in linseed, improves arterial function by increasing the strength, flexibility, and permeability of cell membranes. ALA offers greater protection against heart attacks than oleic acid (found in canola and olive oil). But in one study, ALA was not responsible for the anti-arteriosclerosis effect in Type II flaxseed. ALA comprises only 2% to 3% of the total oil in Type II flaxseed.

  Linolenic acid is a biologic precursor of prostaglandins. Prostaglandins are hormone-like substances that influence serum cholesterol levels, red blood cell aggregation, and smooth muscle function. Omega-3 oils help prevent cancer, stroke, and heart attacks by mediating the actions of prostaglandins. In other research, linseed oil had antibacterial action. Both linolenic acid and hydrolyzed linseed oil blocked the growth of methicillin-resistant strains of *Staphylococcus aureus*.

  Flaxseed is a rich source of lignans. Lignans are platelet-activating factor-receptor antagonists that have recently sparked medical interest because of their role in improving cardiovascular health. The lignans in linseed oil have both estrogenic and anti-estrogenic effects. Phytoestrogens in linseed are thought to favorably reduce certain symptoms of menopause while other lignans act as weak estrogen antagonists.

  There is new evidence that anti-estrogenic activity as well as other mechanisms inhibit carcinogenesis at various stages of tumor development. ALA and other compounds in linseed oil are known to have anti-cancer activity, particularly during the initiation and promotional stages of carcinogenesis. Lignans also suppress colon tumor growth, and it appears that flaxseed has both short-term and long-term protective effects against colon cancer.

  In one investigation, the lignans enterolactone and enterodiol reduced the number of tumors observed in test animals genetically prone to developing mammary tumors. In another study, mice with experimentally-induced melanoma had flaxseed added to their diets. Flaxseed reduced metastasis and suppressed the development of metastatic secondary tumors in the animals. These findings strongly support the use of flaxseed as a complementary nutritional therapy for preventing metastasis in cancer patients. However, it should be noted that the correlations between dietary flaxseed supplements and cancer inhibition at various stages of carcinogenesis have been inconsistent.

Dosage Ranges and Duration of Administration

Recommended dosage:

- Flaxseed: 1 tbsp. whole or bruised (but not ground) seed with 150 ml liquid bid to tid times a day for gastritis and enteritis; 2 to 3 tbsp. bulk seeds taken with 10 times the amount of water as a bulk laxative
- Poultice: 100 g soaked in boiling water for 10 to 15 minutes, strained, placed in cheesecloth and applied
- Decoction: 15 g of whole seed simmered in 1 cup water for 10 to 15 minutes
- Flaxseed oil: 1 tbsp. daily

Cautions

- **Adverse Effects/Toxicology**
  There are no side effects if flaxseed and linseed oil are taken within recommended therapeutic doses. However, large quantities of flaxseed consumed without sufficient fluid can cause ileus (constriction of the small intestine).

- **Warnings/Contraindications/Precautions**
  Contraindications include esophageal stricture, ileus, GI stricture, and acute intestinal inflammation. No contraindications for pregnant or lactating women.

Interactions

Flaxseed can delay the absorption of other drugs if taken simultaneously with them.

Regulatory and Compendial Status

The U.S. FDA classifies flaxseed as a dietary supplement.

References

Allman MA, Pena MM, Pang D. Supplementation with flaxseed oil versus sunflowerseed oil in healthy young men consuming a low fat diet: effects on platelet composition and function. *Eur J Clin Nutr.* 1995;49:169–178.

Bierenbuam ML, Reichstein R, Watkins TR. Reducing atherogenic risk in hyperlipemic humans with flax seed supplementation: a preliminary report. *J Am Coll Nutr.* 1993;12:501–504.

Blumenthal M, ed. *The Complete German Commission E Monographs. Therapeutic Guide to Herbal Medicines.* Boston, Mass: Integrative Medicine Communications; 1998:47,132.

British Herbal Pharmacopoeia. 4th ed. Dorset, England: British Herbal Medicine Association; 1996.

Clark WF, et al. Flaxseed: a potential treatment of lupus nephritis. *Kidney International.* 1995;48:475–480.

Cunnane SC, et al. High alpha-linolenic acid flaxseed *(Linum usitatissimum):* some nutritional properties in humans. Br J Nutr. 1993;69:443–453.

Cunnane SC. Nutritional attributes of traditional flaxseed in healthy-young adults. *Am J Clin Nutr.* 1995;61:62–68.

De Smet P. *Adverse Effects of Herbal Drugs.* New York, NY: Springer-Verlag; 1997.

Grieve M. *A Modern Herbal.* New York, NY: Dover; 1971;1:309–310.

Gruenwald J. Brendler T, Christof J. *PDR for Herbal Medicines.* Montvale, NJ: Medical Economics Company; 1998:940–941.

Prasad K, Mantha S, Muir A, Westcott N. Reduction of hypercholesterolemic arteriosclerosis by CDC-flaxseed with very low alpha-linolenic acid. *Arteriosclerosis.*1998;434:367–375.

Serraino M, Thompson L. The effect of flaxseed supplementation on the initiation and promotional stages of mammary tumorigenesis. *Nutr Cancer.* 1992;25:153–159.

Sung M, Lautens M, Thompson L. Mammalian lignans inhibit the growth of estrogen-independent human colon tumor cells. *Anticancer Research.* 1998;1346:1405–1408.

Thompson L, Richard S, Orcheson L, Seidl M. Flaxseed and its lignan and oil components reduce mammary tumor growth at a late stage of carcinogenesis. *Carcinogenesis.* 1996;434:1373–1376.

Yan L, Yee J, Li D, McGuire M, Thompson L. Dietary flaxseed supplementation and experimental metastasis of melanoma cells in mice. *Cancer Lett.* 1998;61:181–186.

© *Copyright Integrative Medicine Communications*

Garlic

Names

■ **English**
Garlic

■ **Botanical**
Allium sativum

■ **Plant Family**
Alliaceae

■ **Pharmacopeial**
Allii sativi bulbus

Overview

Known for their pungent odor, garlic bulbs have been revered as both a food and medicine in many cultures for millennia. Construction workers who built the Egyptian pyramids were supposedly given huge rations of garlic to sustain their resistance against fevers. Legend has it that gravediggers in early eighteenth-century France drank a concoction of macerated garlic in wine to protect themselves against a plague. And during the two world wars, military physicians gave garlic to their patients as a preventive against gangrene.

The primary active compound in garlic is alliin, an odorless substance derived from the sulfur-containing amino acid, cysteine. However, alliin is found only within the intact cells of garlic. When garlic bulbs are crushed, the cell walls are broken, and an enzyme, allinase, converts alliin into a degradation product called allicin (diallyldisulfide-S-oxide). Allicin is an unstable compound that gives garlic its characteristic odor. Allicin is more active than alliin, and it readily forms other odorous sulfur-containing active constituents.

Macro Description

Native to central Asia, garlic now grows worldwide as a cultivated plant. This perennial reaches a height of 25 to 70 cm (10 to 28 in). Its stem is either erect or crook-like, and its leaves are flat and broad. Topping the stalks are five to seven pale flowers with reddish or greenish white petals arranged in a loose globular cluster. The subterranean compound bulb has 4 to 20 cloves, or secondary bulbs, each one weighing about 1 g. Each clove is covered by a silky white or green skin.

Part Used/Pharmaceutical Designations

- Bulbs

■ **Constituents/Composition**

On average, 0.35% sulfur (1% of the dry weight). Alliin rapidly decomposes to form allicin which comprises 0.25% to 1.15% of garlic cloves. Alliin content is 0.7% to 1.7% in dried bulbous garlic. Other sulfur-containing constituents comprise about 25% to 35% of compounds in garlic after the cells have been damaged.

■ **Commercial Preparations**

Commercial preparations are manufactured from whole fresh bulbous garlic, dried bulbous garlic, or oil of garlic. The quantity of active principles in commercial products varies depending on the method of preparation and percentage of active compounds in fresh garlic cloves. This percentage reportedly varies by a factor of 10. Aged garlic products (garlic fermentation products) are odor-free. However, aged garlic products have limited therapeutic benefits because the active principles in them are usually converted into inert substances. Consumers should use standardized garlic products containing a specified concentration of allicin.

Medicinal Uses/Indications

Historical uses: all infections both internally and as a poultice. Used as a warming herb and as preventive for colds and flu, menstrual pain, mouthwash, and as a douche. Anthelmintic (expels worms).

Traditional actions: antihypertensive, anticholesterolaemic, antilipidaemic, reduces platelet aggregation, vasodilator, expectorant, antihistiminic, antimicrobial.

Clinical Applications: treatment and prevention of atherosclerosis, elevated blood lipids, and thrombosis. Also used to stabilize blood sugar level, and for gastrointestinal infections by positively affecting intestinal flora.

■ **Pharmacology**

Numerous in vitro and in vivo investigations show that garlic has broad spectrum antimicrobial activity against bacteria, viruses, fungi, and intestinal parasites (helminths). Garlic also has immune-enhancing, antioxidant, and vasodilating activity. In both in vitro and in vivo studies, garlic produces anti-inflammatory, blood-sugar lowering (antidiabetic), and anti-cancer effects.

Research on garlic shows unequivocally that it can help prevent atherosclerosis through its effects on elevated lipids and blood pressure. Studies on both animals and humans indicate that garlic favorably shifted the high-density lipoprotein: low-density lipoprotein ratio toward lowered LDL and higher HDL values. It also lowered plasma viscosity and improved both blood fluidity and capillary blood flow. Garlic increased fibrinolytic activity, prolonged bleeding and clotting time, and inhibited platelet aggregations. Garlic consumption reduced blood pressure in hypertensive patients.

Double-blind clinical studies reveal that garlic lowered cholesterol and triglyceride levels in hyperlipidemic patients, and reduced blood pressure. In a 16-week, placebo-controlled trial involving 261 patients, the treatment group had a significant reduction in total cholesterol when compared with the placebo group. This trend has been confirmed by two meta-analyses of investigations on the influence of garlic on blood lipids. Garlic powder administered to patients for a minimum of four weeks resulted in an average decline of either 9% or 12% in total blood cholesterol. The average reduction in triglycerides was 13%.

Findings on the therapeutic effects of commercial garlic preparations were contradictory, presumably due to variable levels of active constituents in the commercial products used in the clinical trials. Garlic preparations can be dried (heated or freeze-dried), distilled, extracted with garlic oils, aged, or deodorized by unspecified processes. Allicin and ajoene (a self-condensation product of allicin) are absent in dried garlic preparations. Furthermore, allinase is unstable in the presence of gastric acids in the stomach. In order to be efficacious, dried garlic products must take the form of enteric-coated capsules or tablets.

Garlic has antioxidant properties, and antitoxic activity against carbon tetrachloride, isoproterenol, and heavy metal poisoning. It inhibits tumor proliferation in sarcoma, bladder tumors, isolated colon carcinoma cells, and liver cell carcinomas. In population studies in Asia, the incidence of stomach cancer deaths was lower in people who ate large quantities of garlic. The active principles in garlic may exert anti-cancer effects by stimulating the immune system to inhibit carcinogenesis.

Allicin probably accounts for antibiotic and antiplatelet activity. Allicin also lowers cholesterol levels by blocking lipid synthesis and by increasing the excretion of neutral and acidic sterols. Ajoene prevents blood clots by inhibiting platelet aggregation in vitro and in vivo in a dose-dependent and reversible manner. By inhibiting platelet aggregation, ajeone has a protective effect against atherosclerosis, coronary thrombosis, and stroke.

Dosage Ranges and Duration of Administration

Recommended dosage (lower doses for prevention, higher doses for infection):

- 1,000 to 3,000 mg daily usually taken in encapsulated form (500 mg capsules)
- Oil: 0.03 to 0.12 ml tid

Cautions

■ **Adverse Effects/Toxicology**

Excessive dietary intake can cause stomach upset, and topical use of garlic can result in both burn-like skin lesions and allergic contact dermatitis.

■ **Warnings/Contraindications/Precautions**

Individuals prone to slow blood clotting should not take therapeutic doses of garlic. Excessive intake of either dietary or nondietary sources of garlic can increase the risk of hemorrhagic complications during surgery and postoperative bleeding. Pregnant and lactating women should also avoid consuming garlic in large quantities since it has abortifacient and uteroactive properties. Garlic can alter the menstrual cycle.

Interactions

Individuals taking anticoagulant drugs such as aspirin should not ingest excessive quantities of garlic.

Regulatory and Compendial Status

The U.S. FDA classifies garlic as a dietary supplement. Bulbous garlic products are sold as nonprescription drugs in France and Germany.

References

Berthold HK, et al. Effect of a garlic oil preparation on serum lipoproteins and cholesterol metabolism. *JAMA.* 1998;279.

Bradley PR, ed. *British Herbal Compendium.* Dorset, England: British Herbal Medicine Association; 1992:1:105–108.

DeSmet PAGM, Keller K, Hnsel R, Chandler RF, eds. *Adverse Effects of Herbal Drugs.* Berlin, Germany: Springer-Verlag; 1997:235–236.

Gruenwald J, Brendler T, Jaenicke C et al, eds. *PDR for Herbal Medicines.* Montvale, NJ: Medical Economics Company 1998:940–941.

Kiesewetter, H; Jung F, Mrowietz C, et al. Effects of garlic on blood fluidity and fibrinolytic activity: a randomised, placebo-controlled, double-blind study. *Br J Clin Pract.* 1990;44:24–29.

Mader FH. Treatment of hyperlipidaemia with garlic-powder tablets. Evidence from the German Association of General Practitioners' multicentric placebo-controlled double-blind study. *Arzneimittelforschung.* October 1990;40:1111–1116.

Murray MT. *The Healing Power of Herbs: The Enlightened Person's Guide to the Wonders of Medicinal Plants.* Second Ed. Rocklin, Calif: Prima Publishing; 1995:121–131.

Newall C, Anderson L, Phillipson J. *Herbal Medicines: A Guide for Health-care Professionals.* London, England: Pharmaceutical Press; 1996:129–133.

Orekhov A, Tertov V, Sobenin I, Pivovorava E. Direct antiatherosclerosis-related effects of garlic. *Ann Med.* 1995;37:63–65.

Schulz V, Hansel R, Tyler V. *Rational Phytotherapy: A Physician's Guide to Herbal Medicine.* 3rd ed. Berlin, Germany: Springer-Verlag; 1998:107–123.

Silagy C, Neil A. Garlic as a lipid lowering agent-a meta-analysis. *JR Coll Physicians Lond.* 1994;28:39–45.

Steiner M, Khan AH, Holbert D, Lin RI. A double-blind crossover study in moderately hypercholesterolemic men that compared the effect of aged garlic extract and placebo administration on blood lipids. *Am J Clin Nutr.* 1996;64:866–870.

Tyler V. *Herbs of Choice: The Therapeutic Use of Phytomedicinals.* Binghamton, NY: Pharmaceutical Products Press; 1994:104–115.

Tyler V. *The Honest Herbal: A Sensible Guide to the Use of Herbs and Related Remedies.* 3rd ed. Binghampton, NY: Pharmaceutical Products Press; 1993:139–143.

Warshafsky S, Kramer RS, Sivak SL. Effect of garlic on total serum cholesterol. *Ann Intern Med.* 1993;119:599–605.

© *Copyright Integrative Medicine Communications*

Ginger

Names

■ **English**
Ginger root

■ **Botanical**
Zingiber officinale

■ **Plant Family**
Zingiberaceae

■ **Pharmacopeial**
Zingiberis rhizoma

Overview

Ginger root relieves nausea and emesis and may prevent or reduce the symptoms of motion sickness and seasickness. While nausea is currently the main indication for use, inhibition of cyclooxygenase and lipoxygenase inflammatory pathways and related prostaglandin synthetase and platelet aggregation support the use of ginger in colds, sore throats, flus, headaches, and some types of arthritis and muscular pain.

As a culinary spice, ginger was known for centuries to reduce flatulence, bloating, and indigestion, and to stimulate the appetite. It was highly sought after by Europeans, who traded with China and India during the sixteenth and seventeenth centuries and used it fresh, powdered, or crystallized in cooking. In 1884, England is said to have imported more than 5 million pounds of ginger.

Native to Asia where its use as a culinary spice spans at least 4,400 years, ginger grows in fertile, moist, tropical soil. It was transported as far west as Jamaica, where it became an export crop as early as 1547. Explorers and settlers brought it to southern Florida and further west to Mexico.

Ginger can be grown at home by planting rhizomes in soils of mixed loam, sand, peat moss, and compost in bright sun with plenty of water. Within a year, gnarled, branched rhizome spread throughout the soil, bearing numerous tubers.

Macro Description

White, yellow, or greenish-yellow flowers, which may have a purplish tint at the edges, form at cone-shaped, three-inch spikes, off erect 6- to 12-inch stalks (cultivated ginger rarely flowers). Above ground leaves are dark green, narrow, lanceolate or linear-lanceolate, with a noticeable rib. The rhizome is light beige, aromatic, and has a sharp, spicy flavor.

Part Used/Pharmaceutical Designations

- Roots (rhizome)

■ **Constituents/Composition**
Volatile oil containing sesquiterpenes (zingiberene, bisabolene); oleoresin with pungent principles (gingerols, shogaols)

■ **Commercial Preparations**
Fresh or dried rhizome prepared as aqueous, aqueous-alcohol, glycerite, or dried powder liquid extracts including tinctures and syrups; oil; rhizome tea; dried, powdered tablets, capsules; crystallized ginger

Medicinal Uses/Indications

Traditional herbal actions: carminative, diaphoretic, antispasmodic, antiemetic, cholagogue, circulatory stimulant, peripheral vasodilator, expectorant, antiseptic, topical rubifacient

Conditions: intestinal colic, flatulence, indigestion, headache, sore throat, arthritis, common cold, flu, delayed menstruation, pelvic congestion, menstrual cramps

Clinical Applications: motion sickness, nausea, vomiting, indigestion, flatulence, common cold, flu, dysmenorrhea; also used topically for arthritis, sore joints, and muscle sprains.

■ **Pharmacology**

Ginger root increases gastric motility, stimulates bile secretion, and is carminative and antiemetic. It promotes bile flow and reduces inflammation through prostaglandin inhibition.

In studies in animals, ginger or its oleoresin or volatile oil components are hypoglycemic, hypo- and hypertensive, anthelmintic (*Anisakis* larvae) in vitro, and positively inotropic. Ginger inhibits cholesterol absorption after time, increases bile flow, and inhibits hydrochloric acid/ethanol-induced gastric lesions. It also inhibits prostaglandin biosynthesis and platelet aggregation in vitro.

In humans, ginger relieves motion sickness comparably to dimenhydrinate (Dramamine), most likely through actions within the gastrointestinal tract and not on the central nervous system, at doses of up to 2 g every four hours or as needed. Its superiority to dimenhydrinate remains equivocal. Currently, at least one formulation awaits FDA approval for over-the-counter status for treating nausea and motion sickness.

High doses of ginger (10 to 20 g of fresh ginger per day, or 500 mg of dried ginger four times a day) were found to significantly reduce migraine intensity and rheumatoid arthritis pain, respectively. Rheumatoid arthritis patients receiving either 5 to 50 g of fresh ginger or 0.1 to 1.0 g of powdered root experienced significant reductions in joint pain and an increase in mobility. These effects may be due to cyclooxygenase and lipoxygenase pathway inhibition.

Dosage Ranges and Duration of Administration

Daily dose:

- 2 to 4 g daily of fresh root (0.25 to 1.0 g of powdered root)

To relieve nausea, flatulence, or indigestion:

- 2 to 4 g daily of fresh root (0.25 to 1.0 g of powdered root) or 1.5 to 3.0 ml tincture daily, relative to the strength and processing of the tincture

To prevent emesis:

- 1 g ginger (1/2 tsp.) every 4 hours as needed
- 2 ginger capsules (1 g) tid
- 1/4 oz. piece of fresh ginger, chewed

To relieve cold symptoms, fever associated with flu, sore throat, menstrual cramps, headache:

- Steep 2 tbsp. of freshly shredded ginger in boiled water, bid to tid.
- Place a drop of ginger oil or a few slices of fresh rhizome in steaming water and inhale.

To relieve arthritis:

- Fresh ginger juice, extract, or tea, 2 to 4 g daily
- Use oil or fresh root in a warm poultice or compress and apply to painful areas. Place a drop of ginger oil in massage oil and rub into painful joints and muscles.

Cautions

■ **Adverse Effects/Toxicology**

American Herbal Products Association safety rating: fresh root, class 1 (safe with appropriate use); dried root, class 2b (not to be used during pregnancy). May cause mild heartburn.

■ **Warnings/Contraindications/Precautions**

Because ginger increases bile flow, gallstones contraindicate use.

The use of ginger to control morning sickness during pregnancy is controversial. Ginger obtained through food is not considered risky during pregnancy. Doses of 1 g dried ginger root to relieve morning sickness has not resulted in any reports of miscarriage or toxicity to either the fetus or the mother. The AHPA does not advise dried root during pregnancy.

Two Japanese studies showed in vitro mutagenicity for one of the pungent principles of ginger. Subsequent studies showed that risk to humans is diminished significantly by antimutagenic properties of other ginger constituents. Some Chinese sources claim that 20 to 28 g of ginger will cause miscarriage, presumably due to its effects on uterine smooth muscle tissue. Pregnant women are advised not to ingest more than normal dietary levels of ginger, such as those found in ginger ale, cookies, breads, and main dishes.

Interactions

In doses exceeding dietary intake, ginger may interfere with cardiac, anticoagulant, or antidiabetic medications due to in vitro actions on platelets and heart muscle and in vivo effects on blood sugar levels.

Regulatory and Compendial Status

Ginger is a GRAS (generally recognized as safe) food additive in the United States and the FDA categorizes it as a dietary supplement. Recently published United States Pharmacopeia (USP) Information Monographs do not recommend therapeutic use of ginger, citing insufficient scientific evidence; OTC approval by the FDA has not yet been granted. In England, ginger is licensed through the General Sales List, and in Germany it is approved as a nonprescription drug for dyspepsia and motion sickness by the Commission E.

References

Awang DVC. Ginger. *Can Pharma J.* 1992:309–311.

Blumenthal M, ed. *The Complete German Commission E Monographs: Therapeutic Guide to Herbal Medicine.* Boston, Mass: Integrative Medicine Communications; 1998.

Blumenthal M, Riggins CW. *American Botanical Council's Popular Herbs in the U.S. Market: Therapeutic Monographs.* Austin, Texas: ABC; 1997:33–240.

Bremness L. Herbs. *The Visual Guide to More than 700 Herb Species from around the World.* London: Dorling Kindersley Limited; 1994.

Duke JA. *The Green Pharmacy.* Emmaus, Pa: Rodale Press; 1997.

USP publishes information monographs on ginger and valerian. *HerbalGram.* 1998;43:30, 57, 71.

Grontved A, et al. Ginger root against seasickness: a controlled trial on the open sea. *Acta Otolaryngol.* 1988;105:45-49.

Kowalchik C, Hylton W, ed. *Rodale's Illustrated Encyclopedia of Herbs.* Emmaus, Pa: Rodale Press; 1998.

McGuffin M, Hobbs C, Upton R, Goldberg A, eds. *American Herbal Products Association's Botanical Safety Handbook.* Boca Raton, Fla: CRC Press; 1997.

Nagabhushan M, Amonkar AJ, Bhide SV. Mutagenicity of gingerol and shogoal and antimutagenicity of zingerone in salmonella/microsome assay. *Cancer Lett.* 1987;36:221–233.

Nakamura H, Yamamoto T. Mutagen and anti-mutagen in ginger, *Zingiber officinale. Mutat Res.* 1982;103:119–126.

Newall CA, Anderson LA, Phillipson JD. *Herbal Medicines: A Guide for Health-care Professionals.* London: The Pharmaceutical Press; 1996:157–159.

Schulick P. The many roles of ginger. *Natural Foods Merchandiser's Nutrition Science News.* 1995:6–7.

Schulz V, Hnsel R, Tyler VE. *Rational Phytotherapy: A Physicians' Guide to Herbal Medicine.* 3rd ed. Berlin, Germany: Springer; 1998.

Yeung H. *Handbook of Chinese Herbs and Formulas.* Los Angeles, Calif: Los Angeles Institute of Chinese Medicine; 1985:1.

© Copyright Integrative Medicine Communications

Ginkgo Biloba

Names

- **English**
  Ginkgo Biloba

- **Botanical**
  Ginkgo biloba

- **Plant Family**
  Ginkgoaceae

- **Pharmacopeial**
  Ginkgo folium

Overview

Ginkgo biloba is one of the oldest living tree species, existing even before the Ice Age. Although Chinese herbal medicine has used both the ginkgo leaf and seed for centuries, modern research has focused on the standardized *Ginkgo biloba* extract (GBE), which is produced from the leaves. This extract is highly concentrated and much more effective than any other use of the leaves. More than 400 published studies have been done on GBE, making it one of the best researched of all herbal medicines. In Germany and France it is the most frequently prescribed herbal medicine and is in the top five of all medical prescriptions written in those countries. GBE is a powerful aid to circulatory problems, particularly cerebral insufficiency and peripheral arterial insufficiency seen most often in the elderly. It has strong antioxidant properties as well, protecting both the central nervous system and the cardiovascular system from damage and the effects of aging.

GBE improves circulation by strengthening the vascular system and inhibiting platelet aggregation, preventing atherosclerosis, which leads to cerebral insufficiency, coronary artery disease, peripheral arterial insufficiency, and strokes. Cerebral insufficiency can cause much of the mental deterioration or dementia associated with aging, including memory loss, vertigo, tinnitus, disorientation, and depression. GBE has been shown to increase blood flow to the brain, resulting in a marked improvement for many patients. It is also used effectively to prevent the onset of mental deterioration for those approaching old age. In a few small studies, GBE seemed to slow and even stop the progress of Alzheimer's disease, particularly in the early stages.

Peripheral arterial insufficiency is caused by arterial narrowing or obstruction and its most common symptom is intermittent claudication, particularly in the calves. GBE has been shown to improve blood flow in the limbs and increase walking tolerance at levels much higher than standard medical treatments. Other peripheral vascular disorders that respond to GBE include diabetic peripheral vascular disease, Raynaud's phenomenon, acrocyanosis, and postphlebitis syndrome. Because of its ability to improve circulation, GBE is being studied as an aid for impotence caused by impaired blood flow. Recent studies have shown good results, which are probably due to GBE's ability to increase blood flow without changing systemic blood pressure. There is evidence that GBE may also reduce certain PMS symptoms, including fluid retention, vascular congestion, and breast tenderness.

Macro Description

Ginkgo biloba is a deciduous tree that can live up to 1,000 years and grow to a height of 120 feet. It has short branches with shoots that have fan-shaped, bilobed leaves. The fruit has a strong, unpleasant odor and is inedible, with an edible inner seed. Once common in North America and Europe, the Ice Age destroyed all but remnants that survived in China. Now grown in Asia, Europe, and North America.

Part Used/Pharmaceutical Designations

- Seeds
- Leaves

- **Constituents/Composition**
  Ginkgo flavone glycosides (quercetin, kaempferol, isorhamnetine, proanthocyandins), several terpene molecules unique to ginkgo (ginkgolides and bilobalide), organic acids

- **Commercial Preparations**
  Ginkgo biloba extract standardized to contain 24% ginkgo flavone glycosides (50:1 extract) and 6% terpene lactones. (There are several different brands of GBE available in the United States, but almost all of the scientific and clinical studies have been performed on the original German formula.) Encapsulated herb and tincture are also available.

Medicinal Uses/Indications

Traditional herbal actions: circulatory stimulant, antidepressant, antithrombotic

Clinical applications: intermittent claudication, allergies, dementia, vertigo, vascular fragility, short-term memory loss, headache, depression, stroke, poor circulation, atherosclerosis, cerebral vascular insufficiency, Alzheimer's disease, tinnitus, cochlear deafness, macular degeneration, diabetic retinopathy, peripheral arterial insufficiency, impotence, PMS, Raynaud's phenomenon

- **Pharmacology**
  GBE strengthens tissue by stabilizing cell membranes, acting as an antioxidant, and inhibiting free radical damage. It also aids cell use of oxygen and glucose. These properties are particularly important for brain cell tissue, which is most vulnerable to free radical damage and oxygen deprivation. Brain cells are also protected by GBE's ability to improve blood circulation to the brain, particularly the hippocampus and striatum, areas most affected by micro-embolization. GBE has also been shown to increase the rate of transmission of information to the nerve cell level, enhancing memory ability. These combined effects allow GBE to reverse mental deterioration caused by vascular insufficiency. The mental deterioration caused by Alzheimer's seems to be significantly delayed by GBE's ability to enhance brain function, along with normalizing the acetylcholine receptors in the hippocamus and increasing cholinergic transmission.

  GBE strengthens the vascular system by focusing on two areas: vascular endothelium and the system that regulates blood vessel tone. As a vasodilator, it stimulates the release of endothelium-derived relaxing factor and prostacyclin. GBE also restricts an enzyme that causes blood vessels to relax and stimulates greater tone throughout the vessels.

  GBE greatly influences platelet function by inhibiting platelet aggregation, platelet adhesion, and degranulation. Along with its powers as an antioxidant, this influence seems to come from GBE's ability to inhibit a substance known as platelet-activating factor (PAF). PAF stimulates platelet aggregation, and causes inflammation and allergic reactions by increasing vascular permeability, activation of neutrophil, smooth-muscle contractions including bronchoconstriction, and reducing coronary blood flow. Higher PAF levels are also associated with aging. Many of GBE's clinical results may come from its ability to inhibit PAF and its effects. The unique terpene lactones in GBE, particularly the ginkgolides, are thought to be the main source of this ability to inhibit PAF.

  The terpene lactones in GBE (ginkgolides and bilobalide) also protect nerve cells from damage during periods of ischemia or hypoxia. This hypoxic tolerance is seen particularly in cerebral tissue, making GBE an effective treatment for people who have suffered strokes or transient ischemic attacks.

Dosage Ranges and Duration of Administration

- Take 120 mg daily in two divided doses of 50:1 extract standardized to 24% flavone glycodises. Patients with more serious dementia or Alzheimer's disease may need to work up to 240 mg daily in two to three divided doses. Results often take four to six weeks, but should continue to accumulate. Some dramatic changes may not appear for six months.
- Capsules of dried herb with 10 mg standardized extract (1 to 3 capsules tid)
- Tincture (1:5): 2 to 4 ml tid
- Fluid extract (1:1): 1 to 3 ml tid

Cautions

- **Adverse Effects/Toxicology**
  GBE is very safe and side effects are rare. In a few cases, gastrointestinal upset, headaches, and dizziness were reported. GBE has been shown not to alter heart rate and blood pressure or to change cholesterol and triglyercides levels. Because it decreases platelet aggregation, there is some concern that ginkgo may increase risk of intracranial hemorrhage. Use with caution in conjunction with other blood-thinning agents (i.e. Coumadin).

■ Warnings/Contraindications/Precautions

The fruit of *Ginkgo biloba* should not be handled or ingested. Ingesting the seed can cause severe adverse effects. The German Commission E reports the only contraindication for GBE is a hypersensitivity to Ginkgo biloba preparations. There are no known contraindications for pregnancy, but pregnant or lactating women should exercise caution since there is a lack of studies showing GBE's effects during pregnancy.

Interactions

None known

Regulatory and Compendial Status

The German Commission E approves specific GBE extracts for use in treating dementia, peripheral arterial insufficiency, vertigo, and tinnitus.

References

Bauer U. Six-month double-blind randomized clinical trial of *Ginkgo biloba* extract versus placebo in two parallel groups of patients suffering from peripheral arterial insufficiency. *Arzneimittelforschung.* 1984;34:716–720.

Blumenthal M, ed. The Complete German Commission E Monographs: Therapeutic Guide to Herbal Medicines. Boston, Mass: Integrative Medicine Communications; 1998.

Brown D. *Herbal Prescriptions for Better Health.* Rocklin, Calif: Prima Publishing; 1996.

Carper J. *Miracle Cures.* New York, NY: HarperCollins, 1997.

DeSmet PAGM, Keller K, Hnsel R, Chandler RF, eds. *Adverse Effects of Herbal Drugs.* Berlin, Germany: Springer-Verlag; 1997.

Kinghorn, A., Ed. *Human Medicinal Agents from Plants.* Washington, DC: American Chemical Society, 1993.

Le Bars PL, Katz MM, Berman N, Itil TM, Freedman AM, Schatzberg AF. A placebo-controlled, double-blind, randomized trial of an extract of *Ginkgo biloba* for dementia. *JAMA.* 1997;278:1327–1332.

Murray M. *The Healing Power of Herbs: The Enlightened Person's Guide to the Wonders of Medicinal Plants.* 2nd ed. Rocklin, Calif: Prima Publishing; 1995.

Newall C, et al. *Herbal Medicines: A Guide for Health-care Professionals.* London, England: Pharmaceutical Press; 1996.

Peters H, Kieser M, Holscher U. Demonstration of the efficacy of *Ginkgo biloba* special extract Egb 761 on intermittent claudication a placebo-controlled, double-blind trial. *Vasa.* 1998;27:105–110.

Schulz V, Hnsel R, Tyler VE. *Rational Phytotherapy: A Physicians' Guide to Herbal Medicine.* Berlin, Germany: Springer-Verlag; 1998.

© *Copyright Integrative Medicine Communications*

Ginseng, American

Names

- **English**
  American ginseng

- **Botanical**
  Panax quinquefolium

- **Plant Family**
  Araliaceae

- **Pharmacopeial**
  Ginseng radix

Overview

American ginseng stimulates convalescence, rehabilitation, stamina and strength through actions that are similar to those of its more famous Asian cousin, *Panax ginseng*. In Asian countries, ginseng is regarded as the king of herbs and is added to many everyday items, including beverages. The Chinese associated ginseng with longevity, virility, strength, and wisdom as early as 1 A.D., according to written accounts. As long as the roots are five or six years old, at which time they contain suitable amounts of active plant chemicals, American ginseng is considered similar enough to Asian ginseng chemically to be used interchangeably.

Ginseng can be difficult to cultivate. It is susceptible to blights, needs loamy, high-humus soil, and prefers 70% shade. This difficulty made it a good export crop early on in American history, because it was plentiful here. In 1718, American ginseng brought five dollars a pound in Canton, China. In 1773, 55 tons of American ginseng were sold to the Chinese. By 1824, 380 tons were exported. Even Daniel Boone traded ginseng.

Ginseng is classified as an adaptogen and antioxidant. Adaptogens increase physiological resistance to stressors. Antioxidants function similarly, reducing the negative consequences of free radicals. Modern research shows that ginseng improves resistance to bacterial, viral, emotional, cognitive, muscular, metabolic, and cardiovascular stressors, and suggests a plethora of ginseng or ginseng constituent actions. While the elderly take it to diminish debility from age-related illness, others take it to enhance physical and cognitive performance. Ongoing studies are looking into ginseng for the treatment of cancer, diabetes, cardiovascular disease, non-AIDS related immune system depression, infertility, aging, and depression.

According to alternative medicine practitioners, American and Asian ginsengs are indicated in stress, fatigue, convalescence and diabetes, and Siberian ginseng in stress, fatigue, atherosclerosis, and impaired kidney function. Confusion regarding which ginseng to use for stress, fatigue, and convalescence (American, Asian, or Siberian) stems from the suggestion that active components in one type are superior to those in another type, e.g., ginsenosides versus eleutherosides. Such superiority has not been demonstrated. Early Russian studies indicated that Siberian ginseng's positive effects exceed those of Asian ginseng's. These results are supported by empirical reports, but are challenged by investigators who question the validity of the studies and the quality of the Siberian ginseng preparation. At this time, all three ginsengs are regarded as adaptogens, all three share contraindication and side effect profiles, and despite qualitative differences, each is used for similar indications. Cost, standardization, and the reputation of the manufacturer may be the deciding points in determining which product to use.

Macro Description

After two years' growth the leaves are five-lobed and palmate; after a few more years, leaflets develop on prongs. Stem grows from a tap root and can reach up to 16 inches in height. Small, greenish-white flowers grow in clusters and produce red berries with two seeds.

Light beige, variably thick, gnarled root can appear similar in shape to the human body, and has offshoots with long stringy hairs that can look like arms and legs. The root is harvested at 4 to 6 years' age; age is determined by the numbers of wrinkles on the neck of the root. The crude drug is prepared from the lateral root and root hairs.

Part Used/Pharmaceutical Designations

- Roots

- **Constituents/Composition**
  Dried root contains ginsenosides (Rb1 as marker); polysaccharide glycans (quinquefolan A, B, and C)

- **Commercial Preparations**
  White ginseng (dried, peeled) is prepared as liquid extracts, powders, or capsules.

Medicinal Uses/Indications

Traditional:

- Adaptogen
- Bitter tonic
- Restorative
- Alterative

Clinical applications:

- Diabetes
- Ulcer
- Edema
- Cancer
- Hypercholesterolemia
- Infertility
- Fatigue
- Frequent colds or viral illness
- Rehabilitation after acute illness
- To increase stamina and well being

- **Pharmacology**
  American ginseng reduces stress and fatigue and improves physical and mental function. In studies in humans, American ginseng improves cholesterol ratios, increases blood alcohol clearance, reduces liver toxicity, improves psychomotor performance, helps control asthma, lowers blood sugar levels, and regulates blood pressure and adrenocorticotropic hormone. Studies in humans also indicate that American ginseng may be used as adjunctive therapy in the treatment of diabetic neuropathy, reactive depression, psychologically-induced impotence, and psychological disorders in children. Many of these studies involve other species of ginseng, in particular, *Panax ginseng* (Asian ginseng). However, while further study is needed for clarification, the two species do exert similar actions.

  Non-insulin-dependant diabetes is perhaps the condition most often used to study the effects of constituents specific to American ginseng. The polysaccharide glycans, quinquefolans A, B, and C are hypoglycemic in mice. Ginsenoside Rb1 reduces concentrations of islet insulin to practically nothing.

Dosage Ranges and Duration of Administration

White ginseng standardized to 0.03% ginsenosides, designated as Rb1. The recommended dose is: 1 to 2 g fresh root, 0.6 to 2 g dried root, or 200 to 600 mg liquid extract daily. Healthy persons using American ginseng for enhanced physical or mental performance or to improve resistance to stressors should take these doses in cycles of 15 to 20 days followed by two-week breaks.

For rehabilitation after an illness, the elderly should take 0.5 g bid 2 for three months; or, take 0.5 g bid for one month, followed by a two-month break, and repeat cycle if desired.

Cautions

- **Adverse Effects/Toxicology**
  American ginseng is not considered to have side effects when used at the recommended daily dose.

  The American Herbal Products Association (AHPA) rates American ginseng as class 2d: 2d indicates that specific restrictions apply; hypertension is the specific restriction.

- **Warnings/Contraindications/Precautions**
  Similar contraindications to those for Asian ginseng may be applicable to American ginseng: patients with acute illness, cardiovascular disease, diabetes, or blood pressure disorders should use caution when taking ginseng. Pregnant women should not take ginseng because its safety during pregnancy has not been determined.

  American ginseng is currently on the United Plant Savers (UpS) at-risk list, meaning that the species is endangered due to overharvesting or lack of habitat. Wisconsin currently produces the most ginseng, which is still sent primarily to

China. In 1905 the state passed a law that made it illegal to dig ginseng roots until after they've been allowed to set seed (August 1). Poaching roots and spreading fungus from cultivated to wild crops are as much of a threat to the species as is overharvesting.

Interactions

American ginseng may increase the effects of caffeine or other stimulants as well as phenelzine (Nardil®), antipsychotics, or blood pressure, anti-diabetic, or steroidal medications.

Regulatory and Compendial Status

The U.S. FDA classifies ginseng as a dietary supplement. In Germany, Asian ginseng root is approved with nonprescription status, and in the United Kingdom it is licensed on the General Sales List.

References

Bahrke M, Morgan P. Evaluation of the ergogenic properties of ginseng. *Sports Medicine.* 1994;18:229–248.

Blumenthal M, ed. *The Complete German Commission E Monographs.* Boston, Mass: Integrative Medicine Communications; 1998.

Blumenthal M, Riggins C. *Popular Herbs in the U.S. Market: Therapeutic Monographs.* Austin, Tex: The American Botanical Council; 1997.

Chen X, et al. The effects of Panax quinquefolium saponin (PQS) and its monomer ginsenoside on heart. *Chung Kuo Chung Yao Tsa Chih.* 1994;19:617–20, 640.

Foster S. *Herbal Renaissance: Growing, Using and Understanding Herbs in the Modern World.* Salt Lake City, Utah: Gibbs-Smith; 1993.

Huang KC. *The Pharmacology of Chinese Herbs.* Boca Raton, Fla: CRC Press; 1993.

Kowalchik C, Hylton W, eds. *Rodale's Illustrated Encyclopedia of Herbs.* Emmaus, Pa: Rodale Press; 1998.

Kwan CY. Vascular effects of selected antihypertensive drugs derived from traditional medicinal herbs. *Clin Exp Pharmacol Physiol.* 1995;(suppl 1):S297–S299. Review.

Li J, et al. Panax quinquefolium saponins protects low density lipoproteins from oxidation. *Life Sci.* 1999;64:53–62.

McGuffin M, Hobbs C, Upton R, Goldberg A. *American Herbal Products Association's Botanical Safety Handbook.* Boca Raton, Fla: CRC Press; 1996.

Murphy LL, et al. Effect of American ginseng (Panax quinquefolium) on male copulatory behavior in the rat. *Physiol Behav.* 1998;64:445–450.

Murray M. *The Healing Power of Herbs: the Enlightened Person's Guide to the Wonders of Medicinal Plants.* Rocklin, Calif: Prima Publishing; 1995.

Newall CA, Anderson LA, Phillipson JD. *Herbal Medicines: A Guide for Health Care Professionals.* London, England: The Pharmaceutical Press; 1996.

Oshima Y. Isolation and hypoglycemic activity of quinquefolans A, B, and C, glycans of *Panax quinquefolium* roots. J Nat Prod. 1987;50:188–190.

Schultz V, Hansel R, Tyler V. *Rational Phytotherapy: A Physician's Guide to Herbal Medicine.* New York, NY: Springer; 1998.

Thornton L. The ethics of wildcrafting. *The Herb Quarterly.* 1998:41–46.

Waki I. Effects of a hypoglycemic component of Ginseng radix on insulin biosynthesis in normal and diabetic animals. *J Pharmacobiodyn.* 1982;5:547–554.

Yuan CS, et al. Modulation of American ginseng on brainstem GABAergic effects in rats. *J Ethnopharmacol.* 1998;62:215–222.

© *Copyright Integrative Medicine Communications*

Ginseng, Asian

Names

- **English**
  Asian ginseng

- **Botanical**
  Panax ginseng

- **Plant Family**
  Araliaceae

- **Pharmacopeial**
  Ginseng radix

Overview

Ginseng is recommended to help the body recover from disease, and to improve mental and physical performance. Benefits attributed to it from over 2,000 years of use have been discussed in numerous studies. In Asian countries, ginseng is regarded as the king of herbs and is added to many every day items, including beverages. The Chinese have associated ginseng with longevity, virility, strength, and wisdom since at least 1 A.D., according to written accounts.

The scientific name given to ginseng by Swedish botanist Carl Linnaeus in 1753 uses the Greek words *pan* (all) and *ax* (akos; cure) to mean the root that cures all ills. More recently, ginseng is classified as an adaptogen and antioxidant. Adaptogens are substances that increase physiological resistance to stressors. Antioxidants function similarly, decreasing circulating free radicals and reducing their negative effects on the body. Modern research shows that ginseng increases the body's ability to fight against bacterial, viral, emotional, cognitive, muscular, metabolic, and cardiovascular stressors.

Elderly persons take ginseng to induce a feeling of well-being, increase stamina, and combat the negative physical and mental effects of recent or chronic age-related degenerative conditions. Younger persons take it to increase athletic strength and sexual virility and to improve intellectual performance. Ongoing studies are looking into the effects of ginseng as adjunctive therapy for cancer, diabetes, cardiovascular disease, non–AIDS related immune system disorders, male and female infertility, aging, menopause, and depression.

American and Asian ginsengs are indicated in stress, fatigue, convalescence and diabetes, and Siberian ginseng in stress, fatigue, atherosclerosis, and impaired kidney function. Confusion regarding which ginseng to use for stress, fatigue, and convalescence (American, Asian, or Siberian) stems from the suggestion that active components in one type are superior to those in another type, e.g., ginsenosides versus eleutherosides. Such superiority has not been demonstrated. Early Russian studies indicated that Siberian ginseng's positive effects exceed those of Asian ginseng's. These results are supported by empirical reports, but are challenged by investigators who question the validity of the studies and the quality of the Siberian ginseng preparation. At this time, all three ginsengs are regarded as adaptogens, all three share contraindication and side effect profiles, and despite qualitative differences, each is used for similar indications. Cost, standardization, and the reputation of the manufacturer may be the deciding points in determining which product to use.

Macro Description

The ginseng root is harvested at 4 to 6 years' age. Mature herbaceous plants bear five-lobed palmate leaves, which circle a stem that grows from a tap root and can reach up to 16 inches in height. At the fourth year, the plant produces a small, greenish-white umbel-shaped flower cluster at the junction of the leaves and stem. These produce red berries.

Light beige, variably thick, gnarled root can appear similar in shape to the human body and has offshoots with long stringy hairs that can look like arms and legs. Age is determined by the numbers of wrinkles around the neck of the root. The crude drug is prepared from the lateral root and root hairs.

Part Used/Pharmaceutical Designations

- Roots

Constituents/Composition

Dried root contains at least 1.5% ginsenosides (Rg1 as marker); glycans (panaxans) up to 0.05% volatile oil; polysaccharide fraction DPG-3-2; peptides; and maltol.

Commercial Preparations

White ginseng (dried, peeled) or red ginseng (unpeeled root steamed before drying) is prepared as aqueous, aqueous-alcohol or alcohol liquid extracts, and as powders or capsules.

Medicinal Uses/Indications

Traditional: adaptogen, tonic, restorative, alterative, anodyne, appetite-stimulant, aphrodisiac, antidepressant, cardiotonic, carminative, expectorant, hormone restorative, nervine, sedative, sialogogue, stimulant, stomachic.

Clinical applications: Rehabilitation; to increase stamina and well-being, particularly in the elderly. German Commission E monograph describes ginseng as a "tonic to counteract weakness and fatigue, as a restorative for declining stamina and impaired concentration, and as an aid to convalescence." Also used to treat diabetes, ulcer, edema, cancer, hypercholesterolemia, infertility, fatigue, frequent colds or viral illness, menopause, and red blood cell depletion.

Pharmacology

In 37 clinical studies published between 1968 and 1990, ginseng improved physical and cognitive performance, mood, or metabolism. Still other studies suggest a plethora of ginseng actions.

- ginseng improves cholesterol ratios
- elevates blood alcohol clearance
- reduces liver toxicity
- improves psychomotor performance
- helps control asthma and chronic respiratory disease (200 mg per day improved respiratory strength, oxygenation capacity, and walking distance in chronic respiratory disease patients)
- lowers blood sugar levels
- regulates blood pressure and adrenocorticotropic hormone
- enhances athletic stamina.

Studies in humans also indicate that ginseng may be used as adjunctive therapy in the treatment of diabetic neuropathy, reactive depression, psychologically-induced impotence, and psychological disorders in children.

Asian ginseng stimulates the central nervous system, neurotransmitters, oxygen metabolism, and glycogen stores. Antidiabetic effects may be due to hypoglycemic actions of panaxans and ginseng polysaccharide fraction DPG-3-2. Virility may be related to increases in both male and female hormones in gonads. The beneficial effects of ginseng in treating cardiovascular disease may be due to decreases in serum levels of cholesterol, triglyceride, and fatty acids, and increases in high-density lipoprotein.

Studies in mice have shown that ginseng elevates antibody levels, improves cell-mediated immunity and natural-killer-cell activity, lymphocytes, phagocytosis, in vitro; stimulates interferon production in the spleen. Polysaccharides in leaves and roots enhance macrophage binding. Also in mice, ginseng extracts inhibit DMBA-, urethane-, and aflatoxin B1-induced tumors; injections of ginseng administered along with radiation prevent radiation-induced bone marrow death and increase liver cell recovery. Ginseng also stimulates red blood cell formation in bone marrow.

Dosage Ranges and Duration of Administration

White or red ginseng standardized to 1.5% ginsenosides, designated as Rg1. The recommended dose is 1 to 2 g fresh root, or 0.6 to 2 g dried root, or 200 to 600 mg liquid extract daily. Healthy persons using ginseng for enhanced physical or mental performance or to improve resistance to stressors should take these doses in cycles of 15 to 20 days followed by two-week breaks.

For rehabilitation after an illnes, the elderly should take 0.5 g bid for three months; or take 0.5 g bid for one month, followed by a two-month break, and repeat cycle if desired.

Cautions

Adverse Effects/Toxicology

The German Commission E cites no adverse effects with recommended daily dose. Agitation, addiction, changes in blood pressure, or "Ginseng Abuse

Syndrome" are no longer associated with the normal use of ginseng. Adulterants, such as caffeine, are thought to cause these effects; NSAID adulterants may cause ginseng-associated Stevens–Johnson syndrome.

The American Herbal Products Association (AHPA) rates ginseng as a class 2d herb. 2d indicates that specific restrictions apply; in the case of ginseng, hypertension is the specific restriction.

■ Warnings/Contraindications/Precautions

Patients with acute illness, cardiovascular disease, diabetes, or blood pressure disorders should use caution when taking ginseng. Pregnant women should not take ginseng because its safety during pregnancy has not been determined.

Interactions

Red ginseng may increase the effects of caffeine or other stimulants. Any ginseng product may increase the effects of phenelzine (Nardil) or other antipsychotics, or blood pressure, antidiabetic or steroidal medications.

Regulatory and Compendial Status

The U.S. FDA classifies ginseng as a dietary supplement. In Germany the ginseng root is approved with nonprescription status, and in the United Kingdom it is licensed on the General Sales List.

References

Bahrke M, Morgan P. Evaluation of the ergogenic properties of ginseng. *Sports Medicine*. 1994;18:229–248.

Blumenthal M, ed. *The Complete German Commission E Monographs*. Boston, Mass: Integrative Medicine Communications; 1998.

Blumenthal M, Riggins C. *Popular Herbs in the U.S. Market: Therapeutic Monographs*. Austin, Tex: The American Botanical Council; 1997.

Choi HK, Seong DH, Rha KH. Clinical Efficacy of Korean red ginseng for erectile dysfunction. *Int J Impotence Res*. 1995;7:181–186.

D'Angelo L, et al. A double-blind, placebo-controlled clinical study on the effect of a standardized ginseng extract on psychomotor performance in healthy volunteer. *J Ethnopharmacol*. 1986;16:15–22.

Dega H, Laporte JL, Frances C, Herson S, Chosidow O. Ginseng as a cause for Stevens-Johnson Syndrome? *Lancet*. 1996;347:1344.

De Smet PAGM, Keller K, Hansel R, Chandler RF, eds. *Adverse Effects of Herbal Drugs*. New York, NY: Springer-Verlag; 1992:1.

Dorling E. Do ginsenosides influence the performance? Results of a double-blind study. *Notabene medici*. 1980;10:241–246.

Foster S. *Asian Ginseng*. Austin, Tex: The American Botanical Council; 1996.

Gross D, Krieger D, Efrat R, Dayan M. Ginseng extract G115 for the treatment of chronic respiratory diseases. *Schweizerische Zeitschrift fur Ganzheits Medizin*. 1995;1(95):29–33.

Huang KC. *The Pharmacology of Chinese Herbs*. Boca Raton, Fla: CRC Press; 1993.

Kowalchik C, Hylton W, eds. *Rodale's Illustrated Encyclopedia of Herbs*. Emmaus, Pa: Rodale Press; 1998.

McGuffin M, Hobbs C, Upton R, Goldberg A. *American Herbal Products Association's Botanical Safety Handbook*. Boca Raton, Fla: CRC Press; 1996.

Murray M. *The Healing Power of Herbs: the Enlightened Person's Guide to the Wonders of Medicinal Plants*. Rocklin, Calif: Prima Publishing; 1995.

Newall CA, Anderson LA, Phillipson JD. *Herbal Medicines: A Guide for Health Care Professionals*. London, England: The Pharmaceutical Press; 1996.

Quiroga HA, Imbriano AE. The effect of *Panax ginseng* extract on cerebrovascular deficits. *Orientacion Medica*. 1979;1208:86–87.

Quiroga HA. Comparative double-blind study of the effect of Ginsana Gii5 and Hydergin on cerebrovascular deficits. *Orientacion Medica*. 1982;1281:201–202.

Choi HK, Seong DH, Rha KH. Clinical efficacy of Korean red ginseng for erectile dysfunction. *Int J Impotence Res*. 1995;7:181–186.

Schultz V, Hansel R, Tyler V. *Rational Phytotherapy: A Physician's Guide to Herbal Medicine*. New York, NY: Springer; 1998.

Sun XB, Matsumoto T, Yamada H. Purification of immune complexes clearance enhancing polysaccharide from the leaves of *Panax ginseng*, and its biological activities. *Phytomedicine*. 1994;1:225–231.

Tang W, Eisenbrand G. *Chinese Drugs of Plant Origin: Chemistry, Pharmacology, and Use in Traditional and Modern Medicine*. New York, NY: Springer; 1992.

You JS, Hau DM, Chen KT, Huang HF. Combined effects of ginseng and radiotherapy on experimental liver cancer. *Phytotherapy Research*. 1995;9:331–335.

© *Copyright Integrative Medicine Communications*

Ginseng, Siberian

Names

■ **English**
Siberian ginseng

■ **Botanical**
Eleutherococcus senticosus/Acanthopanax senticosus

■ **Plant Family**
Araliaceae

■ **Pharmacopeial**
Eleutherococci radix

Overview

Explored in the 1950s as an alternative to Asian ginseng, which was expensive and difficult to grow, Siberian ginseng is used today to increase physical and mental stamina, speed convalescence, and provide resistance to the detrimental effects of stress. Mirroring the functions of Asian and American ginseng, these uses also reflect thousands of years' use by the people of Russia and China.

All three types of ginseng occur in the same plant family, Araliaceae. While their constituents differ, studies conducted in Russia since the late 1950s conclude that like its distant cousins, Siberian ginseng has similar adaptogenic functions. Adaptogens increase physiologic resistance to stressors. They also normalize processes within the body that may have been altered in response to those stressors, and are nontoxic and nonspecific in action. By 1985, studies of Siberian ginseng conducted in the Soviet Union, with the involvement of over 4,300 healthy and diseased subjects, confirmed these effects. In 1962, consequent to approval of 33% alcohol Siberian ginseng extract for human use by the Pharmacological Committee of USSR Ministry of Health, 3 million Soviets were estimated to be taking it regularly. Among these were Soviet astronauts and Olympic team members. Ongoing studies are looking into the effects of ginseng in terms of its adjunctive therapeutic use for diabetes, infertility, atherosclerosis and rheumatic heart disease, cancer, and conditions due to depressed immune function, such as chronic fatigue syndrome.

American and Asian ginsengs are indicated in stress, fatigue, convalescence and diabetes, and Siberian ginseng in stress, fatigue, atherosclerosis, and impaired kidney function. Confusion regarding which ginseng to use for stress, fatigue, and convalescence (American, Asian, or Siberian) stems from the suggestion that active components in one type are superior to those in another type, e.g., ginsenosides versus eleutherosides. Such superiority has not been demonstrated. Early Russian studies indicated that Siberian ginseng's positive effects exceed those of Asian ginseng's. These results are supported by empirical reports, but are challenged by investigators who question the validity of the studies and the quality of the Siberian ginseng preparation. At this time, all three ginsengs are regarded as adaptogens, all three share contraindication and side effect profiles, and despite qualitative differences, each is used for similar indications. Cost, standardization, and the reputation of the manufacturer may be the deciding points in determining which product to use.

Macro Description

Siberian ginseng is cultivated from a shrub that grows one to three meters in height. Palmate leaves with five serrated, thorny-veined leaflets are attached to long petioles that are covered with bristles. Petioles are attached to stems, which are noted for their backward-pointing prickles. Stem bark is gray-brown.

Flowers grow in umbels from a peduncle; male flowers are violet, female flowers, yellow. These produce round black berries.

The Siberian ginseng root is 1.5 to 4 cm long, brown to brownish gray, with lengthwise wrinkles. It is twisted, variably branched with a few rootlets. It smells aromatic and tastes bitter and astringent.

Part Used/Pharmaceutical Designations

• Roots

■ **Constituents/Composition**

Root contains 0.6% to 0.9% eleutheroside components common to many plant species. Many are glycosides. Eleutheroside A is a sterol (daucosterol); B is a phenylopropanoid (syringin); B_1 (isofraxidin) and B_3 are coumarins; C is a monosaccharide (methyl-alpha-D-galactoside); B_4, D, and E (acanthoside D) are lignans; and I, K, L, and M are triterpene saponins. Root also contains aglycones, polysaccharide glycans (eleuthocans A-G) and various sugars, phenylpropanoids, oleanolic acid, dihydroxybenzoic acid (DBA), and volatile oil.

■ **Commercial Preparations**

• Crude drug (bark, whole root and rhizome)
• Aqueous-alcohol liquid extracts
• Solid extracts
• Powders
• Capsules
• Tablets

Medicinal Uses/Indications

Traditional:

• Stimulant
• Tonic
• Diuretic
• To treat insomnia
• To enhance virility
• To increase the body's resistance to stress

Clinical applications:

• Stress
• Fatigue
• Atherosclerosis
• Impaired kidney function
• Lower back/kidney pain
• Anorexia
• Rheumatoid arthritis
• Chronic fatigue syndrome
• Blood pressure disorders
• Symptoms of coronary arteriosclerosis
• Symptoms of radiotherapy- and chemotherapy-induced leukopenia
• ADHD
• Debility
• Diminished capacity for work or concentration
• To help during convalescence

■ **Pharmacology**

Siberian ginseng has normalizing, stress-resistant, and immune stimulant effects. In studies involving over 4,300 subjects, Siberian ginseng was administered orally to determine its effects on disease, or to assess its ability to help the body tolerate stress. Subjects who had atherosclerosis, pyelonephritis, diabetes mellitus, hypertension, hypotension, craniocerebral trauma, neurosis, rheumatic heart disease, chronic bronchitis, and pulmonary tuberculosis noted overall improvements in their condition. Healthy subjects in these studies were exposed to extremes in temperature, sound, working conditions, exercise, and deep-sea diving decompression. They noted enhanced physical labor and stamina, mental concentration and acuity. They were better able to tolerate to extreme conditions, had improved capillary function, and improved resistance to hypoxemia. New blood formation was enhanced in blood donors. In both healthy and nonhealthy subjects, a 33% alcohol extract was used, for up to 39 days followed by a two-to-three week break if the study was to be continued.

Immune stimulant effects, noted through increases in lymphocyte count (particularly T-lymphocytes) were reported in a double-blind, placebo-controlled study of healthy subjects.

In studies in animals, Siberian ginseng polysaccharides were immunostimulating. Intraperitoneal injection resulted in eleutheran-stimulated hypoglycemia in alloxan-induced hyperglycemic mice. DBACK reduced collagen- and ADP- induced platelet aggregation comparably to aspirin.

Infusions of Siberian ginseng increased stress resistance in rats and improved work performance in mice. Intraperitoneal injections increased gonadotrophic action in both male and female mice. Mineralcorticoid, glucocorticoid, and steroid receptor binding was observed. Siberian ginseng had sedative and CNS stimulant effects, and caused both increases and reduction in barbiturate sleeping time. It was antileukemic and reduced toxicity caused by antitumor and antileukimic agents (rybromycin, thio-TEPA, Dopan, 6-mercaptopurine, cyclophosan, ethymidine, benzo-TEPA, sarcolysin; chlorofos s.c., malonic acid).

Dosage Ranges and Duration of Administration

- Dried root (tea, or in capsules): 2 to 3 g daily or equivalent preparations
- Tincture: 5 ml tid
- 33% aqueous-alcohol extract, 2 to 4 ml, one to three times daily
- Solid extract (dried, powdered), with at least 1% eleutheroside F: 100 to 200 mg tid

Note: Take before 3 P.M. to avoid insomnia; A three-month course, followed by a two-to-three week Siberian ginseng–free interval, or occasional use for one month, followed by two-month Siberian ginseng–free intervals, should be observed.

Cautions

■ Adverse Effects/Toxicology

American Herbal Products Association safely rating: class 1 (safe with appropriate use); German Commission E lists no side effects. High doses (4.5 to 5 ml tid) may cause insomnia, irritability, melancholy, anxiety; in studies conducted in the Soviet Union, some patients with rheumatic heart disease noted pericardial pain, high blood pressure, headaches, and palpitations.

■ Warnings/Contraindications/Precautions

Hypertension (>180/90 mm Hg) contraindicates use. Although studies in animals suggest Siberian ginseng is nonteratogenic, its safety during pregnancy has not been determined.

Interactions

Siberian ginseng may potentiate the effects of caffeine and other stimulants and should not be taken with antipsychotic drugs, steroids, or hormones.

Regulatory and Compendial Status

U.S. FDA: dietary supplement; German Commission E: approved for non-prescription use; not licensed through the General Sales List in the United Kingdom.

References

Asano K, et al. Effect of *Eleutherococcus senticosus* extract on human physical working capacity. *Planta Medica.* 1986;3:175–177.

Awang D. Siberian ginseng toxicity may be case of mistaken identity. *Can Med Assoc J.* 1996;155:1237.

Blumenthal M, Riggins C. *Popular Herbs in the U.S. Market: Therapeutic Monographs.* Austin, Tex: The American Botanical Council; 1997.

Blumenthal M, ed. *The Complete German Commission E Monographs.* Boston, Mass: Integrative Medicine Communications; 1998.

Farnsworth N, Wagner H, Kikino H. *Economic and Medicinal Plant Research.* London, England: Academic Press Inc; 1985:1.

Foster S. *Siberian Ginseng (Eleutherococcus senticosus).* Austin, Tex: American Botanical Council; 1990.

Hacker B, Medon P. Cytotoxic effects of *E. sentococcus* aqueous extract against L1210 leukemia cells. *J Pharm Sci.* 1984;73:270–272.

Hebel S, ed. Eleutherococcus. *The Lawrence Review of Natural Products.* Facts and Comparisons; 1996:1–3.

Kaloeva ZD. Effect of glycosides from *Eleutherococcus senticosus* on the parameters of hemodynamics in patients with hypotension. *Farmakol Toksikol.* 1986;49:73.

Leung A, Foster S. *Encyclopedia of Common Natural Ingredients Used in Food, Drugs, and Cosmetics.* 2nd ed. New York, NY: John Wiley & Sons, Inc; 1996.

McGuffin M, Hobbs C, Upton R, Goldberg A. *American Herbal Products Association's Botanical Safety Handbook.* Boca Raton, Fla: CRC Press; 1996.

Murray M. *The Healing Power of Herbs: the Enlightened Person's Guide to the Wonders of Medicinal Plants.* Rocklin, Calif: Prima Publishing; 1995.

Newall CA, Anderson LA, Phillipson JD. *Herbal Medicines: A Guide for Health Care Professionals.* London, England: The Pharmaceutical Press; 1996.

Novozhilov GN, Sil'chenko KI. The mechanism of adaptogenic action of *Eleutherococcus senticosus* extract on the human body under thermal stress. *Fiziol Cheloveka.* 1985;11:303–306.

Schultz V, Hansel R, Tyler V. *Rational Phytotherapy: A Physician's Guide to Herbal Medicine.* New York, NY: Springer; 1998.

Wu Jia Seng: Acanthopanax senticosus [in Chinese]. Heilungkiang Institute of Traditional Chinese Medicine. [No date].

Xiao, P-G. et al. Immunological aspects of Chinese medicinal plants as antiaging drugs. *J Ethnopharmacol.* 1993;38:167–175.

© *Copyright Integrative Medicine Communications*

Goldenseal

Names

- **English**
  Goldenseal

- **Botanical**
  Hydrastis canadensis

- **Plant Family**
  Ranunculaceae

- **Pharmacopeial**
  Hydrastis rhizoma

Overview

Goldenseal was originally a Native American medicinal herb, introduced to early settlers by Cherokee and Iroquois tribes. They used it as a yellow dye, as well as a wash for skin diseases and sore eyes, and various forms of catarrh. It has acquired a considerable reputation as a general bitter tonic, anti-infective, and remedy for various gastric and genitourinary disorders. In recent years it has been over-harvested and is now considered a threatened species. Fortunately, commercial cultivation has alleviated the shortage, but it is still quite expensive.

Goldenseal is an herb that is particularly applicable to disorders and infections of the mucous membranes. It is thought to strengthen the immune system, potentiate the effects of insulin, and cleanse the system. Extensive laboratory research has shown that the alkaloid constituents of goldenseal possess anti-inflammatory and antibiotic properties. One of the main ingredients in goldenseal, berberine, has been shown to have activity against a broad range of microbes, from trichomonas to giardia to candida to tapeworms.

Goldenseal is considered by naturopathic physicians to be astringent and healing to the gut wall and other mucous membranes, making it useful for disorders of the intestine and stomach. It also is considered to act as a digestive stimulant and cholagogue, a laxative, and as a stimulating adjunct to other remedies for the lungs, kidneys, and reproductive tract. Goldenseal may be especially useful for congestion and chronic inflammation of the respiratory and urogenital tracts; catarrhal affliction of the nose; chronic gastritis and enteritis; catarrh of the bladder; hepatic congestion; eye inflammation; inflammation of the vagina, uterus, and urethra; chronic constipation; hemorrhoids; and anal fissures.

Externally, goldenseal is valuable for chronic inflammation of mucous membranes, cracks and fissures of the nipples, indolent ulcers, and as a lotion to stop profuse sweating. It is also useful as an eyewash.

Macro Description

Goldenseal is a small perennial plant, with a single hairy stem producing two five-lobed, serrated leaves and a small single apetalous flower with greenish sepals. These give way to a raspberry-like fruit. The rhizome is a bright yellow-brown in color, twisted, and wrinkled with many fine rootlets attached. This breaks easily to reveal a dark yellow interior. The taste is bitter. Goldenseal can be found growing wild in rich, shady woodlands throughout northern North America. It is now also commercially cultivated.

Part Used/Pharmaceutical Designations

- Root/rhizomes

- **Constituents/Composition**
  Alkaloids: berberine, canadine, corypalmine, hydrastine, reticuline
  Also contains: tannins, vitamins, minerals

- **Commercial Preparations**
  Goldenseal is available in the following forms.
  - Dried root/rhizomes
  - Tablets, various concentrations
  - Powdered root in capsules, various concentrations
  - Alcoholic tinctures
  - Low-alcohol extracts

Medicinal Uses/Indications

Traditional herbal actions: cholagogue, astringent, digestive bitter, vulnerary (heats ulcerated surfaces internally and externally), laxative, anti-pathogenic
Clinical applications:

- For gastric and enteric inflammations (e.g., gastritis, enteritis, diarrhea, peptic ulcers)
- Useful for colds, flu, and glandular swelling
- Acts as a cholagogue, improves digestion and reduces food sensitivities
- May be helpful in diabetes
- Used as a nasal infusion to reduce excess mucous
- As external application for lacerations, abrasions, abscesses, boils, and other skin eruptions
- As a rinse for throat, gum, and mouth inflammation or sores, use extract or tincture as mouthwash, or prepare a rinse as follows: In 1 cup of warm water, mix 1/4 tsp. salt and 1/2 tsp., or the contents of 1 capsule of goldenseal powder. (It will not dissolve completely.)
- For vaginal problems, use tea or extract, or the rinse described above as a douche. (Strain out suspended particles before using.)
- For middle-ear inflammation and congestion, mix with olive oil and use several drops in each ear.
- For mild conjunctivitis or eye irritation, use sterile water to make the rinse above and use as eyewash. (Discard if the solution becomes cloudy, indicating bacterial growth.)

- **Pharmacology**

  - Antibiotic, anti-infective: Berberine has been shown to have antibacterial, antifungal, and antiprotozoal properties. It has been shown to inhibit the growth of *Giardia lamblia, Trichomonas vaginalis,* and *Entamoeba histolytica* in culture, as well as numerous other bacteria and microorganisms, including *Candida, C. vibrio,* and trypanosomes. It may also be an immune stimulant. Hydrastine has been found to kill tapeworms, and also has bactericidal properties. Reticuline has bactericidal properties as well.
  - Anti-diabetic/hypoglycemic: Berberine is known to be effective in lowering blood glucose.
  - Anti-diarrheal: Berberine has been shown to have antidiarrheal properties. In addition to its antimicrobial properties, laboratory studies have shown that it can halt the excessive intestinal secretion of electrolytes caused by endotoxins from bacteria such as *E. coli.*
  - Anti-inflammatory/analgesic: Berberine has been found to have anti-inflammatory properties. One study found that this may arise in part from the inhibition of DNA-synthesis in activated lymphocytes. Berberine and reticuline both have analgesic and antispasmodic properties. Berberine and corypalmine are both antioxidant, which may also help reduce inflammation.
  - Carminative and cholagogue: Berberine has both carminative and cholagogic actions.

Dosage Ranges and Duration of Administration

- Tincture (1:5): 60% alcohol .5 to 1.5 ml tid
- Tablets or powder/capsules: 0.5 to 2 g tid
- Tea, 1/4 tsp. to 1/4 tsp. powdered root per cup, steeped 10 minutes. Up to 2 cups/day.
- Extract: 0.03 to 0.12 g tid

Cautions

- **Adverse Effects/Toxicology**

  In very large doses, goldenseal may cause convulsions and over-stimulation of the nervous system. Long-term use of high dosages have caused elevated white blood cell counts. Signs of toxicity take the form of irritation of the mouth and throat, diarrhea, and vomiting. Ulceration can occur internally and externally with severe overdosing.

- **Warnings/Contraindications/Precautions**

  - Not recommended for use in pregnancy—contains berberine which has abortifacient properties.
  - Not recommended for use in presence of hypertension.
  - Long-term use may weaken the beneficial bacterial flora of the digestive tract. Acidophilus capsules or yogurt should therefore be taken to restore proper balance of probiotic flora.

- Extended consumption of large amounts of this herb have been shown to lower B vitamin absorption and utilization.

Interactions

There is debate as to whether goldenseal acts as a brain tonic when combined with gotu kola.

Regulatory and Compendial Status

Goldenseal has been officially recognized by most Western pharmacopeias. However, a federal interagency committee has recommended that the National Toxicology Program review and possibly test goldenseal for its potential to cause developmental problems or cancer of the reproductive system or both.

References

Balch J, Balch P. *Prescription for Nutritional Healing: A-to-Z Guide to Drug-Free Remedies Using Vitamins, Minerals, Herbs, & Food Supplements.* New York, NY: Avery Publishing Group; 1990.

Duke JA. *Handbook of Phytochemical Constituents of GRAS Herbs and Other Economic Plants.* Boca Raton, Fla: CRC Press; 1992.

Foster S. Goldenseal. *American Botanical Council: Botanical Series No. 309.*

Genest K, Hughes DW. Natural products in Canadian pharmaceuticals, *Hydrastis canadensis. Can J Pharm Sci.* 1969;4.

Kaneda Y, Tanaka T, Saw T. Effects of berberine, a plant alkaloid, on the growth of anaerobic protozoa in axenic culture. *Tokai J Exp Clin Med.* 1990;15:417–423.

Mills SY. *Dictionary of Modern Herbalism: A Comprehensive Guide to Practical Herbal Therapy.* Rochester, Vt: Healing Arts Press; 1988.

Nishino H, et al. Berberine sulfate inhibits tumor-promoting activity of teleocidin in two-stage carcinogenesis on mouse skin. *Oncology.* 1986;43:131–134.

Shideman FE. A review of the pharmacology and therapeutics of Hydrastis and its alkaloids, hydrastine, berberine and canadine. *Comm on Nat Formulary Bull.* 1950;18:3–19.

Sun D, Courtney HS, Beachey EH. Berberine sulfate blocks adherence of Streptococcus pyogenes to epithelial cells, fibronectin, and hexadecane. *Antimicrob Agents Chemother.* 1988;32:1370–1374.

Swanston-Flatt SK, et al. Evaluation of traditional plant treatments for diabetes: studies in streptozotocin diabetic mice. *Acta Diabetol Lat.* 1989;26:51–55.

Zhu B, Ahrens FA. Effect of berberine on intestinal secretion mediated by Escherichia coli heat-stable enterotoxin in jejunum of pigs. *Am J Vet Res.* 1982; 43:1594–1598.

© *Copyright Integrative Medicine Communications*

Grape Seed Extract

Names

- **English**
  Grape Seed

- **Botanical**
  Vitis vinifera

- **Plant Family**
  Vitaceae

Overview

Grapes reach far back into history. Fossilized leaves and seeds from the Miocen and Teriary periods have been unearthed in Europe, Iceland, and North America; in Switzerland from the period of the Bronze Age; and in Egyptian tombs and hieroglyphics. Grapes are noted in the Bible. Homer drank wine made from grapes, circa 700 B.C.

All parts of the plant have been used for medicinal use. Sap was used in Europe for eye and skin ailments. Leaves had astringent and hemostatic actions. Grapes that were not yet ripe were used for sore or infected throats. Raisins had therapeutic applications, too—for instance, in the treatment of consumption, constipation, and thirst. Ripe grapes, however, had a plethora of applications, including cancer, cholera, smallpox, nausea, ophthalmia, and skin, kidney, and liver diseases. Similar and additional applications were prevalent in the Middle East, India, and China. Grapes have also been listed in many pharmacopoeias.

Today, however, grapes are rarely, if ever, used for any of these purposes. Apart from being source materials in the manufacture of food and beverage uses, grapes are harvested because they are a source of oligomeric proanthocyanidins (OPCs), therapeutically active antioxidants. Compared to most botanical products used for their own individual therapeutic properties, grape seed is used for the OPCs it contains. These polyphenolic constituents are also found in green tea and maritime pine bark. Extracts made from each of these plants contain similar OPC values and may be used interchangeably for specific indications, including chronic venous insufficiency and some opthalmologic conditions. Effects have not been evaluated by Germany's Commission E, and in the United States, the use of pine bark (pycnogenol) for OPCs is much more prevalent than grape seed OPCs.

Macro Description

Grapes are the fruit of *Vitis vinifera*, native to Asia but naturalized to most other continents in temperate regions. The perennial consists of a woody, climbing vine. The stem produces a peeling bark, and the large, circular to circular-ovate leaves are dentate or jagged at the margins, pale green on the top, and grayer underneath. Fruits are oval, and may be green, red, or purple. OPCs occur on the outside of the grape seeds as well as on the inner grape skin.

Part Used/Pharmaceutical Designations

- Seeds
- Fruit skin

- **Constituents/Composition**
  OPCs, also called procyandins, consist of a variable number of flavan units, and are dimeric, trimeric, tetrameric, and oligomeric, depending on the length of the bonds that link them. A patented process, developed by French biochemist Jaques Mesquelier in 1970, assures that each of these chains is present in a grape seed product.

- **Commercial Preparations**
  Extracts are standardized to 95% OPC content.

Medicinal Uses/Indications

Grape plants were originally used for purposes described in the overview. Because OPCs were not isolated from grape seed until 1970, there was no traditional folk use of OPCs.

Clinical applications: Results from controlled trials support the use of grape seed OPCs for impaired visual function due to macular degeneration and chronic venous insufficiency. In addition, lymphedema, acrocyanosis, varicose veins, telangiectases, capillary fragility and permeability secondary to diabetes, cancer, premenstrual syndrome, and dental caries are some of the many indications for which grape seed OPCs might prove useful.

- **Pharmacology**
  Pharmacologic activities of OPCs are numerous. In vitro, OPCs' antioxidant activity is 50 times greater than vitamin E's and 20 times greater than vitamin C's, in both lipid and aqueous phases. OPCs significantly and dose-dependently prevent vitamin E loss, and lower blood cholesterol levels through possible reversal of cholesterol transport, and by increasing both intestinal cholesterol absorption and bile acid excretion. OPCs also inhibit angiotensin I converting enzyme, ascorbic acid oxidase, histidine decarboxylase, and prevents histamine release and arterial damage. OPCs are thought to prevent atherosclerosis by inhibiting platelet aggregation and vascular constriction. They stabilize capillary walls and prevent xylene-induced capillary permeability. OPCs also demonstrate anti-mutagenic activity, and inhibit carageenan-induced rat paw edema.

In a double-blind, placebo controlled trial, grape seed extract was an effective prophylactic against post-operative facial swelling. In an open trial, venolymphatic symptoms of premenstrual syndrome in 165 study subjects were relieved with grape seed OTC therapy. Capillary resistance in 28 diabetic and hypertensive patients rose significantly in an open trial that provided patients with 150 mg OPCs daily. It is also effective in relieving upper extremity lymphedema secondary to radical mastectomy.

Dosage Ranges and Duration of Administration

- As a preventive for atherosclerosis, ophthalmologic disorders, or other conditions: 50 mg standardized extract/day.
- For therapeutic purposes: 150 to 300 mg/day.

Cautions

- **Adverse Effects/Toxicology**
  None known

- **Warnings/Contraindications/Precautions**
  None known

Interactions

None known

Regulatory and Compendial Status

In the United States, grape seed OPC is a dietary supplement. It was not reviewed by Germany's Commission E.

References

Amsellem M, et al. Endotelon in the treatment of venolymphatic problems in premenstrual syndrome: multi-center study on 165 patients. *Tempo Medical.* 1987;282.

Ariga TK, Hamano M. Radical scavenging action and its mode in procyanidins B-1 and B-3 from azuki beans to peroxyl radicals. *Agricultural Biological Chemistry.* 1990;54:2499–2504.

Baruch J. Effect of grape seed extract in postoperative edema [in French]. *Ann Chir Plast Esthet.* 1984;4.

Blumenthal M, Riggins C. *Popular Herbs in the U.S. Market: Therapeutic Monographs.* Austin, Tex: American Botanical Council; 1997.

Bombardelli E, Morazzoni P. *Vitis vinifera* L. *Fitoterapia.* 1995; 66:291–317.

Chang WC, Hsu FL. Inhibition of platelet aggregation and arachidonate metabolism in platelets by procyanidins. *Prostagland Leukotri Essential Fatty Acids.* 1989;38: 181–188.

Corbe C, Boissin JP, Siou A. Light vision and chorioretinal circulation: study of the effect of procyanidolic oligomers (Endotelon) [in French]. *J Fr Ophthalmol.* 1988;11:453–460.

Delacrois P. Double-blind study of grape seed extract in chronic venous insufficiency. *La Revue De Med.* 1981;28–31.

Fromantin M. Les oligomeres procyanidoliques dans le traitement de la fragilite capillaire et de la retinopathie chez les diabetiques: a propos de 26 cas. *Med Int.* 1982;16.

Kashiwada Y, et al. Antitumor agents, 129: tannins and related compounds as selective cytotoxic agents. *J Nat Prod.* 1992;55:1033–1043.

Lagrua G, et al. A study of the effects of procyanidol oligomers on capillary resistance in hypertension and in certain nephropathis. *Sem Hop.* 1981;57:1399–1401.

Maffei FR, Carini M, Aldini G, Bombardelli E, Morazzoni P, Morelli R. Free radical scavenging action and anti-enzyme activities of procyanidins from *Vitis vinifera*: a mechanism for their capillary protective action. *Arzneimittelfarichung.* May 1994; 44:592–601.

Maffei FR, Carini M, Aldini G, Bombardelli E, Morazzoni P. Sparing effect of procyanidins from *Vitis vinifera* on vitamin E: in vitro studies. *Planta Med.* 1998;64:343–347.

Masquelier J. Comparative action of various vitamin P related factors on the oxidation of ascorbic acid by cupric ions. *Bulletin de la Societe de Chimie Biologique.* 1951;33:304–305.

Masquelier J. Natural products as medicinal agents. *Planta Med.* 1980;242S–256S.

Meunier M T, et al. Inhibition of angiotensin I converting enzyme by flavonolic compounds: *in vitro* and *in vivo* studies. *Planta Med.* 1987;53:12–15.

Murray M. *The Healing Power of Herbs: the Enlightened Person's Guide to the Wonders of Medicinal Plants.* Rocklin, Calif: Prima Publishing; 1995.

Schultz V, Hnsel R, Tyler V. *Rational Phytotherapy: A Physician's Guide to Herbal Medicine.* New York, NY: Springer-Verlag; 1998.

Schwitters B, Masquelier J. *OPC in Practice: The Hidden Story of Proanthocyanidins, Nature's Most Powerful and Patented Antioxidant.* Rome, Italy: Alfa Omega Publishers; 1995.

Tebib K, et al. Dietary grape seed tannins affect lipoproteins, lipoprotein lipases, and tissue lipids in rats fed hypercholesterolemic diets. *J Nutr.* 1994; 124: 2451–2457.

Tebib K, et al. Polymeric grape seed tannins prevent plasma cholesterol changes in high-cholesterol-fed rats. *Food Chem.* 1994;49:403–406.

Walker, Morton. The nutritional therapeutics of Masquelier's oligomeric proanthocyanidins (OPCs). *Townsend Letter for Doctors and Patients.* 1996;175/76:84–92.

Zafirov D, Bredy-Dobreva G, Litchev V, Papasova M. Antiexudative and capillaritonic effects of procyanidines isolated from grape seeds *(V. vinifera)*. *Acta Physiol Pharmacol Bulg.* 1990;16:50–54.

© *Copyright Integrative Medicine Communications*

Green Tea

Names

- **English**
  Green tea

- **Botanical**
  Camellia sinensis

Overview

Native to eastern Asia, tea was originally grown in China at least 5,000 years ago. Today, tea is widely cultivated in Asia and parts of the Middle East and Africa. Green tea is unfermented, while black tea is fermented. Oolong tea is semifermented. In green tea the fresh leaves are slightly steamed and then quickly dried. This process inactivates enzymes that oxidize polyphenols to derivative compounds.

Polyphenols have antioxidant and anticancer activities, but their conversion products do not. Green tea polyphenols (GTP) surpass vitamins C and E in their antioxidant protective properties. In black teas, the leaves are dried slowly, allowing them to ferment. The polyphenol conversion products in black tea have no significant therapeutic benefits.

Green tea is used in traditional Chinese medicine to promote digestion, counter flatulence, stimulate mental function, improve eyesight, and regulate body temperature. It is also thought to strengthen the arteries, reduce excess fats, clear phlegm, and neutralize poisons. The tannins in green tea have antidiarrhea activity. The longer tea leaves are brewed, the greater the tannin content.

Macro Description

The tea plant is a large shrub with evergreen leaves that can reach a height of 30 feet. However, it is usually pruned to two to three feet. The flowers have five or six white petals and multiple yellow stamens. The branches are smooth and covered by shiny, dark green, hairy leaves. The age of the leaf can be determined by its position on the harvested stem. The leaf buds, young leaves, and stem are the preferred plant parts for making teas.

Part Used/Pharmaceutical Designations

- Leaves
- Leaf buds

Constituents/Composition

Purine alkaloids (caffeine [2.9 to 4.2%], theophylline [0.02 to 0.04%], theobromine [0.15 to 0.2%]; polyphenols (including (+)-catechin, d-catechin, +catechin, (−)-epicatechin (EC), (−)epicatechin gallate (ECG), (−) epigallocatechin (EGC), (−) epigallocatechin-gallate (EGCG), and other catechin derivatives; phenolic acids; terpenoids; indole; anorganic ions.

Commercial Preparations

Commercial preparations consist of dried leaf tea as well as extracts made from the leaves and leaf buds. The leaves are harvested, immediately heated, and then rolled and crushed to prevent enzymatic changes from altering the color and natural constituents. Green tea has 300 to 400 mg polyphenols and 50 to 100 mg caffeine per cup. Decaffeinated products contain concentrated polyphenols (60% to 89% total polyphenols). Both the epigallocatechin and total polyphenol content should be considered when purchasing commercial products.

Medicinal Uses/Indications

Traditional herbal actions: astringent, bronchodilator, antiviral, antiarteriosclerotic, anticholesteremic

Current clinical applications: cancer prevention, coughs, colds, asthma, diarrhea, bacterial dysentery, and adjunct to radiation treatment (reduces tissue damage).

Pharmacology

Green tea taken as a beverage has antioxidant, anticancer, antimutagenic, antibacterial, antifungal, and antiviral properties. Population studies show that green tea use correlated with lowered serum cholesterol totals and triglyceride levels, lowered LDL levels, and increased HDL levels. Green tea probably prevents atheroslerosis by blocking the oxidation of LDL. Purine alkaloids isolated from green tea have a relaxing effect on bronchial smooth muscle. Purine alkaloids also enhance cornary blood flow and simulate cardiac muscle. They may even account for the diuretic effects of green tea. One of the catechins in green tea, EGCG, had an antiplatelet aggregation effect comparable to aspirin.

Other population studies suggest that green tea taken daily as a beverage prevents cancer. Black tea consumption, on the other hand, correlated with increased risk of cancers of the rectum, gallbladder, and endometrium. GTP suppressed the activation and formation of cancer-causing substances. The cancer-prevention effects of green tea are strongest against cancers of the gastrointestinal tract, lung, and breast.

In in vitro experiments, GTP blocked the growth of mammary cancer cell lines. Green tea apparently disrupts interactions among tumor promoters, hormones, growth factors, and their receptors. In animal models, green tea extracts administered to mice in doses comparable to the amount consumed by humans blocked the formation of ultraviolet B (UVB)-induced sunburn lesions and skin tumors. And in both animal and human investigations, green tea beverages ingested with meals inhibited the formation of carcinogenic nitrosamines.

In vivo research revealed that green tea polyphenols (GTP) enhanced the catalytic activity of key enzymes involved in the synthesis of glutathione and quinone in the liver, small intestine, and lungs. EGCG showed potent antitumorigenesis in skin. In human investigations, GTP had significant antimutagenic properties against carcinogens formed through the process the cooking meats and fish. Polyphenols also scavenged free radicals such as hydrogen peroxide and superoxide anions. In other research, epicatechin derivatives decreased lipid peroxidation in epidermal microsomes. And GTP significantly decreased dental carries by inhibiting Streptococcus mutans, the bacterium that causes dental cavities.

Dosage Ranges and Duration of Administration

Green tea is not usually prescribed as a medication even though it has therapeutic benefits.

Recommended dosage:

- Tea beverage: 3 cups/day (3 g soluble components, or 240 to 320 g polyphenols)
- Standardized green tea extract (80% total polyphenols and 55% epigallocatechin): 300 to 400 mg/day.
- Capsules and liquid preparations are also available.

Cautions

Adverse Effects/Toxicology

Quantities of greater than 5 cups of tea consumed as a beverage (equivalent to more than 300 mg caffeine taken daily) are considered overdoses. Intake above this level can produce side effects of restlessness, tremor, and heightened reflex excitability. Long-term daily dosage beyond 1.5 g of caffeine can induce irritability, insomnia, palpitation, vertigo, vomiting, diarrhea, loss of appetite, and headache. Vomiting and abdominal spasm are indications of potential caffeine overdose.

Warnings/Contraindications/Precautions

Individuals who have sensitive stomachs should limit their intake of green tea. The chlorogenic acid and tannins in tea can cause hyperacidity, gastric irritation, reduced appetite, and diarrhea. Tea should also be used with caution by people who have cardiovascular complications, kidney disorders, overactive thyroids, and a tendency toward spasm. Because caffeine overdoses can lead to anxiety attacks, persons prone to panic or other similar psychiatric disorders should exercise caution in drinking tea.

Pregnant women should avoid caffeine. At the very least, they should limit their intake to a maximum of 200 mg/day, or 3 cups taken at evenly spaced intervals during the day. Nursing mothers who drink tea put their infants at risk for sleep disorders.

Interactions

Individuals taking alkaline drugs should not use tea products. Tea beverages can delay the resorption of alkaline medications because tannins bind with alkaline compounds.

Regulatory and Compendial Status

The U.S. FDA classifies green tea as a dietary supplement. Green tea is not usually sold as an herbal medicine. It is approved as a nonprescription traditional diuretic in Belgium.

References

Ali M, et al. A potent thromboxane inhibitor in green tea. *Prostaglandins Leukot Essent Fatty Acids.* 1990;40:281–283.

Blumenthal M, ed. *The Complete German Commission E Monographs.* Therapeutic Guide to Herbal Medicines. Boston, Mass: Integrative Medicine Communications; 1998:47, 132.

Bradley P, ed. *British Herbal Compendium.* Dorset, England: British Herbal Medicine Association; 1992:1:96–98.

Heinerman J. *Heinerman's Encyclopedia of Fruits, Vegetables and Herbs.* Englewood Cliffs, NJ: Prentice Hall; 1988:112–113.

Imai K, Nakachi K. Cross sectional study of effects of drinking green tea on cardiovascular and liver diseases. *BMJ.* 1995;310:693–696.

Murray M. *The Healing Power of Herbs: The Enlightened Person's Guide to the Wonders of Medicinal Plants.* Second Ed. Rocklin, Calif: Prima Publishing; 1995.

Poppel Piet A, van den Brandt. Consumption of black tea and cancer risk: a prospective cohort study. *J Natl Cancer Inst.* 1996;88:93–100.

Shim JH, Kang MG, Kim YH, Roberts C, Lee IP. Chemopreventive effect of green tea (*Camellia sinensis*) among cigarette smoke. *Cancer-Epidemio-Biomarkers-Prev.* 1995;Jun; 4(4): 387–91.

Sirving K. Drinking black tea may cut risk of stroke. *AMA Arch Intern Med.* March 25, 1998.

Snow J. Camellia sinensis (L.) Kuntze (Theaceae). *The Protocol Journal of Botanical Medicine.* 1995;1:47–51.

Tamozawa H, et al. Natural antioxidants I. Antioxidant components of tea leaf (Thea sinensis L.). *Chem Pharm Bull.* 1984;32:2011–2014.

Tyler V. *Herbs of Choice: The Therapeutic Use of Phytomedicinals.* Binghamton, NY: Haworth; 1994.

Wang Z, et al. Antimutagenic activity of green tea polyphenols. *Mutation Research.* 1989;223:273–285.

Windridge C. *The Fountain of Health. An A-Z of Traditional Chinese Medicine.* London, England: Mainstream Publishing; 1994:259.

© Copyright Integrative Medicine Communications

Hawthorn

Names

- **English**
  Hawthorn berry/hawthorn flower/hawthorn leaf/hawthorn leaf with flower

- **Botanical**
  Crataegus monogyna/Crataegus laevigata

- **Plant Family**
  Rosaceae

- **Pharmacopeial**
  Crataegi fructus/crataegi flos/crataegi folium/crataegi folium cum flore

Overview

Hawthorn improves cardiac function in patients with New York Heart Association stage II heart failure. Clinical trials support a minimum dose of 300 mg hawthorn extract to reduce debility from cardiac insufficiency. Various tolerance markers (standard bicycle ergometry, spiroergometry, radionucleotide ventriculography, and subjective complaints) support this conclusion. Further study is required to determine the effects of hawthorn on other cardiovascular conditions (hypertension, arteriosclerosis, angina pectoris, and paroxysmal tachycardia) considered by herbalists to be indications for hawthorn therapy.

Macro Description

Hawthorn is a thorny, deciduous shrub up to five feet tall, found in deciduous forests of North America, Europe, North Africa, and western Asia. Flower clusters, which bloom in May, have five petals, five sepals, and numerous stamens. Leaves are variable, toothed or lobed, and alternate. Oval or round fruit (haws), which are red when ripe, contain five nutlets. Crude drug is prepared from leaves, white flowers, and berries.

Part Used/Pharmaceutical Designations

- Flowers
- Leaves
- Fruit

- **Constituents/Composition**
  Flavonoids (e.g., hyperoside, vitexin rhamnoside, rutin, vitexin, kaempferol, apigenin); oligomeric procyanidins (e.g., epicatechin, catechin).
  Leaves and flowers in crude drug contain about 1% flavonoids (hyperoside as marker), 1% to 3% oligomeric procyanidins (epicatechin as marker); berries in crude drug contain about 0.1% hyperoside.

- **Commercial Preparations**
  Aqueous, aqueous-alcohol, solid, glycerite, dried (powdered), and compounded extracts are available as liquid, tablet, or capsule, standardized to flavonoid/oligomeric procyanidin content.

Medicinal Uses/Indications

Traditional: cardiotonic, hypotensive, coronary vasodilator, mild diuretic, astringent

Conditions: coronary artery disease, congestive heart failure, essential hypertension, angina pectoris, postmyocardial infarction rehabilitation, cardiac weakness following infectious disease, antiarrythmias, possibly varicose veins, thrombosis

Clinical applications: for diminishing or deteriorating cardiac capacity due to stage II heart failure, according to New York Heart Association standards

- **Pharmacology**
  Animal studies originated with a 1966 genetic experiment that focused on gypsy moths. The colony, about to die due to inbreeding and a diet of alder leaves, recovered completely when fed hawthorn leaves, and also became stronger and larger. Subsequent in vivo and in vitro animal experiments showed that hawthorn extracts increase coronary blood flow, cause vasodilation (and hypotension), reduce peripheral resistance, benefit peripheral blood flow (and circulation), and have positive inotropic effects (increasing rat myocyte efficiency more than isoprenaline). Hawthorn extracts also block beta-adrenoceptors, are antiarrhythmic, and, in rat hearts subject to ischemia and reperfusion, increase recovery rate, reduce lactate release, reduce ventricular fibrillation, and prolong survival.

In humans, hawthorn, a positive inotropic agent, increases the refractory period that cardiac glycosides shorten, reducing the probability of arrhythmia while stabilizing heart rhythm. Also a peripheral vasodilator, hawthorn reduces blood pressure and increases coronary flow. It has positive dromotropic effects and negative bathmotropic effects, and increases coronary and myocardial circulatory perfusion. Actions may be due to cAMP (cyclic adenosine monophosphate)—or TXA_2 (thromboxane$_2$)—inhibition or to other undetermined actions.

Dosage Ranges and Duration of Administration

To decrease NYHA stage II cardiac insufficiency:

- 160 to 900 mg standardized (4 to 20 mg flavonoids/30 to 160 mg oligomeric procyanidins) fluid crude extract daily for at least six weeks
- 120 to 240 mg extract, standardized to 1.8% vitexin rhamnoside/10% procyanidins three times daily for at least six weeks.

Cautions

- **Adverse Effects/Toxicology**
  American Herbal Products Association (AHPA) safety rating: class 1 (safe with appropriate use).
  Infrequent side effects: Two of 367 subjects in placebo-controlled trials reported nausea, headache, migraine, palpitations, and soft stools.
  Toxicity: After IP dosing of 3 g per kg body weight (rats and mice), toxicity was indicated by sedation, difficulty breathing, and tremors, but not death. Oral doses—30, 90, or 300 mg per kg body weight administered to rats and dogs for 26 weeks and 300 to 600 mg per body weight administered for one month—were nonfatal and nontoxic.

- **Warnings/Contraindications/Precautions**
  Advise patients not to self-medicate. If symptoms do not improve after six weeks of treatment, reevaluate the condition. Encourage frequent follow-ups. Take appropriate precautions regarding potential heart failure, imminent surgery, and prescription change.
  Patients should not use hawthorn during pregnancy.

Interactions

Hawthorn may increase the effects of digitalis. Hawthorn is sometimes combined with other supplements and herbs for stronger effect.

Regulatory and Compendial Status

In the United States, the FDA classifies hawthorn as a dietary supplement; in Canada, it has new-drug status and is not approved for self-treatment of cardiovascular disease. Hawthorn is not licensed through the General Sales List (GSL) in England, and while the Commission E in Germany approves the use of hawthorn leaf and flower for the treatment of NYHA stage II heart failure, it does not approve the use of hawthorn berry.

References

Bahorun T, Gressier B, Trotin F, et al. Oxygen species scavenging activity of phenolic extracts from hawthorn fresh plant organs and pharmaceutical preparations. *Arzneimittelforschung*. 1996;46:1086–1089.

Blumenthal M, ed. *The Complete German Commission E Monographs: Therapeutic Guide to Herbal Medicines*. Boston, Mass: Integrative Medicine Communications; 1998.

Blumenthal M, Riggins C. *American Botanical Council's Popular Herbs in the U.S. Market. Therapeutic Monographs*. Austin Tex: ABC; 1997.

Chaterjee SS. In vitro and in vivo studies on the cardioprotective action of oligomeric procyanidins in a crataegus extract of leaves and blooms. *Arzneimittelforschung*. 1997;47:821–825.

The Criteria Committee of the New York Heart Association I. *Diseases of the Heart and Blood Vessels: Nomenclature and Criteria for Diagnosis*. 6th ed. Boston, Mass: Little, Brown; 1964.

Hoffmann D. Hawthorn: The Heart Helper. *Alternative & Complementary Therapies*. 1995;4:191–192.

Kowalchik C, Hylton W, eds. *Rodale's Illustrated Encyclopedia of Herbs*. Emmaus, Pa: Rodale Press; 1998.

Leuchtgens H. Crataegus special extract WS 1442 in NYHA II heart failure. A placebo controlled randomized double-blind study [in German]. *Fortschr Med.* 1993;111:352-354.

Loew D, Albrecht M, Podzuweit H. Efficacy and tolerability of a Hawthorn preparation in patients with heart failure stage I and II according to NYHA—a surveillance study. Presented at the Second International Congress on Phytomedicine; 1996; Munich, Germany.

McGuffin M, Hobbs C, Upton R, Goldberg A. *American Herbal Products Association's Botanical Safety Handbook.* Boca Raton, Fla: CRC Press; 1997.

Nasa Y, Hashizume AN, Hoque E, Abiko Y. Protective effect of crataegus extract on the cardiac mechanical dysfunction in isolated perfused working rat heart. *Arzneimittelforschung.* 1993;42II(9):945-949.

Newall CA, Anderson LA, Phillipson JD. *Herbal Medicines: A Guide for Health Care Professionals.* London, England: The Pharmaceutical Press; 1996.

Nikolov N, Wagner H, Chopin J, Della Monica G, Chari VM, Seligmann O. Recent investigations of crataegus flavonoids. Proceedings of the International Bioflavonoid Symposium; 1981; Munich, Germany.

Popping S, Rose H, Ionescu I, Fischer Y, Kammermeier H. Effect of a hawthorn extract on contraction and energy turnover of isolated rat cardiomycocytes. *Arzneimittelforschung.* 1995;45:1157-1161.

Schmidt U, Kuhn U, Ploch M, Hubner WD. Efficacy of the hawthorn (crataegus) preparation LI 132 in 78 patients with chronic congestive heart failure defined as NYHA functional class II. *Phytomedicine.* 1994;1:17-34.

Schultz V, Hansel R, Tyler V. *Rational Phytotherapy: A Physician's Guide to Herbal Medicine.* Heidelberg: Springer; 1998.

Schussler M, Holzl J, Fricke U. Myocardial effects of flavonoids from crataegus species. *Arzneimittelforschung.* 1995;45:842-845.

Tauchert M, Ploch M, Hubner WD. Effectiveness of hawthorn extract LI 132 compared with the ACE inhibitor Captopril: Multicenter double-blind study with 132 NYHA stage II. *Muench Med Wochenschr.* 1994;136 (suppl):S27-S33.

Vibes J, Lasserre B, and Gleye J. Effects of a methanolic extract from *Crataegus oxycantha* blossoms on TXA2 and PGI2 synthesizing activities of cardiac tissue. *Med Sci Res.* 1993;21:534-436.

Vibes J, Lasserre B, Gleye J, Declume C. Inhibition of thromboxane A2 biosynthesis I vitro by the main components of *Crataegus oxyacantha* (hawthorn) flower heads. *Prostaglandins, Leukotrienes and Essential Fatty Acids.* 1994;50:174-175.

Weikl A, Assmus KD, Neukum-Schmidt A, et al. Crataegus special extract WS 1442. Assessment of objective effectiveness in patients with heart failure. *Fortschr Med.* 1996;114:291-296.

Weiss R F. *Herbal Medicine.* Beaconsfield, England: Beaconsfield Publishers, Ltd; 1988:162-169.

Werbach M. *Botanical Influences on Illness.* Tarzana, Calif: Third Line Press; 1994.

Zapfe G, Assmus KD, Noh HS. Placebo-controlled multicenter study with Crataegus special extract WS 1442: clinical results in the treatment of NYHA II cardiac insufficiency. Presented at the Fifth Congress on Phytotherapy; June 11, 1993; Bonn, Germany.

© Copyright Integrative Medicine Communications

Horsetail

Names

- **English**
  Horsetail

- **Botanical**
  Equisetum arvense

- **Plant Family**
  Equisetaceae

- **Pharmacopeial**
  Equiseti herba

Overview

Horsetail belongs to *Equisetum*, the only genus in the family Equisetaceae. It is a descendant of a large, primeval plant that thrived 400 million years ago during the Paleozoic geological period. The genus name, *Equisetum*, comes from two Latin words which mean "bristle horse." It bears this name because its stems are rich in silica and silicic acids. As the plant dries, silica crystals form on the walls of cells in the stems and branches. These crystals give the ground plant material a scratching effect. It is for this reason that horsetail historically has been used to polish metal, particularly pewter. Horsetail is also known as "scouring rush" and "pewterwort," appropriate synonyms in light of these traditional uses for the plant.

Studies on the flavonoid compounds in *Equisetum arvense* reveal that this species has two discrete chemotypes, or chemical subspecies. One chemotype is native to North America and the Far East, including China, Japan, and Siberia, while the other is indigenous to Europe. Horsetail is now widespread throughout parts of Europe, Asia, the Middle East, and North America.

Closely related to the ferns, horsetail is a non-flowering weed that flourishes on clay-filled, sandy soils. It is technically a pteridophyte and, as in the case of ferns, reproduces through spores. Pteridophytes are flowerless plants that have two distinct and alternating generations. The first is a non-sexual, spore-bearing generation of relatively larger plants. The second generation is sexual, and composed of smaller plants that lack well-differentiated stems and leaves. *Equisetum* species can also propagate non-sexually through stolons and tubers.

Best known as a mild diuretic, the aerial parts of horsetail are used medicinally for numerous ailments. The astringent properties of this plant render it a valuable treatment for kidney and bladder complaints, as well as an external therapy for bleeding wounds. Although horsetail is also indicated for dropsy, rheumatic conditions, and tuberculosis, there is no pharmacological evidence that it is effective in treating conditions other than mild water retention.

While horsetail remedies prepared from *Equisetum arvense* are basically safe, other *Equisetum* species such as *Equisetum palustre* contain poisonous alkaloidal constituents. Every effort should thus be made to ensure that horsetail herbal preparations are made from *Equisetum arvense*. The authenticity of *Equisetum arvense* should be confirmed by both morphological and chemical studies using microscopy and thin layer chromatography (TLC).

Macro Description

Horsetail is a perennial with the two distinct forms of stems. Between March and April, red-brown to straw-yellow fertile stems grow up to 20 cm in height. These pencil-slim stems bear brown, scale-like leaves arranged in whorls. At the tip of each stem is a scaly head containing a spore that is easily transported by the wind to other plants for sexual reproduction.

By early summer, usually during May and June, longer, sterile green stems appear that form a pale green brush up to 35 cm high. These barren stems give of multiple branches arranged in whorls at the nodes. The sterile stems and branches are characterized by deep grooves, a square-shape, and a rough texture. Both the fertile and barren stems are erect, jointed, and brittle. However, only the sterile stems are used medicinally.

Part Used/Pharmaceutical Designations

- Herb (fresh or dried sterile, green shoots).

- **Constituents/Composition**
  Flavonoids (particularly quercetin 3-glucoside and its 6"-malonyl ester are found in both chemotypes; also kaempferol-, luteolin-, genkwanin-3-O-glucosides; 5-O-, 7-O-glucosides; and diglucosides); caffeic acid ester (chlorogenic acid, dicoffeoyl-meso-tartaric acid); silicic acid (partially water-soluble); styrolpyrone glucoside (equisetumpyron); pyridine alkaloids (nicotine in trace amounts). The purported presence of equisetonin, a saponin of unknown structure, requires confirmation.

- **Commercial Preparations**
  Available as dried herb and liquid preparations made from the fresh or dried, green, sterile shoots of *Equisetum arvense*. Horsetail preparations should be stored in well-sealed containers to ensure protection from light.

Medicinal Use/Indications

Traditional uses: tuberculosis; nasal, pulmonary, and gastric hemorrhages; brittle fingernails and hair loss; rheumatic diseases; gout; catarrh for kidney and bladder areas; hematostatic (a therapeutic agent that stops bleeding) for profuse menstruation; stubborn wounds and ulcers, swelling and fracture; frostbite.

Conditions:

- Internal: inflammation or mild infections of the genito-urinary tract, kidney stones, bladder stones
- External: wounds, burns, poorly healing wounds, rheumatic conditions, fractures, sprains

Clinical applications:

- Internal: post-traumatic and static edemal, flushing-out (irrigation) treatment for bacterial and inflammatory diseases of the lower urinary tract; kidney stones
- External: supportive therapy for poorly healing wounds

- **Pharmacology**
  Although pharmacological investigations on *Equisetum arvense* are limited, this herb has been shown to have mild diuretic, hemostatic (arresting the blood flow), and vulnerary (wound-healing) properties. In addition, horsetail induces mild leucocytosis (a transient increase in white blood cell count).

  In vivo studies confirm that horsetail has weak diuretic action, but research findings have been inconsistent. Flavonoids presumably account for the diuretic effect, which apparently does not involve an increase in electrolyte excretion. However, other evidence suggests that the diuretic activity of horsetail results from the combined pharmacological action of flavone glycosides and the saponin.

  In other animal studies, horsetail was shown to produce a hemostatic effect. Therapeutic claims that horsetail and its active constituents, silica and silicic acid derivatives, promote tissue repair of bleeding pulmonary tubercular lesions have not been fully substantiated. However, in other research, the silicic acid content of horsetail reportedly had a strengthening and regenerative effect on connective tissues.

Dosage Ranges and Duration of Administration

- Internal: 6 g per day
- Herbal infusion: 4 oz. tid
- Tincture (1:5): 1 to 4 ml tid
- External (compresses): 10 g of herb per 1 liter water per day

Adequate fluid should be taken when using oral horsetail preparations for irrigation therapy. A tea is prepared by pouring boiled water over 2 to 3 g horsetail herb, boiling for five minutes, and then straining after 10 to 15 minutes. Drink during the day between meals. An infusion for internal use is made by adding 1.5 g of horsetail herb to 1 cup of boiling water. Let steep 30 to 40 minutes.

Cautions

- **Adverse Effects/Toxicology**
  Health risks and side effects have not been reported for horsetail when taken in recommended therapeutic doses. However, it is advisable to consult a health care practitioner when using fresh horsetail as a bath additive to treat major skin lesions, acute skin lesions of unknown origin, feverish and infectious diseases, or hypertonia (increased muscle resistance to passive stretching).

■ **Warnings/Contraindications/Precautions**

Horsetail is contraindicated in patients who have edema concomitant to cardiac or renal dysfunction. A related species, *Equisetum palustre,* is potentially toxic since it contains lapustrin, a poisonous alkaloid.

Interactions

None reported.

Regulatory and Compendial Status

Horsetail herb is approved by the German Commission E. In the United Kingdom, horsetail is on the General Sale List, Schedule 2, Table A (R1a).

References

Allaby M, ed. *Concise Oxford Dictionary of Botany.* Oxford/New York: Oxford University Press; 1992: 337–338.

Blumenthal M, ed. *The Complete German Commission E Monographs. Therapeutic Guide to Herbal Medicines.* Boston: Integrative Medicine Communications; 1998: 150–151.

Bradley P, ed. *British Herbal Compendium.* Vol. I. Dorset (Great Britain): British Herbal Medicine Association; 1992: 92–94.

Dorland's Illustrated Medical Dictionary. 25th ed. Philadelphia: W.B. Saunders; 1974.

Grieve M. *A Modern Herbal.* Vol. I. New York: Dover; 1971: 419–421.

Gruenwald J, Brendler T, Christof J. *PDR for Herbal Medicines.* Montvale, NJ: Medical Economics Company; 1998: 830–831.

Harnischfeger G, Stolze H. Equisetum arvense - Ackerschachtelhalm. In: *Bewahrte Pflanzendrogen in Wissenschaft und Mediizin.* Bad Homburg/Melsungen, Germany: Notamed Verlag; 1983: 119–127.

Hoppe HA. *Drogenkunde.* 8th ed. Vol. 2. Berlin: Waler de Gruyter; 1977: 173–176.

Kreitmair H. *Die Pharmazie.* 1953; 8:298–300.

Steinegger E, Hansel R. *Lehrbuch der Pharmakognosie.* 3rd ed. Berlin: Springer-Verlag; 1972: 214.

Thomson WA. *Medicines from the Earth: A Guide to Healing Plants.* Alfred Van Der Marck Ed. Maidenhead, England: McGraw-Hill Book company; 1978: 62.

Tyler V. *The Honest Herbal: A Sensible Guide to the Use of Herbs and Related Remedies.* 3rd ed. New York: Pharmaceutical Products Press; 1993: 179–180.

Vollmer H, Hubner K. Nauyn-Schmiedebergs. *Archiv fur experimentelle Pathologie und Pharakologie.* 1937; 186: 565–573, 592–605.

© *Copyright Integrative Medicine Communications*

Jamaica Dogwood

Names

- **English**
  Jamaica Dogwood

- **Botanical**
  Piscidia erythrina/Piscidia piscipula

- **Plant Family**
  Fabaceae

- **Pharmacopeial**
  Piscidiae radicis cortex

Overview

Piscidia erythrina is indigenous to Central America, Florida, and the West Indies, and is now found in Texas, Mexico, and the northern part of South America. *Piscidia erythrina* and *Piscidia piscipula* are generally considered synonyms for the same species. *Piscidia erythrina* provides a valuable source of charcoal and wood for building boats. The roots, pounded leaves, and branches of this plant have traditionally been employed in fish poisons (piscicides). Jamaica dogwood, or the dried root bark, is used medicinally to treat a variety of ailments.

In Belize, a decoction made from the bark of the Jamaica dogwood tree is taken internally for dysentery, diarrhea, and dysmennorhea (painful menstruation). Bark decoctions are known to have astringent action. Belizeans use them as a mouthwash for bleeding gums, and as an external wash for wounds, rashes, and other skin problems.

However, Jamaica dogwood is best known as a traditional remedy for treating neuralgia, menstrual pain, migraine, insomnia, and nervous tension. As early as 1844, Western scientists discovered that Jamaica dogwood had narcotic, analgesic, and sudorific (sweat-promoting) properties. Recent pharmacological studies have shown unequivocally that bark extracts of this plant produce sedative and narcotic effects in animals. Scientific findings such as these have helped to substantiate many of the traditional uses of this species.

Although Jamaica dogwood is an effective herbal remedy, it is also known to have potentially adverse side effects. Experts stress that Jamaica dogwood should be cautiously administered only by trained and qualified health care practitioners who understand the pharmacology, toxicology, and proper herbal preparation of this plant.

Macro Description

Jamaica dogwood has a foliage similar to that of *Lonchocarpus*. Its characteristic pods bear four projecting longitudinal wings. The bark is yellow or grayish brown on the outer surface, and either lighter colored or white on the inner surface. If the bark becomes damp, the inner surface turns to a peculiar shade of blue. The inner texture of the bark is quite fibrous. Its distinctly acrid and bitter taste causes a burning sensation in the mouth. The bark also gives off a noticeably unpleasant odor similar to that of broken opium.

Part Used/Pharmaceutical Designation

- Root bark (dried)
- Stem bark

- **Constituents/Composition**

  - Acids: piscidic acid (p-hydroxybenzyltartaric) plus its mono and diethyl esters, fukiic acid and its 3'-O-methyl derivative; malic acid, succinic acid, tartaric acid.
  - Isoflavonoids of varied structure: include ichthynone, jamaicin, piscerythrone, piscidone; milletone, isomilletone, dehydromilletone, rotenone, sumatrol (a rotenoid), lisetin (coumaronochrome)
  - Glycosides: piscidin (crystallizable substance that is reportedly a mixture of two compounds), saponin glycoside (unidentified)
  - Other constituents: alkaloid (unidentified, present in stem), resin, volatile oil (0.01%), beta-sitosterol, tannin (unspecified)

- **Commercial Preparations**

  The bark is sold commercially in quilled pieces about one to two inches in length and 1/8 inch in thickness. However, there is considerable variation in the chemical constituents of Jamaica dogwood from different geographical regions. For example, chemical analysis of root bark material from Mexico revealed the presence of certain active principles (1% piscidone, 0.8% piscerythrone, 0.8% erythbigenin, 0.6% ichthynone, and 0.5% rotenone), but a total lack of jamaicin and only a minute quantity of lisetin. Jamaicin and lisetin are chief active principles in the bark from trees grown in Jamaica. This suggests that there may be chemical races (chemotaxonomic subspecies) of Jamaica dogwood. The geographical origin of bark material from *Piscidia erythrina* should thus be authenticated to ensure that it contains a maximal quantity of all active constituents, including jamaicin and lisetin.

Medicinal Uses/Indications

Traditional uses: neuralgia, nervous debility, insomnia accompanying neuralgia; migraine, dysmenorrhea, violent toothache, whooping-cough, antispasmodic for asthma, dysmenorrhea, agent for dilating the pupil, piscicide, anodyne (analgesic), cardiotonic, diuretic, sedative, spasm

Conditions: sedative and narcotic actions for treating neuralgia, nervous debility, insomnia, migraine, dysmenorrhea

Clinical applications: sleep disorders (e.g., insomnia), neuralgia, dysmenorrhea, migraine, sedative, antitussive, spasmolytic, anti-inflammatory

- **Pharmacology**

  In several in vivo pharmacological studies, bark extracts of Jamaica dogwood showed sedative, antitussive, antispasmodic, antipyretic, anti-inflammatory, hypotensive, and weak cannabinoid activity. In a comparative investigation of vegetable extracts on CNS activity in the mouse, oral dosing of *Piscidia erythrina* produced pharmacological effects intermediate between the sedative action of *Valeriana officinalis* and the anxiolytic (anti-anxiety) activity of *Passiflora incarnata*. In another study, *Piscidia piscipula* was one of several plants used in Guatemalan traditional medicine that elicited in vitro inhibition of dermatophytoses (microbial agents causing skin infections), including fungal pathogens.

  Rotenone is an isoflavone isolated from the wood of Jamaica dogwood. It is one of the piscicidal constituents of the bark of this plant. Although rotenone is virtually nontoxic to warm-blooded animals, it is reportedly carcinogenic. However, in other research, rotenone exhibited anticancer action against lymphocytic leukemia and human epidermoid carcinoma of the nasopharynx.

  Rotenone is also presumably responsible for the antispasmodic activity of Jamaica dogwood on uterine smooth muscle. Both in vitro and in vivo findings reveal that the antispasmodic properties of Jamaica dogwood bark extract are either equal to or, in some cases, even greater than those of papaverine.

Dosage Ranges and Duration of Administration

- Dried root bark: 0.5 to 2 g (or equivalent in decoction) tid
- Fluid extract: (1:1 in 30% alcohol): 1 to 2 ml tid; or 2 to 8 ml per day (1:1, 60% ethanol)
- Tincture (1:5 in 45% ethanol): 5 to 30 drops (1 to 2 ml) tid

Cautions

- **Adverse Effects/Toxicology**

  Jamaica dogwood is known to have irritant and toxic effects in humans. Overdosing with this plant can produce adverse symptoms such as numbness, tremors, salivation, and sweating.

  In one study, Jamaica dogwood extract was toxic to rats and rabbits when given parenterally but nontoxic when administered orally. The test animals in this study were able to tolerate oral doses greater than 90 g dried extract/kg. An unidentified saponin isolated from the bark and administered intravenously to mice showed a LD_{50} of 75 g/kg b.w.

- **Warnings/Contraindications/Precautions**

  Although Jamaica dogwood shows low toxicity in some animal species, it can have irritant and toxic effects in humans. In some human subjects, Jamaica dogwood reportedly produces adverse side effects of gastric distress and nausea. In both in vitro and in vivo studies, extracts of this plant were shown to have potential depressant activity. Jamaica dogwood should be administered only by qualified health care practitioners, and excessive use should be avoided. Under no circumstances should this plant be used during pregnancy and lactation.

Interactions

Jamaica dogwood should not be taken concurrently with narcotic-like drugs or substances since it can potentially enhance the sedative activity of both pharmaceutical agents and herbal remedies.

Regulatory and Compendial Status

In the United Kingdom, Jamaica dogwood is listed as a licensed product in Schedule 1, Table A of the General Sale List (GSL). The Council of Europe does not approve of Jamaica dogwood as a natural food flavoring because of its potential toxicity to humans. Powdered Jamaica dogwood is listed in the *British Herbal Pharmacopeia* as complying with requirements for identification and quantitative standards. The herb has not been approved by the German Commission E.

References

Arvigo R, Balick M. *Rainforest Remedies:One Hundred Healing Herbs of Belize.* Twin Lakes, Wis: Lotus Press; 1993:97.

Aurousseau M, et al. Certain pharmacodynamic properties of *Piscidia erythrina*. *Ann Pharm Fr.* 23:251–257.

British Herbal Pharmacopoeia. 4th ed. Great Britain: Biddles Ltd, Guildford and King's Lynn; 1996:139–141.

Caceres A, Lopez BR, Giron MA, Logemann H. Plants used in Guatemala for the treatment of dermatophytic infections. 1. Screening for antimycotic activity of 44 plant extracts. *J Ethnopharmacol.* 1991;51(5):263–276.

Costello CH, Butler CL. An investigation of *Piscidia erythrina* (Jamaica dogwood). *J Am Pharm Assoc.* 1948;37:89–96.

Della Loggia, R, Tubaro A, Redaelli C. Evaluation of the activity on the mouse CNS of several plant extracts and a combination of them. *J Ethnopharmacol.* 1991;31:263–276.

Dorland's Illustrated Medical Dictionary. 25th ed. Philadelphia, Pa: WB. Saunders; 1974.

Duke JA. Phytochemical Database, USDA–ARS–NGRL, Beltsville Agricultural Research Center, Md. Available at www.ars-grin.gov/cgi-bin/duke

Grieve M. *A Modern Herbal.* Vol. I. New York, NY: Dover; 1971:261–262.

Mabberley DJ. *The Plant-Book: A Portable Dictionary of the Higher Plants.* England: Cambridge University Press; 1987: 457.

Newall C, Anderson L; Phillipson J. *Herbal Medicines: A Guide for Health-care Professionals.* London, England: Pharmaceutical Press; 1996: 174–175.

Pilcher JD, et al. The action of the so-called female remedies on the excised uterus of the guinea-pig. *Arch Int Med.* 1916;18:557–583.

Pilcher JD, Mauer RT. The action of female remedies on the intact uteri of animals. *Surg Gynecol Obstet.* 1918;97–99.

© *Copyright Integrative Medicine Communications*

Kava Kava

Names

- **English**
  Kava kava

- **Botanical**
  Piper methysticum

- **Plant Family**
  Piperaceae

- **Pharmacopeial**
  Piperis methystici rhizoma

Overview

Kava root preparations reduce stress-related anxiety and the effects of anxiety disorders. Studies show that these antianxiety effects are significant, superior to placebo, and similar to effects of benzodiazepines used in the treatment of anxiety without causing similar adverse side effects. Kava also reduces anxiety associated with or precipitated by menopause, and it is a topical oral anaesthetic. Kava promotes sleep in larger doses and a state of calm in smaller doses. The effects of kava are relaxing, not stupefying; it disposes users to sociability, not hostility.

The kava plant comes from Oceania, the geographical area of Polynesia, Micronesia, and Melanesia in the Pacific Ocean. Kava consumption among native peoples was first discovered during Captain James Cook's *Endeavour* voyage (1768 to 1771). The Swedish botanists who accompanied Captain Cook recorded kava as an indigenous intoxicant. Tribes used kava as a ceremonial as well as social drink, with different purposes and rituals surrounding its use, including which members were allowed to drink it. Despite the efforts of the 19th century Christian missionaries to quash kava use, today kava is available at kava bars on some islands and provides a good living for exporters, who cultivate kava commercially. It is often presented as a gift of honor and goodwill to dignitaries and foreigners at welcoming ceremonies. President and Mrs. Lyndon B. Johnson, Hillary Rodham Clinton, and Pope John Paul II have participated in kava ceremonies.

Kava was available in some parts of Germany by the late 19th century, but it was rare. Despite its long-standing use in Hawaii, Kava has caught on only recently in the mainland U.S. as a popular herbal medicine. In the past three years, kava has been the subject of intense marketing and may soon exceed South Pacific supply. Its safety and regulation are also current points of controversy. While side effects effects are mild (the most frequently reported are GI discomfort, headache, dizziness, or skin rash, and these occur in a small percentage of study participants), excess amounts of kava impair driving ability. Yellowing of the skin, hair, and nails, and drying and cracking of the skin, is seen in some chronic users, as is disturbance to vision or oculomotor equilibrium. And because so many recovered substance abusers are taking kava daily, its addictive potential is still under question, despite the lack of demonstrable evidence from a 1994-addiction potential study.

Macro Description

Kava is an erect, branching shrub with prominent, succulent leaves. It grows up to six meters in damp tropical climates. The heart-shaped green leaves are smooth and pointed; erect yellow-green inflorescence develops at axils. The rhizome is harvested when it is five to eight cm thick, after three to five years' growth, when the plant is two to two and a half meters tall. Numerous long, bundled, tuberous hairs grow from the rhizome.

Part Used/Pharmaceutical Designations

- Roots[rhizome]

- **Constituents/Composition**
  Dried herb contains 3.5% kavapyrones, including 1% to 2% kawain, 0.6% to 1% dihydrokawain, 1.2% to 2% methysticin, and 0.5% to 0.8% dihydromethysticin.

- **Commercial Preparations**
  In some cultures, the method of preparation involved chewing the root and spitting the juice into a bowl; saliva served as a macerate. Today, manufacturers use alcohol-water or acetate macerations or percolations to extract kava's active constituents from ground rhizome. Kava is available as aqueous-alcohol extracts and encapsulations, standardized to 70% kavalactone content, and as tinctures, tablets, and dried root.

Medicinal Uses/Indications

Traditional Actions: Antispasmodic, nervine, relaxant, anti-anxiety, anaestetic, diuretic. Historically used for gonorrhea, chronic cystitis or other urinary tract symptoms, menstrual disorder and migraines, but it is not used for this now. Currently used as a relaxant of skeletal muscles for pain and stiffness, anxiety, insomnia, menopausal anxiety, uncontrolled epilepsy, pain, and jet lag.

Conditions: anxiety, insomnia

Clinical Applications: stress-related anxiety, anxiety disorder, phobias, restlessness, insomnia

- **Pharmacology**
  By 1998, six human double-blind, controlled trials on kava's therapeutic effects had been conducted. These trials demonstrate consistent, significant antianxiety effects of kava, although the methodologies of some are questionable. One recent study (1997) found a standardized, 70% kavalactone kava extract superior to placebo in treating non-psychotic patients. Of 101 outpatients who met DSM-III-R criteria and participated in the study, 52 received kava, and symptoms in the majority of this group improved throughout the 25-week study, some noting improvements by week eight. Results from the Hamilton Anxiety Scale, somatic and psychic anxiety, Clinical Global Impression, Self-Report Symptoms Inventory, and Adjective Mood Scale not show only kava's superiority to placebo in the treatment of non-psychotic anxiety, but also support kava's use in lieu of tricyclic antidepressants and benzodiazepine drugs.

  Individual effects of kava constituents have also been investigated. The kavapyrones (kawain, dihydrokawain, methysticin, dihydromethysticin) are anticonvulsant, central muscle relaxants (similar to mephenesin) and locally anesthetic. They are also superior to strychnine antagonists in preventing strychnine poisoning in animal tests. In rabbits, these constituents diminish excability to the limbic system similar to benzodiazepines, and are also neuroprotective in mice and rats. In addition, nine studies have analyzed the effects of isolated dihydrokawain (DL-kawain) in anxiety disorder, with results similar to those of whole extract preparations.

Dosage Ranges and Duration of Administration

To relieve anxiety and insomnia, and reduce stress, standard dose is 2.0 to 4.0 g as decoction up to three times daily, or standardized formulas (containing 70% kavalactones) for a daily intake of 60 to 600 mg kavalactones. Treatment length varies: it may take four weeks to reach peak therapeutic effect. In Germany and Australia, patients are advised not to continue dosing longer than three months.

Cautions

- **Adverse Effects/Toxicology**
  Typical side effects are mild, and include allergy (skin rash), headache, gastrointestinal distress, and dizziness. The American Herbal Products Association recommends that kava not be used during pregnancy or while breast-feeding (class 2b and 2d); also, do not drive when using excessive dosages (class 2d).
  Extreme doses of 13 liters per day—300 to 400 g dried rhizome per week—resulted in yellowing of the skin, ataxia, rash, hair loss, and changes in vision, appetite, and respiration. This dose exceeds recommended doses by 100 times.

- **Warnings/Contraindications/Precautions**
  Do not use during pregnancy or while breast-feeding. Do not exceed recommended dose or length of treatment.

Interactions

May potentiate effects of barbiturates or alcohol.

Regulatory and Compendial Status

Kava is a dietary supplement in the U.S. and approved for use by the German Commission E in the treatment of anxiety and restlessness. Not approved in Canada for non-medicinal inclusion in oral preparations.

References

Blumenthal M, ed. *The Complete German Commission E Monographs: Therapeutic Guide to Herbal Medicines*. Boston, Mass: Integrative Medicine Communications; 1998.

Foster S. *101 Medicinal Herbs*. Loveland, Colo: Interweave Press; 1998.

Kinzler E, Kromer J, Lehmann E. Effect of a special kava extract in patients with anxiety-, tension, and excitation states of non-psychotic genesis. Double blind study with placebos over four weeks [in German]. *Arzneimforsch*. 1991;41:584–588.

Lehmann E, et al. Efficacy of special kava extract *(Piper methysticum)* in patients with states of anxiety, tension and excitedness of non-mental origin—A double blind placebo controlled study of four weeks treatment. *Phytomedicine*. 1996;3:113–119.

Lindenberg Von D, Pitule-Schodel H. D, L-Kavain in comparison with oxazepam in anxiety states. Double-blind clinical trial. *Forschr Med*. 1990;108:50–54.

McGuffin M, Hobbs C, Upton R, Goldberg A. *American Herbal Products Associations's Botanical Safety Handbook*. Boca Raton, Fla: CRC Press; 1996.

Munte TE, Heinze HJ, Matzke M, et al. Effects of oxazepam and an extract of kava roots *(Piper methysticum)* on event-related potentials in a word recognition task. *Neuropsychobiology*. 1993;27:46–53.

Schulz V, Hnsel R, Tyler V. *Rational Phytotherapy: A Physician's Guide to Herbal Medicine*. New York, NY: Springer-Verlag; 1998.

Singh YD, Blumenthal M. Kava: An overview. *HerbalGram*. 39:34–55.

Volz HP, Kieser M. Kava-kava extract WS 1490 versus placebo in anxiety disorders—a randomized placebo-controlled 25-week outpatient trial. *Pharmacopsychiatry*. 1997;30:1–5.

Warnecke G. Psychosomatic dysfunction in the female climacteric. Clinical effectiveness and tolerance of kava extract WS 1490 [in German]. *Fortschr Med*. 1991;109:119–122.

© *Copyright Integrative Medicine Communications*

Lavender

Names

- **English**
  Lavender

- **Botanical**
  Lavandula angustifolia

- **Plant Family**
  Lamiaceae

- **Pharmacopeial**
  Lavandulae

Overview

Lavender is native to the mountainous zones of the Mediterranean where it grows in sunny, stony habitats. Long heralded for its aromatic fragrance, this scented plant is now widely cultivated throughout southern Europe. The oil extracted from the flowers is used primarily in perfumery and, to a lesser extent, in medicinal remedies. The aromatic odor of English lavender is supposedly more delicate than French lavender, rendering the English variety more expensive.

Historically, lavender oil has been touted as a natural remedy for insomnia, nervousness, depression, and mood disturbances. As a tonic for the nervous system, lavender oil is used in aromatherapy or inhalation therapy, to treat nervous debility and exhaustion. A growing number of pharmacological and human serial case studies indicate that lavender essential oil produces significant sedative, calming, and anticonvulsive effects. Several investigations evaluating aromatherapy of the volatile oil from lavender in both test animals and humans subjects have shown unequivocally that this mode of administration yields measurable clinical benefits. According to some research, lavender essential oil may be as effective as certain barbiturates in treating sleep disorders.

Macro Description

Lavender is a heavily branched shrub that grows to a height of 60 cm. Its broad rootstock bears woody branches with erect, rod-like, leafy, green shoots. A silvery down covers the gray-green narrow leaves which are oblong-lanceolate, sessile, and involute.

The small blue-violet labiate flowers have a characteristic scent due to the presence of volatile oil. The flowers are arranged in whorls of 6 to 10 blossoms and form interrupted terminal spikes above the foliage. The amethyst-colored tubular calyx consists of uneven tips that are sealed by a lid-like appendage after the flower unfolds.

Part Used/Pharmaceutical Designation

- Flowers (fresh, dried)

- **Constituents/Composition**
  Volatile (essential) oil (1% to 5%) (v/w) contains linalyl acetate (30% to 40%), linalool (20% to 50%), camphor, borneol, B-ocimene, 1,8-cineoil, terpene-4-ol, beta-caryophyllene, lavandulyl acetate, cineole (eucalyptol). Also contains about 12% tannins unique to Lamiaceae; hydroxycoumarins (e.g., umbelliferone, herniarin, coumarin, dihydrocoumarin); caffeic acid derivatives (e.g., rosmaric acid), triterpenes (e.g., ursolic acid), flavonoids (e.g., luteolin).

- **Commercial Preparations**
  Lavender oil is extracted from fresh flower tops and inflorescences through a process of steam distillation. The essential oil is found only in the flowers and lower stalks. The most valuable raw drug consists of dried flowers collected just before the flower has completely unfolded. Raw plant material that contains a substantive amount of stem and leaf is commercially less valuable. Similarly, the value of lavender raw drug material declines if it is adulterated with related species such as *Lavendula intermedia* (Lavendin) and *Lavendula latifolia*.

  Lavender is sold commercially as dried flower, dried herb, essential oil, and tincture.

Medicinal Uses/Indications

Traditional uses: mild sedative, antiflatulent, cholagogue choleretic (stimulates bile production by liver) and cholagogic effects (stimulates bile flow to duodenum). Used externally as rubefacient (reddens the skin).

Internal use: mood disturbances, sedative (restlessness, insomnia), antiflatulent, functional abdominal complaints (e.g., nervous stomach discomfort, abdominal gas)

External use: balenotherapy used for functional circulatory disorders; liniment used for rheumatic ailments

Conditions: restlessness, insomnia, functional abdominal complaints, rheumatism

Clinical applications: loss of appetite; nervousness, insomnia

- **Pharmacology**

Lavender oil diluted (1:60) with olive oil produced sedative activity when administered orally to mice. In combination with 40 mg/kg pentobarbital I.P., 0.4 mg/kg lavender oil given in multiple oral doses elicited a significant potentiating effect. The time of sleep onset increased and the duration of sleeping time decreased in the test animals compared to a control group. In another investigation, lavender oil reduced the twitch response in a phrenic nerve diaphragm preparation of skeletal muscle isolated from the rat.

Other research showed that inhalation of lavender oil reduced motility in laboratory mice. Motility correlated with serum levels of linalool, one of the main active principles in lavender essential oil. The structure-activity relationship between diminished motility and elevated linalool serum level offers experimental support for folk medicinal claims about the sedative properties of this essential oil. In this study, lavender oil completely blocked caffeine stimulation while its active constituents, linalool and linalyl acetate, abrogated caffeine stimulation by 50% in mice. Lavender oil administered I.P. to test animals receiving electric shock produced anticonvulsant activity. Recent findings on the anticonvulsive effects of inhaling lavender oil suggest that the mechanism underlying the sedative and calming effect may involve the neurotransmitter GABA.

In a human study, volatile oil of lavender flowers was evaluated for its effects on lipid peroxidation-antioxidant defense and lipid metabolism in bronchitis patients. The essential oil helped normalize total lipids levels, as well as the ratio of total cholesterol to its alpha-fraction. In other research, inhalation of lavender oil significantly lowered selective EEG potentials associated with vigilance, expectancy, and alertness in seven human subjects. In contrast to nitrazepam, lavender essential oil did not affect reaction time or heart rate. In addition, it showed relaxing and sedative properties when compared to other substances.

Four geriatric patients who had discontinued their use of benzodiazepines and neuroleptics for sleep disorders were given lavender oil aromatherapy after a two-week "washout period." Although their sleep time initially decreased after stopping the synthetic medication, they showed significant improvement, including prolonged sleeping time, during aromatherapy with lavender oil.

While the mechanism of action of lavender oil has not been fully elucidated, there is experimental evidence available for the calming and relaxing effects of lavender flowers and lavender oil.

Dosage Ranges and Duration of Administration

Internal use:

- Tea: 1 to 2 tsp. whole herb per cup of water
- Lavender oil: 1 to 3 drops may be taken on sugar cube (however, other authorities advise against taking lavender oil internally)
- Tincture (1:4): 20 to 40 drops tid

External use:

- Inhalation: 2 to 4 drops in 2 to 3 cups of boiling water; inhale vapors for headache, depression, or insomnia.
- Topical application: lavender oil is one of the few oils that can be safely applied undiluted. For ease of application, add 1 to 4 drops per tablespoon of base oil.

Cautions

- **Adverse Effects/Toxicology**
  None reported, although there is a slight risk for sensitization in certain individuals.

■ Warnings/Contraindications/Precautions

None reported when administered according to designated therapeutic dosages. The volatile oil possesses a weak potential for sensitization. Caution with internal use of lavender oil.

Interactions

None reported.

Regulatory and Compendial Status

Lavender flower is listed as an approved herb in *The Complete German Commission E Monographs*.

References

Atanassova-Shopova S, Roussinov KS. On certain central neurotropic effects of lavender essential oil. *Bull Inst Physiology*. 1970;8:69–76.

Blumenthal M, ed. *The Complete German Commission E Monographs*. Boston, Mass: Integrative Medicine Communications; 1998.

Dorland's Illustrated Medical Dictionary. 25th ed. Philadelphia, Pa: W.B. Saunders; 1974.

Gamez MJ, Jimenez J, Navarro C, Zarzuelo A. Aromatherapy: evidence for sedative effects of the essential oil of lavender after inhalation. *Z Naturforsch*. 1991;46c:1067–1072.

Grieve M. *A Modern Herbal*. Vol. I. New York, NY: Dover; 1971.

Gruenwald J, Brendler T, Jaenicke C. *PDR for Herbal Medicines*. Montvale, NJ: Medical Economics Company; 1998.

Guillemain J, Rousseau A, Delaveau P. Effets neurodepresseurs de l'huile essentielle de Lavandula angustifolia Mill. *Ann Pharmaceutiques Francaises*. 1989;47:337–343.

Hardy M, Kirk-Smith MD. Replacement of drug treatment for insomnia by ambient odor. *Lancet*. 1995;346:701.

Lis-Balchin M, Hart S. A preliminary study of the effect of essential oils on skeletal and smooth muscle in vitro. *J Ethnopharmacol*. 1997;58(4):183–187.

Schulz V, Hansel R, Tyler V. *Rational Phytotherapy: A Physicians' Guide to Herbal Medicine*. 3rd ed. Berlin, Germany: Springer; 1998.

Siurin SA. Effects of essential oil on lipid peroxidation and lipid metabolism in patients with chronic bronchitis. *Klin Med* (Mosk). 1997;58(4):43–45.

Thomson WA, ed. *Medicines from the Earth: A Guide to Healing Plants*. Maidenhead, England: McGraw-Hill Book Company; 1978.

Yamada K, Mimaki Y, Sashida Y. Anticonvulsive effects of inhaling lavender oil vapour. *Biol Pharm Bull*. 1994;17(2):359–360.

© Copyright Integrative Medicine Communications

Lemon Balm

Names

- **English**
  Lemon balm

- **Botanical**
  Melissa officinalis

- **Plant Family**
  Lamiaceae

- **Pharmacopeial**
  Melissae folium

Overview

Lemon balm—mildly sedating, antiviral, and carminative—is used commonly as tea, tincture, and ointment throughout Western Europe, where it was named Europe's plant of the year in 1988. In the United States, herbalists recommend lemon balm for a broad range of indications, including insomnia, dyspepsia, infant colic, anxiety, depression, and chronic fatigue syndrome.

Lemon balm is also used to reduce the pain and swelling of arthritis; to alleviate headaches; to desensitize individuals prone to allergy, eczema, and asthma; to relax uterine smooth muscle tissue during premenstrual syndrome; and to regulate hot flashes during menopause. While many of these uses have not been corroborated with controlled trials, studies with laboratory animals and tissue cultures have supported the empirical results of traditional uses of lemon balm.

In the 1970's, lemon balm volatile oil was demonstrated to exact nonspecific sedative actions. Its effects on the gastrointestinal tract are apparently due to smooth muscle relaxation. Studies also demonstrate modulation of thyroid stimulating in relation to lemon balm administration. And current research supports its use for cold sores or lesions due to herpes virus types 1 and 2.

Lemon balm has been used for thousands of years. The Greek physician Dioscorides used it for dog and scorpion bites. In the Middle Ages, Eau de Melissa was commonly used as a sedative. The 17th century English herbalist, Nicholas Culpepper, claimed that lemon balm could lift spirits, prevent faint-ing, stimulate clear thinking, and precipitate menstruation. American eclectic physicians used lemon balm during the 19th century as a mild stimulant. European colonists used it to sweat out fevers. Lemon balm's scientific name, Melissa, is derived from the Greek word for bee: bees are attracted to its odor. It is added to cosmetics, furniture polish, insect repellant, and food.

Macro Description

Erect perennial, growing up to two feet in height, with branching, hairy, square stems. Oval/heart shaped leaves, wrinkled, opposite, broad, toothed, grow one to three inches long, and smell like lemon. White-yellow flower clusters bloom at leaf axils July through September and sometimes become light blue. Native to Southern Europe and North Africa. Cultivated around the world.

Part Used/Pharmaceutical Designations

- Leaves

- **Constituents/Composition**
  Leaves contain a minimum of 0.05% volatile oil, with citronellal, citral a and b, geraniol, neral, caryophyllene, linalool, and limonene primary terpenoid constituents; also, phenol carboxylic acids and estimated 4% rasmarinic acid; and bitter principles, flavonoids, and tannins.

- **Commercial Preparations**
  Dried leaf, tea, capsules, extracts, creams, and oil, and combined with other sedative or carminative botanical preparations.

Medicinal Uses/Indications

Traditional: carminative, diaphoretic, febrifuge; essential oil is sedative, spasmolytic, antibacterial; poultices used for sores, tumors, headaches, stomach and menstrual complaints, insect bites

Conditions: catarrh, influenza, painful or delayed menstruation, nervous unrest or insomnia, gastrointestinal discomfort (internal administration); wounds or lesions (topical application)

Clinical applications: Lemon balm leaf preparations are approved in Germany as treatment for nervous sleep disorders, appetite loss, and for symptoms of functional gastrointestinal disorders (flatulence, abdominal bloating). There is promise of potential usefulness in treatment of cold sore/ Herpes simplex symptoms

- **Pharmacology**
  Components in lemon balm essential oil cause mild, nonspecific sedation when given at dosage ranges of 3 to 100 mg/kg (laboratory animals). Citronellal, a terpene in the volatile oil, may be the primary sedating constituent. In a study to determine the effects of 178 herbal extracts on herpes, influenza, and polio viruses, lemon balm's phenol constituents showed significant antiviral effects. The oil also has antibacterial activity, and tannins are currently considered the antiviral agents that speed healing from cold sores and herpes.

  A multicenter, double-blind study showed that a concentrated ointment (700 mg crude drug per g ointment), applied bid to qid for 5 to 10 days, began to relieve symptoms by the second day of treatment. By the fifth day, 50% more participants applying lemon balm versus placebo noted full symptom relief, and recovery involved less scabbing than with placebo. Both patients and their doctors preferred the lemon balm treatment. Lemon balm ointment at this level of concentration is not currently available in the United States. Tea can be used when cooled and applied topically.

  Freeze-dried liquid extracts are both antithyrotropic and antigonadotropic in laboratory tests. Lemon balm extract interferes with thyroid stimulating hormone binding with Graves' immunoglobulin (Graves'-specific IgG), and consequent thyroid activation, a finding that supports lemon balm's use in the treatment of Grave's disease.

  Eugenol, geraniol, and nerol, constituents in many plant volatile oils in addition to lemon balm's, have been evaluated individually. Eugenol, which is used in dentistry as an antiseptic and anesthetic, has convulsant, antioxidant, hypothermic, spasmolytic, central nervous system depressant, and platelet aggregation suppressant actions. Spasmolytic actions pertained to general smooth muscle activity in both human and animal experimental models; platelet aggregation provoked by arachidonate, adrenaline, and collagen was blocked in vitro. Geraniol's antiseptic actions are seven times more potent than phenol. Antibacterial actions of both geraniol and nerol are under investigation.

Dosage Ranges and Duration of Administration

- For difficulty in sleeping, or to reduce symptoms of gastrointestinal distress: 1.5 to 4.5 g dried herb as tea several times daily or as directed by physician, or tincture, 2 to 5 ml tid, or equivalent in fluid extract or encapsulated form.
- For cold/herpes sores: Steep 2 to 4 tsp. dried leaf in 1 cup boiling water for 10 to 15 minutes, cool, apply topically throughout the day.

Cautions

- **Adverse Effects/Toxicology**
  The American Herbal Products Association safety rating for lemon balm is class 1, safe with appropriate use. The German Commission E cites no associated toxicity or side effects.

- **Warnings/Contraindications/Precautions**
  Emmenagogue; do not use during pregnancy.

Interactions

May interfere with thyroid treatments, other Graves' disease therapy.

Regulatory and Compendial Status

Dietary supplement in U.S.; leaf preparations are approved for use as tea in the treatment of functional digestive distress and insomnia by the German Commission E.

References

Auf'mkolk M, Ingbar JC, Kubota K, et al. Extracts and auto-oxidized constituents of certain plants inhibit the receptor-binding and the biological activity of Graves' immunoglobulins. *Endocrinology*. 1985;116:1687–1693.

Auf'mkolk M; H; Hesch RD; Ingbar SH Ingbar JC; Amir SM; Winterhoff H; Sourgens. Inhibition by certain plant extracts of the binding and adenylate cyclase stimulatory effect of bovine thyrotropin in human thyroid membranes. *Endocrinology*.1984;115: 527–534.

Blumenthal M, ed.*The Complete German Commission E Monographs*. Boston, Mass: Integrative Medicine Communications; 1998.

Bremness L. *Herbs*. New York, NY: DK Publishing, 1994.

Castleman M. *The Healing Herbs*. Emmaus, Pa: Rodale Press; 1991.

Duke JA. *The Green Pharmacy*. Emmaus, Pa: Rodale Press; 1997.

Foster S. *Herbal Renaissance: Growing, Using and Understanding Herbs in the Modern World*. Salt Lake City, Utah: Gibbs-Smith; 1993.

Kowalchik C and Hylton W, eds. *Rodale's Illustrated Encyclopedia of Herbs.* Emmaus, Pa: Rodale Press; 1998.

Leung A, Foster S. *Encyclopedia of Common Natural Ingredients Used in Food, Drugs, and Cosmetics*. 2nd ed. New York, NY: Wiley & Sons; 1996.

May G, Willuhn G. Antiviral effect of aqueous plant extracts in tissue culture [In German]. *Arzneimittelforschung*. 1978;28:1–7.

McCaleb R. Melissa relief for herpes sufferers. *HerbalGram*. 1995;34.

McGuffin M, Hobbs C, Upton R, Goldberg A. *American Herbal Products Associations's Botanical Safety Handbook*. Boca Raton, Fla: CRC Press; 1996.

Perry EK, et al. Medicinal plants and Alzheimer's disease: Integrating ethnobotanical and contemporary scientific evidence. *J Altern Complement Med*.1998;4:419–428.

Schultz V, Hansel R, Tyler V. *Rational Phytotherapy: A Physician's Guide to Herbal Medicine*.New York, NY: Springer-Verlag; 1998.

Soulimani R, et al. Neurotropic action of the hydroalcoholic extract of *Melissa officinalis* in the mouse. *Planta Med.* 1991;57:105–109.

Tagashira M, Ohtake Y. New Antioxidative 1,3-Benzodioxole from *Melissa officinalis*. *Planta Med.* 1988;64:555–558.

Taylor L.*Herbal Secrets of the Rainforest*.Rocklin, Calif: Prima Publishing; 1998.

Tyler VE. Phytomedicines in Western Europe: their potential impact on herbal medicine in the United States. Presented at: Human Medicinal Agents from Plants, The American Chemical Society, 1992. *HerbalGram* 30, 67.

Vogt HJ, Tausch I, Wbling RH, Kaiser PM. Melissenextrakt bei Herpes simplex. *Der Allgemeinarzt.* 1991;13:832–841.

Wbling RH, Leonhardt K. Local therapy of herpes simplex with dried extract from *Melissa officinalis*. *Phytomedicine*. 1994;1:25–31.

© *Copyright Integrative Medicine Communications*

Licorice

Names

- **English**
  Licorice

- **Botanical**
  Glycyrrhiza glabra

- **Plant Family**
  Fabaceae

- **Pharmacopeial**
  Liquiritiae radix

Overview

Glycyrrhiza glabra, or Spanish licorice, grows wild in some areas of Europe and Asia. It is one of several important medicinal plant species belonging to the *Glycyrrhiza* genus. Numerous pharmacological studies conducted over the past 50 years show that licorice has both therapeutic uses and adverse side effects.

Glycyrrhizin, one of the active components in licorice root, consists of glycyrrhizic acid in a mixture of potassium and calcium salts. Glycyrrhizin is 50 times sweeter than sugar and gives licorice its characteristic sweet taste. The active ingredient in licorice root is glycyrrhetic acid, a triterpene glycoside with saponin-like properties formed from the hydrolysis of glycyrrhizin. Both glycyrrhizin and glycyrrhetic acid are efficacious in treating peptic ulcers. However, both compounds can also cause mineralocorticoid side effects, including lethargy, headache, sodium and water retention, excess potassium excretion, and high blood pressure.

Macro Description

Spanish licorice is a perennial that grows three to seven feet in height. It has a root system comprised of taproots, branch rootstock, and runners, or underground woody stems that grow horizontally. The long, cylindrical roots are straight pieces of wrinkled, fibrous wood 14 to 20 m in length and 5 to 20 mm in diameter. The rootstock has a yellowish-brown exterior and yellow interior.

Part Used/Pharmaceutical Designations

- Roots (rhizome): rhizome, root, and stolon

Constituents/Composition

Terpenoids (glycyrrhizic acid [yields glycyrrhetinic acid and glucuronic acid upon hydrolysis], glycyrrhetol, glabrolide, licoric acid, liquiritic acid, beta-amyrin); coumarins (glycyrin, heniarin, liqcoumarin, umbelliferone, GU-7); flavonoids (flavonols, isoflavones); volatile oil; amino acids, amines, sterols, gums, lignin.

Commercial Preparations

Licorice products are made from both peeled and unpeeled dried roots, and the underground roots, stolons, and rhizomes of several varieties of *Glycyrrhiza glabra*. Commercial preparations consist of powdered root, finely cut roots, dry extracts, and liquid extracts. Deglycyrrhizinated licorice (DGL) is usually manufactured as an extract. DGL is free of adverse side effects and is used to treat gastric and duodenal ulcers.

Medicinal Uses/Indications

Traditional herbal actions: expectorant (cough remedy), demulcent (soothing topical medication), antispasmodic, anti-inflammatory, laxative, adaptogen, antihepatatoxin, antiviral, antitumor, antipyretic, relaxing expectorant. It is also used to normalize immune function.

Clinical applications: allergies, autoimmune conditions, especially those that affect connective tissue (for example, lupus scleroderma), bronchitis, peptic ulcer, chronic gastritis, rheumatism, arthritis, primary adrenocortical insufficiency, chronic esophageal and gastric inflammation, asthma, used as antimicrobial and antiviral.

Pharmacology

In in vivo research, glycyrrhizin had antitoxic activity against diphtheria, tetanus, and tetrodotoxin. The isoflavonoid constituents account for the in vitro antimicrobial effects of licorice alcohol extracts against *Staphylococcus aureus*, *Streptococcus mutans*, *Mycobacterium smegmatis*, and *Candida albicans*. In other in vivo investigations, glycyrrhetic acid blocked free radical formation that can lead to chemically-induced liver toxicity.

In in vitro experiments, glycyrrhizin and its derivative showed antimicrobial activity against numerous bacteria, fungi, and viruses (including HIV, hepatitis A, and several herpes viruses). Glycyrrhetinic acid significantly reduced tumor promoter activity both in vitro and in vivo, and it inhibited the growth of various cancer cell lines.

Glycyrrhizin and glycyrrhetic acid have moderate binding affinity for glucocorticoid and mineralocorticoid receptors, and weak affinity for estrogen, sex-hormone-binding globulin, and corticosteroid-binding globulin. Licorice inhibits estrogen metabolism when estrogen levels are high, and it enhances estrogen metabolism when estrogen levels are low. The estrogenic activity of licorice probably comes from isoflavones.

The steroid-like activity of glycyrrhizin and glycyrrhetic acid is responsible for the anti-inflammatory properties of licorice root. Licorice extends the half-life of cortisol by suppressing the metabolism of cortisol in the liver. In studies in humans, oral intake of glycyrrhizin increased the plasma levels of prednisolone administered intravenously. And glycyrrhetinic acid enhanced the pharmacological activity of hydrocortisone on the lungs. Topical glycyrrhetinic acid enhances the action of hydrocortisone on inflammatory conditions of the skin.

In other human research, glycyrrhizin products taken intravenously resolved at least some liver function damage in about 40% of hepatitis patients. Both oral and topical licorice preparations have been shown to be effective in treating canker sores, eczema and psoriasis, herpes simplex, premenstrual syndrome, and Addison's Disease. Other studies reveal that the efficacy of DGL in treating gastric ulcers can be comparable to that of Tagamet and Zantac.

Licorice achieves its anti-ulcer effect by accelerating the secretion rate of mucus by the gastric mucosa. Glycyrrhetic acid in particular has a therapeutic effect on peptic ulcers. It helps maintain high levels of prostaglandin in the stomach by blocking the activity of two crucial enzymes involved in the metabolism of prostaglandins E and F_2-alpha. This is a key mechanism since elevated prostaglandin levels in the stomach protect the gastric mucosa.

The pharmacological activity of DGL is due to flavonoids, and unlike glycyrrhizin and licorice extracts, DGL is virtually free of the adverse mineralocorticoid side effects.

Dosage Ranges and Duration of Administration

Recommended dosage:

- Dried root: 1 to 5 g as infusion or decoction tid
- Licorice tincture 1:5: 2 to 5 ml tid
- DGL extract: 0.4 to 1.6 g tid for peptic ulcer
- DGL extract 4:1: in chewable tablet form 300 to 400 mg 20 minutes before meals for peptic ulcer

Cautions

- **Adverse Effects/Toxicology**

Oral intake of more than 20 g/day of licorice can cause adverse effects. Excessive consumption of glycyrrhizin causes pseudoaldosteronism, a condition characterized by over-sensitization to the hormone aldosterone from the adrenal cortex. Pseudoaldosteronism produces the mineralocorticoid symptoms of headache, lethargy, hypertension, sodium and water retention, elevated potassium secretion, and sometimes even cardiac arrest. Symptoms usually manifest within one week if the daily ingestion is over 100 g. The adverse effects of licorice resemble symptoms associated with injections of deoxycorticosterone (ACTH) given in large doses.

Death occurs only rarely from ingesting licorice, but side effects such as lethargy and muscular weakness may occur with excess consumption. Muscle pain occurs about one third of the time, and numbness in the extremities is seen about one fourth of the time with moderate intake. Other side effects include weight gain and, on rare occasions, myoglobinuria.

- **Warnings/Contraindications/Precautions**

Persons who consume large quantities of licorice, chew tobacco, or use other licorice-flavored products are at risk for licorice toxicity. Adverse reactions to ingesting licorice products have been reported for individuals who have hypertension, kidney or heart disorders, hypokalemia, cirrhosis of the liver or cholestatic liver diseases, and hypertonia. Licorice is also contraindicated for pregnant women. High doses of licorice products should not be used for longer than four to six weeks.

Interactions

Interactions with thiazide diuretics can cause potassium loss, which can lead to increased sensitivity to digitalis glycosides.

Regulatory and Compendial Status

The U.S. FDA classifies licorice root as a dietary supplement. The German Commission E approves the herb for use in catarrhs of the upper respiratory tract and for gastric/duodenal ulcers.

References

Acharya SK; Dasarathy S, Tandon A, Joshi YK, Tandon BN. A preliminary open trial on interferon stimulator (SNMC) derived from *Glycyrrhiza glabra* in the treatment of subacute hepatic failure. Indian *J Med Res.* 1993;98:69–74.

Arase Y, et al. The long term efficacy of glycyrrhizin in chronic hepatitis C. *Cancer.* 1997;79:1494–1500.

Blumenthal M, ed. *The Complete German Commission E Monographs: Therapeutic Guide to Herbal Medicines.* Boston, Mass: Integrative Medicine Communications; 1998:161–162.

Bradley P, ed. *British Herbal Compendium.* Dorset, England: British Herbal Medicine Association; 1992:1:145–148.

Chen M, et al. Effect of glycyrrhizin on the pharmokinetics of prednisolone following low dosage of prednisolone hemisuccinate. *J Clin Endocrinol Metab.* 1990;70:1637–1643.

De Smet PAGM, Keller K, Hnsel R, Chandler RF, eds. *Adverse Effects of Herbal Drugs.* Berlin, Germany: Springer-Verlag; 1997:67–87.

Gruenwald J, Brendler T, Christof J, Jaenicke C, eds. *PDR for Herbal Medicines.* Montvale, NJ: Medical Economics Co.; 1998:875–879.

Hattori T, et al. Preliminary evidence for inhibitory effect of glycyrrhizin on HIV replication in patients with aids. *Antiviral Research.* 1989;II:255–262.

Heinerman J. *Heinerman's Encyclopedia of Fruits, Vegetables and Herbs.* Englewood Cliffs, NJ: Prentice Hall; 1988.

Kinghorn A, Balandrin M, eds. *Human Medicinal Agents from Plants.* Washington DC: American Chemical Society; 1993: chap 3.

Mori, K. et al. Effects of glycyrrhizin (SNMC: stronger neo-minophagen C) in hemophilia patients with HIV-I infection. Tohoku *J. Exp. Med.* 1990;162:183–193.

Murray MT. *The Healing Power of Herbs: The Enlightened Person's Guide to the Wonders of Medicinal Plants.* 2nd ed. Rocklin, Calif: Prima Publishing; 1995:228–239.

Newall CA, Anderson LA, Phillipson JD, eds. *Herbal Medicines: A Guide for Health-care Professionals.* London: Pharmaceutical Press; 1996:183–186.

Ohuchi K, et al. Glycyrrhizin inhibits prostaglandin E2 formation by activated peritoneal macrophages from rats. *Prostagland Med.* 1981; 7:457–463.

Snow JM. Glycyrrhiza glabra L. (Leguminaceae). *Protocol J Botan Med.* 1996;1:9–14.

Turpie A, Runcie J, Thomson T. Clinical trial of deglycyrrhizinate liquorice in gastric ulcer. *Gut.* 1969;10:299–303.

Tyler VE. *Herbs of Choice: The Therapeutic Use of Phytomedicinals.* Binghamton, NY: Pharmaceutical Products Press; 1994:197–199.

© Copyright Integrative Medicine Communications

Linden

Names

■ **English**
Linden charcoal/Linden Flower/Linden Leaf/Linden Wood

■ **Botanical**
Tilia cordata/Tilia platyphyllos

■ **Plant Family**
Tiliaceae

■ **Pharmacopeial**
Tiliae carbo/Tiliae flos, Tiliae folium/Tiliae lignum

Overview

Various species of *Tilia*, or lime trees, have been used in European folk medicine for centuries to treat a wide range of health conditions. Also known as basswood, *Tilia* species are native to the northern temperate regions. Lime trees are valued not only as raw material for botanical therapies, but also as a commercial source of wood and charcoal.

Most linden herbal remedies consist of the flowers, but the leaves, wood, and charcoal are also used medicinally. The light charcoal is administered for gastric and dyspeptic complaints while powdered charcoal is applied topically to burns. A honey made from linden flowers is highly touted for its flavor and quality.

Linden flower tea is traditionally used as a diaphoretic (promotes perspiration). Precise structure-activity relations for the diaphoretic properties of *Tilia* species have not yet been elucidated. However, the diaphoretic activity has been attributed to *p*-coumaric acid and several flavonoid constituents, including quercetin- and kaempferol-derivatives.

Linden flower formulas typically call for either *Tilia cordata*, the small-leafed European linden, or *Tilia platyphyllos*, the large-leafed linden. These two species furnish the bulk of commercial linden flowers. A related species, *Tilia tomentosa*, the silver linden, is sometimes employed in linden leaf preparations, but not in linden flower remedies. *Tilia cordata*, also called the winter linden, flowers about two weeks earlier than *Tilia platyphyllos*, the early-blooming summer linden. Both species are frequently planted as ornamental trees along city streets.

Linden flower tea is a popular remedy for treating headaches, indigestion, hysteria, and diarrhea. It reportedly has antispasmodic, hypotensive, emollient, and mildly astringent properties. In addition, linden flower possesses opposing pharmacological activities, acting as both a sedative and stimulant.

Linden tea has a pleasing taste, presumably because of the interaction of astringent tannins with mucilage and an aromatic volatile oil in the flowers. Since the slightest amount of moisture decreases their aromatic effects, the fragrant flowers must be quickly dried in the shade after they are collected during late spring.

The taste of linden tea can also influence its therapeutic effects. Taste is crucial because large quantities of the tea must be consumed to promote perspiration, for example, during feverish colds. Patients are more likely to drink linden teas that are more palatable, and the better-tasting teas are those with a relatively higher tannin (minimum 2.0%) and a lower mucilage content. *Tilia cordata* and *Tilia platyphyllos* are preferable sources of linden flower because they contain larger quantities of tannin and lower amounts of mucilage than other *Tilia* species such as the silver linden.

Macro Description

Linden species are large deciduous trees that can grow to a height of 25 to 33 meters. The yellowish-white flowers of *Tilia cordata* are arranged in clusters of 5 to 11 in cymes that hang from slender stalks. Their potent and sweet fragrance contrasts with the profusely rich scent of *Tilia tomentosa*. The dried inflorescences are mildly sweet and mucilaginous to the palate, while the fruit has a somewhat sweet, slimy, and dry taste.

The long-petioled leaves of linden are broadly cordate with an uneven base. *Tilia platyphyllos* is characterized by obliquely heart-shaped, broad leaves that are paler on the underside and dark green on the upperside. The bark of linden trees is fissured and either gray-brown or black-gray. *Tilia cordata* has a relatively shorter trunk and tougher leaves than does *Tilia platyphyllos*. *Tilia cordata* can live to 1,000 years, and its smooth brown bark roughens with age.

Part Used/Pharmaceutical Designations

- Fresh and dried flowers
- Dried leaves
- Wood

■ **Constituents/Composition**

- Leaves *(Tilia spp.)*: flavonoids, including linarin (acacetin-7-rutinosides); tannins, mucilage
- Flowers *(Tilia spp.)*: flavonoids, including rutin, hyperoside, quercitrin, isoquercitrin, astragalin, tiliroside; mucilage, volatile oil containing linalool, geraniol, 1,8-cineole, 2-phenyl ethanol; caffeic acid derivatives, tannins
- Flowers *(Tilia tomentosa)*: flavonoids, including hyperoside; hydroxycoumarins, including calycanthoside, aesculin; caffeic acid derivatives (chlorogenic acid); mucilage
- Charcoal *(Tilia spp.)*: source of exceedingly absorbent charcoals
- Wood *(Tilia spp.)*: mucilage, sterols, triterpenes

■ **Commercial Preparations**

Linden preparations are made primarily from the dried flower, particularly of *Tilia cordata* and *Tilia platyphyllos*. Flowers should always be stored in airtight, light-resistant containers in order to preserve their maximum fragrance. Commercial preparations manufactured from authenticated *Tilia cordata* and *Tilia platyphyllos* are considered superior.

Medicinal Use/Indications

- Flowers: colds, cough, bronchitis, diaphoretic to promote sweating during feverish common colds and infectious diseases; also used as diuretic, stomachic, antispasmodic, sedative
- *Tilia tomentosa* flowers: respiratory tract catarrhs, antispasmodic, expectorant, diaphoretic, diuretic
- Leaf: diaphoretic
- Charcoal: (internal) intestinal complaints; (external) crural (leg-related) ulcers
- Wood: liver and gallbladder disorders, cellulitis
- Mild hypertension
- Tension headaches

Conditions: upper respiratory catarrh, common cold, irritable cough, hypertension, restlessness, headache, migraine; topically for skin ailments.

Clinical applications: diaphoretic; flowers incorporated into some standardized urological, antitussive, and sedative preparations.

■ **Pharmacology**

Pharmacological investigations on *Tilia species* are limited. In earlier in vivo research, flower extracts administered i.v. to test animals produced hypotensive and vasodilative effects, increased pulse rate, and decreased cardiac tone. While specific mechanisms of action have not been determined for pharmacological activity, some general structure-activity relationships have been described. Flavonoids, glycosides, and phenolic acids are reportedly responsible for the diaphoretic action of linden flower.

Since mucilages are known to elicit emollient effects, these compounds may account for the antitussive activity of linden flower tea. The wound-healing effects are probably due to the astringent properties of the tannins in linden. Although the volatile oil contains only a small quantity of farnesol, this active principle may stimulate the sedative and antispasmodic effects of linden.

Other research suggests that the diaphoretic activity of linden flower tea derives in part from thermal influences, especially the heated beverage itself and the bodily warmth that comes from bed rest. In one study, diaphoresis seemed to have a diurnal pattern. Profuse perspiration was associated with heat applied in the afternoon and evening, but not in the morning.

Dosage Ranges and Duration of Administration

Tea (infusion): 1 to 2 tsp. flowers in 8 oz. water; steep covered 20 minutes; drink three cups/day hot
Fluid extract (1:1, 25% ethanol): 2 to 4 ml tid
Tincture (1:5, 30% ethanol): 4 to 10 ml tid

Cautions

■ **Adverse Effects/Toxicology**
None reported for either flower or leaf.

■ Warnings/Contraindications/Precautions

The flower and leaf are considered safe when used as directed. However, since excessive use of linden flower tea may cause cardiac complications, this plant should be avoided by persons with heart problems. An account stating that tea from very old linden flowers may induce narcotic intoxication has not been substantiated and should be considered invalid.

Interactions

Non reported.

Regulatory and Compendial Status

German Commission E lists linden flower as an approved herb, and linden leaf as an unapproved herb. Although the clinical effectiveness of leaf preparations has not been documented, German Commission E permits the use of the leaves as a filler in tea mixtures.

In the United Kingdom, linden flower appears on the General Sale List, Schedule 2, Table A [R1a]. Linden is recognized as safe in the United States, and the Council of Europe has approved its use as a flavoring.

References

Benigni R, Capra C, Cattorini P. Piante Medicinali - Chimica. *Farmacologia e Terapia.* Vol. 1,1962; Vol 2.1964; 2:1606–1614.

Bzanger-Beauquesne L, Pinkas M, Torck M, Trotin F. *Plantes Mdicinales des Rgions Temprés*. Paris: Maloine S.A.; 1980.

Bradley P, ed. *British Herbal Compendium*. Vol. I. Dorset (Great Britain): British Herbal Medicine Association; 1992: 142–144.

Blumenthal M, ed. *The Complete German Commission E Monographs. Therapeutic Guide to Herbal Medicines.* Boston: Integrative Medicine Communications; 1998: 163, 343.

Dorland's Illustrated Medical Dictionary. 25th ed. Philadelphia: W.B. Saunders; 1974.

Glasl H, Becker U. Flavonol-O-Glykoside: Photometrische Gehaltsbestimmung. *Disch Apoth Ztg.* 1984; 124:2147–2152.

Grieve M. *A Modern Herbal.* Vol. II. New York: Dover; 1971: 485–486.

Gruenwald J, Brendler T, Christof J. *PDR for Herbal Medicines.* Montvale, NJ: Medical Economics Company; 1998: 1185–1187.

Hildebrandt G, Engelbrecht P, Hildebrandt-Evers G. Physiologische Grundlagen fur eine tageszeitliche Ordnung der Schwitzprozeduren. *A Klin Med.* 1954; 152:446–468.

Kanschar H, Lander C. Welche Aussagerkraft besitzt die Quellungszahl (QZ) als Wertbestimmungs-methode bei Tilliae flos DABS? *Pharm Ztg.* 1984; 129:370–373.

Schmersahl KJ. Uber die Wirkstoffe der diaphoretischen Drogen des DAB 6. Naturwissenschaften.1964; 51:361.

Schulz V, Hansel R, Tyler V. *Rational Phytotherapy: A Physician's Guide to Herbal Medicine.* 3rd ed. Berlin: Springer; 1998.

Thomson WA. *Medicines from the Earth: A Guide to Healing Plants.* Alfred Van Der Marck ed. Maidenhead, England: McGraw-Hill Book company (UK); 1978:105.

Tyler V. *The Honest Herbal: A Sensible Guide to the Use of Herbs and Related Remedies.* 3rd ed. New York: Pharmaceutical Products Press; 1993: 203–204.

© *Copyright Integrative Medicine Communications*

Lobelia

Names

■ **Botanical**
Lobelia inflata

■ **Plant Family**
Campanulaceae

Overview

Lobelia inflata is indigenous to the flora of Canada, Kamchatka, and the northeastern United States. It has a long history of medicinal use as a respiratory stimulant, antiasthmatic, antispasmodic, expectorant, and emetic therapy. Well-known to Native Americans, this acrid-tasting plant is also called Indian tobacco. It was also highly touted by the Thomsonians, a group of nineteenth-century health care practitioners sarcastically labeled "lobelia doctors." Herbalists have traditionally combined lobelia with other medicinal plants such as cayenne pepper, lungwort, Ma Huang, or licorice. American Indians historically smoked lobelia as a treatment for asthma. More recently, individuals have smoked dried lobelia herb as a recreational euphoriant drug.

At one time, lobelia was approved by the FDA for use as a major ingredient in antismoking, herbal preparations. Lobelia reportedly alleviated symptoms of nicotine withdrawal during smoking cessation. However, the rationale for doing this was eventually called into question since lobelia possesses many of the same pharmacological properties of nicotine. The crude drug is now considered unsafe both as an antismoking agent and as a treatment for asthma and bronchitis. Many authorities in plant drug research claim that the risk of potential toxicity from the alkaloids present in lobelia outweigh its benefits.

Pharmacological support for the effectiveness of lobelia as a therapeutic agent (other than as a sedative) and euphoriant is weak. Although lobelia has a favorable stimulatory action on the respiratory center, it is metabolized too quickly to be considered an efficacious respiratory analeptic (restorative).

Macro Description

Lobelia is a visually attractive, annual or sometimes biennial herb that grows to a height of 50 cm. It erect, hairy stem is angular, branching at the top, and characteristically green with a tinge of violet. The pale green or yellowish leaves are narrow, lance-shaped, and short-stemmed. They are alternate or oblong, with hairy veins and irregularly toothed margins. The leaves have an acrid taste and a slightly irritating odor. The sparse, small, two-lipped flowers are pale violet-blue outside and pale yellow inside. The flowers grow in a terminal spike on long pedicles in the leaf axils.

Part Used/Pharmaceutical Designations

- Herb (aerial parts), leaves, tops, seeds.

■ **Constituents/Composition**
Piperidine-type alkaloids (0.48%): lobeline, lobelanine, lobelanidine, norlobelanine, lelobanidine, norlelobanidine, norlobelanidine, lobinine; bitter glycoside (lobelacrin), chelidonic acid, fats, gum, resin, volatile oil.

■ **Commercial Preparations**
Available for oral intake as dried herb and liquid preparations, including tinctures; and for topical use in ointments, lotions, suppositories, and plasters.

Medicinal Use/Indications

Traditional uses: Taken internally for angina pain, bronchitic asthma, chronic bronchitis, particularly spasmodic asthma with secondary bronchitis, and symptoms of smoking withdrawal; applied externally for myositis and rheumatic nodules.
Conditions: Asthma, spasmodic asthma with secondary bronchitis, chronic bronchitis, spastic colon, spastic muscle conditions, pneumonia.
Clinical applications: Respiratory stimulant, spasmolytic, expectorant.

■ **Pharmacology**
The pharmacological effects of lobelia are attributed primarily to piperidine-type alkaloid constituents, particularly lobeline. Although lobeline is less potent than nicotine, its actions on the peripheral and central nervous (CNS) systems are similar to those of nicotine. According to other research, however, the principle pharmacological activity of lobeline is not nicotinic agonism. Rather, lobeline may affect CNS activity by altering the dopamine chemistry of the brain. Lobeline has been shown to be more potent than d-amphetamine in blocking dopamine uptake into synaptic vesicles.

In normal doses, lobeline functions as a CNS stimulant that dilates the bronchioles, thereby increasing respiration. However, the initial bronchial dilation is often followed by an adverse effect of respiratory depression, particularly during overdosing.

Lobeline induces reflex stimulation of the respiratory center by acting on the chemoreceptors of the glomus caroticus. This medicinal plant presumably exerts its antiasthma activity by stimulating the adrenal glands to release epinephrine, which in turn binds to beta-2 receptors. The net effect of this physiological property is relaxation of the airways. Lobelia also affects gastrointestinal function by stimulating the vomiting center in the reticular formation of the medulla oblongata at the base of the brain.

In an in vivo experiment, a crude methanolic leaf extract of *Lobelia inflata* produced antidepressant effects in mice. The active constituent responsible for this activity was identified as beta-amyrin palmitate. In another study, the in vivo actions of beta-amyrin palmitate on central nervous system activity were compared with those of two antidepressant drugs, mianserin and imipramine. Beta-amyrin palmitate (administered at 5, 10 and 20 mg kg/1) produced a dose-related decrease in locomotor activity of mice and had an antagonistic effect on methamphetamine-induced locomotor stimulation.

In addition, beta-amyrin palmitate at these same doses exhibited potentiating action on chemically-induced narcosis in test animals. Beta-amyrin palmitate was milder than mianserin but more potent than imipramine in eliciting the potentiating effect. These findings offer pharmacological evidence for the sedative properties of lobelia. However, since oral preparations of lobeline are metabolized so rapidly that their effects are only transitory, topical applications may be more efficacious.

Dosage Ranges and Duration of Administration

- Dried herb (infusion or decoction): to tsp. herb in 8 oz. water, preferably mixed with other herbs; steep 30 to 40 minutes. Take 2 oz. qid. (This method is not preferred because of lobelia's acrid taste.)
- Liquid extract (1:1 in 50% alcohol): 0.2 to 0.6 ml tid
- Tincture of lobelia: 0.6 to 2.0 ml
- Vinegar tincture of lobelia (1:5 in dilute acetic acid): 1 to 4 ml tid

Some practitioners recommend starting dosage at 7 to 8 drops, adding a drop with every dose. If the patient experiences nausea, cut back the dosage.

Note: Therapy should begin with the use of lower level dosages and increased appropriately depending upon individual patient response.

Cautions

■ **Adverse Effects/Toxicology**
Both lobelia and its main active principle, lobeline, can produce undesirable symptoms of nausea, vomiting, diarrhea, coughing, dizziness, disturbed hearing and vision, mental confusion, and weakness. All these symptoms resemble toxic reactions to nicotine.

Overdosage of lobelia may cause adverse side effects of shivering, profuse sweating, tachycardia, convulsion, hypothermia, hypotension, coma, and, in extreme cases, death due to respiratory failure. Ingestion of 0.6 to 1 g of lobelia leaves is reportedly toxic.

Note: In cases of acute toxicity from lobelia, atropine (2 mg) should be administered subcutaneously as an antidote.

■ **Warnings/Contraindications/Precautions**
Lobelia should not be consumed in excessive amounts because of the toxicity of its potent alkaloid compounds. As in the case of nicotine, lobelia and lobeline are contraindicated during pregnancy and lactation.

Interactions

None reported.

Regulatory and Compendial Status

Lobelia has not been designated as an approved herb, or an unapproved herb, by the German Commission E. In the United Kingdom, lobelia (in doses of up to 65 mg per single dose) is on the General Sale List, Schedule 1, Table A. Higher oral doses of up to 200 mg per dose (600 mg per day) and external preparations containing quantities of not more than 10% lobelia are reserved for pharmacy use only in the United Kingdom. Herbal practitioners are exempt from this regulation.

References

Bradley P, ed. *British Herbal Compendium.* Vol. I. Dorset (Great Britain): British Herbal Medicine Association; 1992: 149–150.

Dorland's Illustrated Medical Dictionary. 22th ed. Philadelphia: W.B. Saunders; 1974.

Ganong WF. *Review of Medical Physiology.* 17th ed. Norwalk, CT: Appleton and Lange; 1995: 211.

Grieve M. *A Modern Herbal. Vol. II* New York: Dover; 1971: 494–495.

Gruenwald J, Brendler T, Christof J. *PDR for Herbal Medicines.* Montvale, NJ: Medical Economics Company; 1998: 943.

Murray, MT. *The Healing Power of Herbs: The Enlightened Person's Guide to the Wonders of Medicinal Plants.* 2nd ed. Rocklin, CA: Prima Publishing; 1995: 240–242.

Murray MT, Pizzorno J. *Encyclopedia of Natural Medicine.* 2nd ed. Rocklin, CA: Prima Publishing; 1998: 270.

Newall C, Anderson L, Phillipson J. *Herbal Medicines: A Guide for Health-care Professionals.* London: Pharmaceutical Press; 1996: 187.

Subarnas A, Tadano T, Oshima Y, Kisara K, Ohizumi Y. Pharmacological properties of beta-amyrin palmitate, a novel centrally acting compound, isolated from *Lobelia inflata* leaves. *J Pharm Pharmacol.* 1993; 45(ISS 6):545–550.

Subarnas A, Oshima Y, Sidik, Ohizumi Y. An antidepressant principle of Lobelia inflata L. (Campanulaceae). *J Pharm Sci.* 1992; 53(7): 620–621.

Teng L, Crooks PA, Dwoskin LP. Lobeline displaces [3H] dihydrotetrabenazine binding and releases [3H]dopamine from rat striatal synaptic vesicles: comparison with d-amphetamine. *J Neurochem.* 1998; 71(1): 258–265.

Thomson WA. *Medicines from the Earth: A Guide to Healing Plants.* Alfred Van Der Marck eds. Maidenhead, England: McGraw-Hill Book company (UK); 1978: 78–79.

Tyler V. *Herbs of Choice: The Therapeutic Use of Phytomedicinals.* Binghamton, NY: Haworth; 1994: 95.

Tyler V. *The Honest Herbal: A Sensible Guide to the Use of Herbs and Related Remedies.* 3rd ed. New York: Pharmaceutical Products Press; 1993: 205–206.

© *Copyright Integrative Medicine Communications*

Marshmallow

Names

- **English**
  Marshmallow

- **Botanical**
  Althaea officinalis

- **Plant Family**
  Malvaceae

- **Pharmacopeial**
  Althaea

Overview

Native to southern and western Europe, marshmallow has been used for centuries as both a food and a medicine. Althaea, the generic name for mallow plants, comes from the Greek word "altho," which means "to cure." Dioscorides revered the medicinal virtues of mallows, while Pliny advised taking a spoonful of mallows every day to be spared sickness. The Arabs used poultices made from the leaves of marshmallow as an anti-inflammatory. The Romans, Chinese, Egyptians, and Syrians used mallows as a source of food.

The high mucilage content in both the leaves and root, particularly the root, make marshmallow an excellent demulcent (soother) and emollient (skin softener and soother). Several pharmacological studies have shown that mucilaginous herbs generally act as demulcents. While the soothing properties of marshmallow have been substantiated, the pharmacological rationale for other therapeutic uses of marshmallow remains questionable.

Macro Description

Marshmallow is found in southern and western Europe, western Asia, and the northeastern region of North America. It originally grew on salty soils but now thrives in moist uncultivated ground. Its fleshy, erect stems reach a height of 3 to 4 feet. The stems give off simple branches or at most, a few lateral branches. The pale yellow roots are tapered, long, and thick, with a noticeably tough and pliant exterior. The short-stemmed leaves are roundish and ovate-cordate, with irregularly toothed margins and three to five lobes. A soft and velvety down of stellate hairs covers the leaves and stem. The flowers have five reddish-white petals. The whole plant, especially the perennial root, is filled with a mild mucilage.

Part Used/Pharmaceutical Designation

- Flowers
- Leaves
- Roots

- **Constituents/Composition**
  Mucilages (supposedly range between 25% and 35%, but may actually be closer to 5% to 11%): major components include galacturonic acid, glucoronic acid, and rhamnose; also arabinose, galactose, glucose, mannose, and xylose. Flavonoids: hypolaeton 8-glucoside, isoscutellarein. Other constituents: asparagine (2%), calcium oxalate, pectin (11%), starch (37%), fat (1.7%), sucrose (10%), tannin, phenolic acids (caffeic, ferulic, syringic).

- **Commercial Preparations**
  Both marshmallow leaf and root are used in commercial preparations. Herbal preparations for internal use are made from either the dried leaf or ground dried root (unpeeled or peeled). The medicinal effects are due to the mucilage content, which becomes lower during late autumn and winter. The roots are typically harvested during the fall from plants that are at least two years old. The actual mucilage content of the commercial product may vary, depending upon time of collection.

Medicinal Uses/Indications

Expectorant, emollient, soothing diuretic, antilithic (prevents formation of stones or calculi), vulnerary (promotes wound healing), demulcent, anti-inflammatory.

Traditional internal uses: respiratory catarrh, cough, peptic ulceration, inflammation of the mouth and pharynx, enteritis, urethritis, and urinary calculus (stone)

Traditonal external uses: topical treatment for abscesses, boils, varicose and thrombotic ulcers; emollient, vulnerary

Conditions: gastroenteritis, peptic and duodenal ulceration, common and ulcerative colitis, enteritis, topical mouthwash or gargle for inflammation of mouth and pharynx; poultice or ointment/cream in furunculosis, eczema, and dermatitis

Clinical applications: irritation of the oral and pharyngeal mucosa, and concomitant dry cough, mild inflammation of the gastric mucosa

- **Pharmacology**
  Many mucilaginous herbs such as marshmallow leaves and roots have demulcent properties. Both the root and leaf of marshmallow are effective demulcents because they reduce local irritation that causes acute gastritis.

  Studies show that marshmallow root suppresses mucociliary action and stimulates phagocytosis. Marshmallow exhibits antimicrobial activity in vivo against *Pseudomonas aeruginosa*, *Proteus vulgaris*, and *Staphlococcus aureus*. When given intraperitoneally to nondiabetic mice, the mucilage from this plant produced significant hypoglycemic activity. In another investigation, however, marshmallow failed to show anti-inflammatory effects during the carrageenan rat paw edema test.

  In one study, coughing was mechanically stimulated in unanesthetized cats. Marshmallow complex extract (100 mg/kg b.w.) and a polysaccharide (50 mg/kg b.w.) isolated from marshmallow roots was given to the test animals. The polysaccharide elicited an antitussive (cough preventive) effect comparable to that of non-narcotic cough suppressants, but the extract was less effective. Mucilaginous herbs such as marshmallow root inhibit coughing by forming a protective coating on the mucosal surface of the respiratory tract that shields it from irritants.

Dosage Ranges and Duration of Administration

- Leaf: 5 g or equivalent preparations daily
- Flowers: 5 g mallow prescribed as gastrointestinal tea XII according to German Standard Registration
- Root: infusion or cold-water maceration (2% to 5%): 150 ml (1 to 2 tsp.) taken to soothe cough and sore throat
- Dried root: 2 to 6 g or equivalent preparations taken daily (cold infusion tid)
- Tincture: 5 to 15 ml (1:5, 25% ethanol) tid
- Marshmallow syrup (from root): 2 to 10 g per single dose (syrup contains sugar, which should be considered by diabetics)
- Root topical preparations: 5% to 10% drug in ointment or cream base

Cautions

- **Adverse Effects/Toxicology**
  No adverse side effects have been reported (leaf and root)

- **Warnings/Contraindications/Precautions**
  No adverse side effects have been reported (leaf and root). There are no precautions concerning either the medicinal or food use of marshmallow since its constituents are declared safe. This plant reportedly poses no problem for use during pregnancy or lactation. Marshmallow has considerable blood-sugar-lowering effects because of its abundant mucilage. However, the mucilage may interfere with the therapeutic actions of other hypoglycemic drugs.

Interactions

No interactions have been reported (leaf and root). Mucilage in marshmallow may cause a delay in the absorption of other drugs and substances taken concurrently. In particular, marshmallow may impede the effectiveness of antidiabetic medications.

Regulatory and Compendial Status

In the United Kingdom, marshmallow root is listed in Schedule 2, Table A of the General Sale List (GSL), and is also accepted in reviewed medicines for internal use. The root is accepted for specified indication in Belgium and France, and listed by the Commission E in Germany. It is permitted as a flavoring by the Code of Federal Regulations (CFR) in the United States, and by the Council of Europe.

References

Blumenthal M, ed. *The Complete German Commission E Monographs.* Boston, Mass: Integrative Medicine Communications; 1998:166–167.

British Herbal Pharmacopoeia. 4th ed. Great Britain: Biddles Ltd, Guildford and King's Lynn; 1996: 151–152.

Dorland's Illustrated Medical Dictionary. 25th ed. Philadelphia, Pa: WB. Saunders; 1974.

Franz G. Polysaccharides in pharmacy. Current Applications and future concepts. *Planta Med.* 1989; 55:493–497.

Grieve M. *A Modern Herbal. Vol. II.* New York, NY: Dover; 1971: 507–508.

Gysling E. *Leitfaden zur Pharmakotherpie.* Vienna: Huber, Bern Stuttgart; 1976:86.

Hahn HL. Husten: Mechanismen, pathophysiologie und therapie. *Disch Apoth A.* 1987;127(suppl 5):3–26.

Kurz H. 1989 Antitussiva und Expektoranzien. *Wissenschaftliche.* Verlagsgesellschaft Stuggart; 1989.

Mascolo N, et al. Biological screening of Italian plants for anti-inflammatory activity. *Phytotherapy Res.* 1987;I:28–31.

Newall C, Anderson L, Phillipson J. *Herbal Medicines: A Guide for Health-care Professionals.* London, England: Pharmaceutical Press; 1996:188.

Nosl'ova G, Strapkov A, Kardsov A, Capek P, Zathureck L, Bukovsk E. Antitussive action of extracts and polysaccharides of marsh mallow (*Althea officinalis* L., var. robusta). *Pharmazia* 1992;47(3): 224–226.

Recio MC, et al. Antimicrobial activity of selected plants employed in the Spanish Mediterranean area. Part II. *Phytotherapy Res.* 1989;3:77–80.

Schulz V, Hansel R, Tyler V. *Rational Phytotherapy: A Physicians' Guide to Herbal Medicine.* 3rd ed. Berlin, Germany: Springer; 1998:150,183.

Thomson WA. *Medicines from the Earth: A Guide to Healing Plants.* Maidenhead, England: McGraw-Hill Book Company; 1978:41.

Tomoda M, Norika S, Oshima Y, Takahashi M, Murakami M, Hikino H. Hypoglycemic activity of twenty plant mucilages and three modified products. *Planta Med.* 1987;53:8–12.

© *Copyright Integrative Medicine Communications*

Milk Thistle

Names

■ **English**
Milk thistle fruit/milk thistle herb

■ **Botanical**
Silybum marianum

■ **Plant Family**
Asteraceae

■ **Pharmacopeial**
Cardui mariae fructus/Cardui mariae herba

Overview

Milk thistle seed protects the liver and restores the liver's ability to detoxify harmful substances. Used for centuries in the ancient world, milk thistle was touted by Greek and Medieval physicians as a remedy for snakebites, jaundice, and other liver diseases. Its uses in Western folk medicine were versatile, and nursing mothers took milk thistle leaf to increase their milk flow. Extensive research conducted over the past 30 years shows that milk thistle seed extract is an effective treatment for cirrhosis of the liver, hepatitis, and inflammatory liver conditions.

Silymarin is a group of flavonoid-like compounds extracted from the small hard fruits (kenguil seeds) of milk thistle. The liver-protecting and liver-repairing functions of silymarin are due to two main actions: antioxidant and protein-restoring activities. The antioxidant activity of silymarin is ten times more powerful than vitamin E. Antioxidants scavenge free radicals that damage cells and cause lipid peroxidation. In lipid peroxidation, unstable free radicals attack the cell membrane. Silymarin prevents toxic and foreign substances from penetrating liver cells by stabilizing the outer membrane of liver cells. The active constituents displace toxins by binding to proteins and receptors on the cell membrane. Silymarin also stimulates protein synthesis in ribosomes so that new liver cells can grow and damaged liver cells can be replaced. Because silymarin acts mainly on the liver and kidneys, it is an effective antidote against poisonous substances that accumulate in the liver.

Macro Description

Native to the Mediterranean, milk thistle is now widespread in many areas, including eastern Europe, Asia, the eastern United States, and California. It grows wild in dry sunny areas with well-drained soils, but is usually cultivated in northern regions. This biennial or annual stout thistle has broad, wavy, lanceolate leaves; large, prickly, leaves marbled with white; and red-purple flowers. The stem branches at the top, reaching heights of 4 to 10 feet. The small, hard-skinned fruits are brown, spotted, and shiny. This plant is easy to grow, and it matures rapidly, usually in less than a year.

Part Used/Pharmaceutical Designations

- Flowers
- Stems
- Seeds
- Leaves
- Fruits (kenguel seed or compressed achenes)

■ **Constituents/Composition**
Fruit contains 1.5% to 3% silymarin (flavonolignans, consisting of 50% silybarin [silybin] and lesser amounts of isosilybin, dehydrosilybin, silydianin, silychristin); tyramine, histamine, essential oils, lipids (20% to 30%), sugars, alkaloids, saponins, mucilages, vitamins C, E, and K, flavonoids.

■ **Commercial Preparations**
Milk thistle is prepared for oral use as capsules of concentrated extract of standardized dried herb (70% to 80%, or about 140 mg silymarin); tincture (liquid extract). There are several teas containing the standardized extract. Silymarin must be concentrated because it is poorly absorbed from the gastrointestinal tract.

Medicinal Uses/Indications

- Traditional herbal actions: promotes milk production; jaundice; cholalogue and choleretic (promotes bile production for obstructive liver and gallbladder disorders); hepato-restorative, galactagogue, and demulcent.
- Clinical applications: for chronic liver and gallbladder disorders such as cirrhosis, damage from harmful chemicals and alcohol abuse, cholangitis, pericholangitis, gallstones, and chronic hepatitis B, C, D, E, and as a supportive in acute hepatitis A; for topical use in skin conditions such as psoriasis, eczema, aging skin, erythema, burns, wounds, and sores.

■ **Pharmacology**
Milk thistle extract (silymarin) has a liver-protecting effect against toxic chemicals (carbon tetrachloride, galactosamine, praseodymium, thioacetamide, acetaminophen). It is the most important antidote in modern medicine to poisoning from deathcap mushroom (*Amanita phalloides*). Milk thistle extract is so effective that it counteracts *Amanita* toxins even if it is taken 10 minutes after mushrooms are consumed.

Silymarin has antioxidant effects in both in vitro and in vivo studies. Glutathione is an antioxidant that helps the liver detoxify harmful chemicals, drugs, and hormones. Silymarin keeps glutathione levels from dropping too low, and in healthy humans it raises glutathione levels in the liver by as much as 35%.

In several experiments, silymarin protected against ulcers and gastrointestinal problems, relieved allergies by blocking histamine release, and decreased the activity of tumor-promoting agents. Silymarin also increased the movement of human polymorphonuclear leukocytes (PML's) blocked by harmful substances. And a silymarin-phospholipid complex had anti-inflammatory activity.

In humans, milk thistle seed extract improved fatty liver caused by chemical and alcohol damage. And in several double-blind, placebo-controlled studies, milk thistle extract improved liver dysfunction in patients with hepatitis B, chronic alcoholic liver disease, alcohol-induced liver disease, chronic exposure to organophosphates, toxic liver disorders, and chronic hepatitis. Silymarin also lowered the death rate of alcoholic patients compared to controls over a two to four year period, and it reduced the symptoms of hepatitis (abdominal upset, decreased appetite, fatigue). Silymarin increased serum bilirubin levels and liver enzymes when compared to controls, and it had a favorable effect on Type II hyperlipidemia, low platelet count, and psoriasis. Benefits of milk thistle extract have been reported for subclinical cholecstasis of pregnancy, cholangitis, and pericholangitis.

Dosage Ranges and Duration of Administration

- Recommended dosage: 1 to 4 g dried fruit (seeds), (200 to 400 mg silymarin)
- Protective dosage for healthy people: silymarin 120 mg bid; Tincture (1:5): L 2 to 6 ml tid
- Restorative dosage for people with liver disorders: silymarin 120 mg tid. Silymarin-phosphatidylcholine complex (in 1:1 ratio) is absorbed better and has more clinical benefits than silymarin alone. (Phosphatidylcholine is a key element in cell membranes.) Decoction: 1 to 4 g of fruit in 500 ml water tid
- Recommended dosage for complex: 100 to 200 mg bid

Cautions

■ **Adverse Effects/Toxicology**
No toxicity has been reported for long-term use in test animals (20 g/kg in mice; 1 g/kg in dogs), and long term use does not seem to pose any danger. Milk thistle occasionally has a mild laxative effect due to increased bile flow and secretion. Dietary fiber (guar gum, psyllium oat bran, pectin) can be taken to stop loose stools and mucosal irritation.

■ **Warnings/Contraindications/Precautions**
Alcohol-based extracts are not recommended for severe liver problems.

Interactions

None noted

Regulatory and Compendial Status

The U.S. FDA classifies milk thistle as a dietary supplement. In Germany, milk thistle is used as a nonprescription drug for inflammatory liver disease and cirrhosis.

References

Alarcn de la Lastra A, Martn M, Motilva V, et al. Gastroprotection induced by silymarin, the hepatoprotective principle of Silybum marianum in ischemia-reperfusion mucosal injury: role of neutrophils. *Planta Med.* 1995;61:116–119.

Dorland Newman WA, ed. Dorland's Illustrated Medical Dictionary. 25th ed. Philadelphia, Pa: WB Saunders. 1974.

Feher J, Deak G, Muzes G, Lang I, Neiderland V, Nekan K, et al. Hepatoprotective activity of silymarin therapy in patients with chronic alcoholic liver disease. *Orv Hetil.* 1990;130:51.

Ferenci P, Dragosics B, Dittrich H, Frank H., Benda L, Lochs H, et al. Randomized controlled trial of silymarin treatment in patients with cirrhosis of the liver. *J Hepatol.* 1989;9:105–13.

Flora K, Hahn M, Rosen H, Benner K. Milk thistle (Silybum marianum) for the therapy of liver disease. *Am J Gastroenterol.* 1998;93:139–43.

Hobbs C. *Milk Thistle: The Liver Herb.* 2nd ed. Capitola, Calif: Botanica Press; 1992.

Hocking G. A Dictionary of Natural Products. Medford, NJ: Plexus; 1997.

Kinghorn A, Balandrin M, eds. *Human Medicinal Agents from Plants*. Washington, DC: American Chemical Society; 1993.

Magliulo E, Gagliardi B, Fiori GP. Results of a double blind study on the effect of silymarin in the treatment of acute viral hepatitis, carried out at two medical centres. *Med Klinik.* 1978;73:1060–1065.

Morazzoni P, Bombardelli E. *Silybum marianum (Carduus marianus). Fitoterapia.* 1995;LXVI.

Murray M. *The Healing Power of Herbs: The Enlightened Person's Guide to the Wonders of Medicinal Plants.* 2nd ed. Rocklin, Calif: Prima Publishing; 1995.

Murray M, Pizzorno J. *Encyclopedia of Natural Medicine.* 2nd ed. Rocklin, Calif: Prima Publishing; 1998.

Palasciano G, Portincasa P, Palmieri V, Ciani D, Vendemiale G, Altomare E. The effect of silymarin on plasma levels of malon-dialdehyde in patients receiving long-term treatment with psychotropic drugs. *Curr Therapeut Res.* 1994;55(5):537–545.

Schulz V, Hansel R, Tyler V. *Rational Phytotherapy: A Physician's Guide to Herbal Medicine.* 3rd ed. Berlin, Germany: Springer-Verlag; 1998.

Tyler V. *The Honest Herbal: A Sensible Guide to the Use of Herbs and Related Remedies.* 3rd ed. New York, NY: Pharmaceutical Products Press; 1993:chap 3.

© Copyright Integrative Medicine Communications

Passionflower

Names

- **English**
  Passionflower

- **Botanical**
  Passiflora incarnata

- **Plant Family**
  Passifloraceae

- **Pharmacopeial**
  Passiflorae herba

Overview

Indigenous to the tropical regions of North America, passionflower is now cultivated throughout Europe. This plant was supposedly given the name passionflower because its corona resembles the crown of thorns worn by Christ during the crucifixion.

The dried flowering and fruiting tops of passionflower are used in traditional herbal remedies for nervousness, insomnia, and convulsion. During the early twentieth century, this plant was a popular sedative and calmative, and was listed in the United States National Formulary between 1916 to 1936. In 1978, the U.S. FDA banned the use of passionflower in OTC preparations, citing the lack of valid evidence to support its safety or efficacy in the treatment of nervousness or insomnia.

A survey conducted in 1986 indicated that passionflower was utilized more frequently in Britain than any other ingredient in herbal sedatives. In Germany, Commission E has approved the use of this herb as a tranquilizer. Commission E's decision was based on evidence showing that passionflower reduced mobility in laboratory animals. A number of sedative-hypnotic pharmaceutical preparations sold in Europe, including a sedative chewing gum, contain passionflower extract.

Scientific research confirms that passionflower has an in vivo motility-inhibiting effect. However, the active principles responsible for this effect have not been unequivocally established. Passionflower contains C-glycoside flavonoid constituents and small quantities (up to 0.01%) of harmala-type indole alkaloids. The sedative effects are presumably not due to these compounds, however, since harmala-type alkaloids tend to act as stimulants rather than depressants.

Macro Description

Passionflower is a perennial climbing vine with herbaceous shoots and a sturdy woody stem that grows to a length of nearly 10 m. The three-lobed leaves are alternate, petiolate, and finely serrated. The flowers are characteristically yellow or flesh-colored, with tinges of purple and a sweet fragrance. Each flower has five petals varying in color from white to pale red. Inside the petals is a secondary corolla composed of four thread wreaths. These form rays that surround the axis of the flower. The ripe fruit is an orange-colored, multi-seeded, ovoid berry containing an edible, sweetish yellow pulp.

Part Used/Pharmaceutical Designation

- Flowers
- Leaves
- Stems
- **Other:** above-ground (aerial) parts; herb

- **Constituents/Composition**
  Flavonoids (up to 2.5%): C-glycosylflavones (isovitexin-2"-glucoside, schaftoside, isoschaftoside, isoorientin, isoorientin-2"-glucoside, vicenin-2, lucenin-2), apigenin, luteolin glycosides (e.g., orientin, homoorientin, lucenin); kaempferol, quercetin, rutin. Cyanogenic glycosides: gynocardine (less than 0.1%). Indole-type alkaloids (up to 0.01%): harman, harmaline, harmalol, harmine, harmol (putative constituent). Other constituents: maltol (0.05%), ethylmaltol, passicol (a polyacetylene), fatty acids, formic acid, butyric acid, sitosterol stigmasterol, gum, volatile oil (trace). Root contains coumarins (scopoletin and umbelliferone).

- **Commercial Preparations**
  Passionflower commercial preparations are made from the fresh or dried aerial parts. Both whole and cut raw plant material are used in teas and infusions. For optimal results, flowering shoots, growing 10 to 15 cm above the ground, are harvested after the first fruits have matured and then either air-dried or hay-dried. Some (but not all) experts recommend collecting the shoots two times each year to coincide with maximum quantity of flavonoids. The content of harman alkaloids also fluctuates, and plant material containing more than 0.01% harman alkaloids should be avoided.

Medicinal Uses/Indications

Traditional uses: used internally as sedative, mild hypnotic, antispasmodic, and anodyne (analgesic) for nervous agitation, insomnia, hysteria, diarrhea, dysentery, neuralgia, generalized seizures, nervous tachycardia, spasmodic asthma, dysmennorhea; used externally for hemorrhoids. Also incorporated into homeopathic preparations.
Conditions: nervousness, insomnia
Clinical applications: nervous restlessness and agitation, insomnia, nervous gastrointestinal conditions

- **Pharmacology**
  In in vitro studies, passicol, one of the main active constituents in passionflower, showed antimicrobial action against several pathogens, including bacteria such as hemolytic *Streptococci* and *Staphylococcus aureus,* yeasts such as *Candida albicans,* and molds.

  Several experiments have clearly demonstrated that passionflower has psychotropic activity. In in vivo studies, passionflower extract and some of its constituents significantly prolonged sleeping time and decreased locomotor activity. An in vivo investigation evaluated the effects of lyophilised hydroalcoholic and aqueous extracts of passionflower as well as its active principles on behavioral parameters in mice. While the hydroalcoholic extract exhibited anxiolytic (anti-anxiety) effects, the aqueous extract showed sedative action. The aqueous extract also extended sleeping time in mice previously given a sub-hypnotic dose of pentobarbital.

  Maltol is a pyrone derivative isolated from an alkaloid fraction of passionflower. Japanese researchers reported that maltol produced depression and other sedative effects in mice. In other animal studies, a high dose of maltol and ethylmaltol exhibited anticonvulsant effects while a low dose of these same compounds reduced spontaneous motor activity. Both maltol and ethylmaltol had sedative action on the CNS and both potentiated sleeping time induced by hexobarbitone. However, other investigators did not attribute these effects to either the flavonoid or alkaloids in passionflower. It is also thought that maltol and ethylmaltol may mask the CNS stimulant effects of the harman alkaloids.

  Expert opinion on the chemical constituents responsible for the sedative action of passionflower is divided. Even though maltol appears to be a likely candidate, some researchers have called for further studies confirming the pharmacological effects of specific active constituents. In addition, clinical investigations on the effects of passionflower on humans are urgently needed.

Dosage Ranges and Duration of Administration

- Infusion: 2 to 5 g dried herb tid
- Fluid extract (1:1 in 25% alcohol): 0.5 to 1.0 ml tid
- Tincture (1:5 in 45% alcohol): 0.5 to 2.0 ml tid

Cautions

- **Adverse Effects/Toxicology**
  No side effects reported. The value for acute toxicity of passionflower fluid extract (I.P.) was greater than 900 mg/kg in mice. Toxic cyanogenic glycosides have been isolated from related *Passiflora* species, but not for *Passiflora incarnata.*

- **Warnings/Contraindications/Precautions**
  Although passionflower extracts and preparation are generally devoid of contraindications, only limited toxicity data are available. Excessive oral intake may induce sedative effects and potentiate existing MAOI therapy. For this reason, passionflower should not be consumed in quantities higher than recommended doses. This herb should be completely avoided during pregnancy and lactation since harman and harmaline have been shown to have in vivo uterine-stimulant action in some studies.

Interactions

Excessive dosing may lead to sedation and potentiate the action of MAOI medications.

Regulatory and Compendial Status

In 1978, the U.S. FDA banned passionflower as an ingredient in OTC sedative preparations. In Britain, passionflower is on the General Sale List (GSL), and in Germany, it is authorized by Commission E for use in remedies. The Council of Europe approves passionflower as a natural source of food flavoring (category N3) that can be added to foodstuffs. However, the Council also notes that the potential toxicity of passionflower cannot be fully assessed because current information is insufficient.

References

Aoyagi N, Kimura R, Murata T. Studies on *Passiflora incarnata* dry extract. I. Isolation of maltol and pharmacological action of maltol and ethyl maltol. *Chem Pharm Bull.* 1974;22:1008–1013.

Blumenthal M, ed. *The Complete German Commission E Monographs.* Boston, Mass: Integrative Medicine Communications; 1998: 179–180.

Dorland's Illustrated Medical Dictionary. 25th ed. Philadelphia, Pa: WB Saunders; 1974.

Grieve M. *A Modern Herbal.* Vol. II. New York, NY: Dover; 1971:618.

Gruenwald J, Brendler T, Jaenicke C. *PDR for Herbal Medicines.* Montvale, NJ: Medical Economics Company; 1998:1015–1016.

Kimura R, et al. Central depressant effects of maltol analogs in mice. *Chem Pharm Bull.* 1980;28:2570–2579.

Mabberley DJ. *The Plant-Book: A Portable Dictionary of the Higher Plants.* England: Cambridge University Press; 1987:434.

Newall C, Anderson L, Phillipson J. *Herbal Medicines: A Guide for Health-care Professionals.* London, England: Pharmaceutical Press; 1996: 206–207.

Nicholls JM, et al. Passicol, an antibacterial and antifungal agent produced by *Passiflora* plant species: qualitative and quantitative range of activity. *Antimicrob Agents Chemother.* 1973;3:110–117.

Soulimani R, Younos C, Jarmouni S, Bousta D, Misslin R, Mortier F. Behavioural effects of *Passiflora incarnata* L. and its indole alkaloid and flavonoid derivatives and maltol in the mouse. *J Ethnopharmacol.* 1997;57(1):11–20.

Minghetti A. Neuropharmacological activity of extracts from *Passiflora incarnata. Planta Med.* 1988;54:488–91.

Tyler V. *Herbs of Choice: The Therapeutic Use of Phytomedicinals.* Binghamton, NY: Pharmaceutical Products Press; 1994:119.

Tyler V. *The Honest Herbal: A Sensible Guide to the Use of Herbs and Related Remedies.* 3rd ed. New York, NY: Pharmaceutical Products Press; 1993:237–238.

© *Copyright Integrative Medicine Communications*

Pau d'Arco

Names

- **English**
  Pau d'arco

- **Botanical**
  Tabebuia avellanedae

- **Plant Family**
  Bignoniaceae

Overview

Pau d'arco is the name of a tea derived from the bark of several *Tabebuia* species. There are over 100 species of evergreen trees and shrubs in the *Tabebuia* genus, all of them native to tropical regions of Central and South America. Pau d'arco often comes from *Tabebuia avellanedae,* a tree found in the Amazonian rain forest. However, according to some, the correct scientific name for pau d'arco is *Tabebuia impetiginosa.* Other sources claim that *Tabebuia chrysata* is also marketed in the United States as pau d'arco.

Traditional herbalists in the Brazilian Amazonian rain forest make an infusion from either *Tabebuia avellanedae* or *Tabebuia altissima* to treat ulcers, diabetes, rheumatism, cancer, and ringworm. The popularity of this tree for treating cancer, malignant tumors, and Candida fungal infections has soared over the past decade. Increasing demand for pau d'arco has only intensified stripping the bark from the trees, making *Tabebuia* one of the most exploited plant groups in the Amazon. *Tabebuia* species are now seriously threatened by extinction.

Extracts of *Tabebuia avellanedae* have anti-inflammatory, antimicrobial, and anticancer effects. The inner part of the bark supposedly contains lapachol, an active principle that has been shown to be an effective anticancer agent. However, the scientific evidence for the anticancer effects of pau d'arco is weak. While the bark of *Tabebuia* species does contain lapachol derivatives, only trace amounts of the anticancer compound, lapachol, are actually present. To further complicate matters, most of the research on the chemistry of *Tabebuia* has been done on the heartwood rather than the bark. But it is the bark that is medicinally important. Critics point out that the relatively high cost and lack of evidence to support therapeutic claims, combined with the fact that pau d'arco is potentially an endangered species, make it a less-than-desirable herbal supplement.

Macro Description

Most species in the *Tabebuia genus* are broad-leaf evergreen trees. *Tabebuia avellanedae* grows to a height of 125 feet and is distinguished by rose-to-violet colored flowers. It has exceptionally hard wood that is disease-resistant and does not easily decay.

Part Used/Pharmaceutical Designations

- Inner bark

- **Constituents/Composition**
  Tabebuia avellanedae heartwood: naphthoquinones (lapachol, 2 to 7%; menaquinone-1, deoxylapachol, beta-lapachone, alpha-lapachone, dehydro-alpha-lapachone); anthraquinones (2-methylanthraquinone, 2-hydroxymethylanthraquinone, 2-acetoxymethylanthraquinone, anthraquinone-2-aldehyde, 1-hydroxyanthraquinone, 1-methoxyanthraquinone, 2-hydroxy-3-methylquinone, tabebuin).

- **Commercial Preparations**
  Pau d'arco products are not usually standardized for lapachol or naphthoquinone content. Some pau d'arco herbal teas are not authentic, but are derived from the bark of *Tecoma curialis*. Since *Tabebuia* and *Tecoma* species are in the same botanical family (Bignoneaceae), they often contain some of the same active principles. Consequently, remedies made from *Tecoma* and *Tabebuia* tree bark sometimes have similar therapeutic activities.

Medicinal Uses/Indications

Traditional use: tonic, blood builder, rheumatism, cystitis, prostatitis, bronchitis, gastritis, ulcers, liver disorders, asthma, gonorrhea, ringworm, hernias; breast, liver, and prostate cancers

Traditional herbal actions: immune tonic, antimicrobial, antifungal, antineoplastic, antiviral

Clinical applications: cancer, *Candida albicans* infections (used internally and topically for internal and topical vaginal candidiasis), oral thrush candidiasis, infections of the genito-urinary tract (cystitis, prostatitis), herpes, stomatitis, lupus, Hodgkins disease

- **Pharmacology**
  In the mid 1950s, Brazilian researchers reported that lapachol isolated from *Tabebuia avellanedae* had antimicrobial effects against gram-positive and acid-fast bacteria. Lapachol also showed strong antimicrobial effects against Brucella, and it had fungistatic (fungus-inhibiting) properties. However, these effects decreased as the extract was progressively purified to yield a higher content of lapachol but lower quantity of other constituents. Ongoing studies have since confirmed that *Tabebuia avellanedae* extracts contain not only lapachol, but other active constituents as well. These additional compounds include active quinones such as alpha-lapachone, beta-lapachone, and xyloidone.

  Lapachol and other quinones in *Tabebuia avellanedae* showed antiviral activity against herpes simplex types I and II, influenza virus, poliovirus, and vesicular stomatitis virus. Beta-lapachone produced an antiviral effect by blocking crucial viral enzymes, including DNA and RNA polymerases, as well as retrovirus reverse transcriptase.

  Lapachol also had antiparasitic activity against the larvae that cause schistosomiasis, a water-borne disease. When taken orally, lapachol is secreted into the skin where it provides a barrier to the larvae of schistosomes. Beta-lapa-chone destroys the parasite responsible for trypanosomiasis (Chagas' disease).

  In other studies, pau d'arco extracts were effective in reducing inflammation associated with cervicitis and cervicovaginitis. Although extracts reportedly had low toxicity in several investigations, lapachol is known to be toxic when administered as an isolated active principle. Lapachol destroys vitamin K activity. Interestingly, pau d'arco contains a vitamin K–like compound that probably compensates for the anti–vitamin K action of lapachol. This may explain why remedies made from the whole plant do not interfere with vitamin K activity.

  In in vivo studies, lapachol exhibited anticancer effects against Walker 256 carinosarcoma, Yoshida sarcoma, and Murphy-Sturm lymphosarcoma. Despite these promising results, lapachol is not a practical cancer therapy. When given at therapeutically effective doses, lapachol produces the adverse side effects of nausea, vomiting, anemia, and a tendency to bleed. Monkeys given daily doses of 0.0625 to 0.25 g/kg of lapachol developed severe anemia, especially during the initial two weeks of treatment.

  Lapachol seemed to be a promising new drug when Phase I clinical trials on its safety were first launched at the National Cancer Institue (NCI) in 1968, but researchers soon discovered that therapeutic doses produced mildly toxic side effects. There have been no clinical investigations on the efficacy of lapachol for treating cancer and other diseases because this compound is too toxic for human consumption. However, the anthraquinones in pau d'arco exhibited vitamin K–like activity. It is possible that anti–vitamin K adverse side effects may not have occurred in the NCI study had the whole plant been used instead of lapachol, the isolated compound.

Dosage Ranges and Duration of Administration

- One cup decocted bark 2 to 8 times/day (1 tsp. pau d'arco boiled in 1 cup water 5 to 15 min)
- Tincture 1:5: 1 ml tid or qid
- Capsules: 1,000 mg tid

Cautions

- **Adverse Effects/Toxicology**

  - Large doses can cause nausea.
  - Whole bark decoctions do not appear to be toxic for human consumption even though lapachol, one of the active constituents, causes adverse side effects.

- **Warnings/Contraindications/Precautions**
  Individuals prone to blood-clotting conditions should consult with their health care practitioner before using pau d'arco.

Interactions

No interactions have been reported.

Regulatory and Compendial Status

The U.S. FDA classifies pau d'arco as a dietary supplement.

References

Anesini C, et al. Screening of plants used in Argentine folk medicine for antimicrobial activity. *J Ethnopharmacol.* 1993;39:119–128.

Block J, Sterpick A, Miller W, Wiernik P. Early clinical studies with lapachol (NSC-11905). *Cancer Chemother Rep* 1974;4(part 2):27–28.

Gershon H, Shanks L. Fungitoxicity of 1,4-naphthoquinones to *Candida albicans* and *Trichophyton mentagrophytes. Can J of Microbio.* 1975;21:1317–1321.

Duke J, Vasquez R. *Amazonian Ethnobotanical Dictionary.* Boca Raton, Fla: CRC Press; 1994:164.

Kinghorn AD, Balandrin MA, eds. *Human Medicinal Agents from Plants.* Washington, DC: American Chemical Society; 1993:16–17.

Murray MT. *The Healing Power of Herbs: The Enlightened Person's Guide to the Wonders of Medicinal Plants.* 2nd ed. Rocklin, Calif: Prima Publishing; 1995:220–227.

Nakona K, et al. Iridoids From *Tabebuia Avellanedae Phytochemisty.* 1993;32:371–373.

Perez H, et al. Chemical Investigations and in Vitro Antimalarial Activity of *Tabebuia ochracea* ssp. Neochrysanta. *International Journal of Pharmacognosy.* 1997;35:227–231.

Schultes RE, Raffauf RF. *The Healing Forest: Medicinal and Toxic Plants of the Northwest Amazonia.* Portland, Ore: Dioscorides Press; 1990:107–109.

Shealy CN. *The Illustrated Encyclopedia of Healing Remedies.* Dorset UK: Element Books; 1998:132.

Tyler VE. *Herbs of Choice: The Therapeutic Use of Phytomedicinals.* Binghamton, NY: Pharmaceutical Products Press; 1994:180.

Tyler VE. *The Honest Herbal: A Sensible Guide to the Use of Herbs and Related Remedies.* 3rd ed. Binghamton, NY: Pharmaceutical Products Press; 1993:239–240.

Ueda S, et al. Production of anti-tumour-promoting furanonaphthoquinones in *Tabebuia avellanedae* cell cultures. *Phytochemistry.* 1994;36:323–325.

© *Copyright Integrative Medicine Communications*

Peppermint

Names

- **English**
  Peppermint leaf/peppermint oil

- **Botanical**
  Mentha x piperita

- **Plant Family**
  Lamiaceae

- **Pharmacopeial**
  Menthae piperitae folium/Menthae piperitae aetheroleum

Overview

Peppermint is widely used for its antispasmodic, antiseptic, carminative, anaesthetic, and choleretic properties. It aids digestion and is held to be helpful for many stomach problems, irritable bowel syndrome, nausea, morning sickness, dysmenorrhea, diarrhea, constipation, and flatulence. In larger doses, it may have an emmenagogic effect. Studies show that peppermint oil acts as a choleretic, stimulating the flow of bile, which improves digestion. Peppermint oil also has antiviral properties, inhibiting many viruses that cause digestive problems.

Menthol, a major constituent of peppermint oil, is well known for its external analgesic counterirritant effects. It cools as well as numbs the skin, producing effective relief from the itching caused by hives and poison ivy. A combination of peppermint oil's analgesic and antispasmodic properties also make it an effective remedy for headaches. Studies suggest that correct use of the oil can be as effective as taking 1 g of acetaminophen.

Peppermint and menthol appear most frequently in cold medicines, where they are effective as decongestants. The strong antiviral properties of peppermint are most concentrated in the tea form, and drinking it will restrict the growth of many cold and flu viruses. It is also very effective for a dry cough, because it calms the throat muscles, and as an expectorant, because menthol thins the mucus.

Macro Description

Square stems grow up to two feet tall. Flowers are tiny, purple, in whorls and terminal spikes, with four stamens. Leaves are opposite, simple, toothed, and very fragrant. It blooms from July through August. Peppermint is native to Europe and Asia; some types are indigenous to South Africa, South America, and Australia. It is naturalized in North America and cultivated primarily in Oregon, Washington, and Wisconsin.

Part Used/Pharmaceutical Designations

- Flower
- Leaves
- Oil

- **Constituents/Composition**
  The herb consists of the leaves and flowering tops of *Mentha x piperita* (family Lamiaceae) and is made up of volatile oil (0.5% to 4%) composed of 50% to 78% menthol and 5% to 20% menthol esterfied with various organic acids, such as acetic and bovaleric. Also flavonoids (luteolin, menthoside), phenolic acids, and triterpenes.

- **Commercial Preparations**
  Packaged peppermint tea is widely available or may be made from dried fresh peppermint leaves.
  Tinctures: Peppermint spirit is an alcoholic solution containing 10% peppermint oil and 1% peppermint leaf extract. To make a tincture, add one part peppermint oil to nine parts pure grain alcohol.
  Enteric-coated capsules (0.2 ml of peppermint oil per capsule)
  Creams or ointments (should contain 1% to 16% menthol): Mentholatum or Vicks VapoRub

Medicinal Uses/Indications

Traditional: antispasmodic, carminative, choleretic, antibacterial, decongestant, external analgesic, antiemetic, aromatic, emmenagogue, antiparasitic, stimulant

Conditions: irritable bowel syndrome, nausea, morning sickness, diarrhea, dysmenorrhea, constipation, flatulence, gallstones, headache, hives, nasal congestion, dry cough

Clinical applications: spastic complaints of gastrointestinal tract and bile ducts, irritable colon, catarrhs of respiratory tract, inflammation of oral mucosa, myalgic and neuralgic conditions

- **Pharmacology**
  Peppermint's primary active component is menthol, the focus of most scientific experiments, which have determined it to be effective internally as an antispasmodic, carminative, choleretic, decongestant, and antibacterial, and externally as an analgesic.

  Peppermint's carminative properties work by relaxing the esophageal sphincter, allowing gas pressure to escape the stomach. Because of this, peppermint should not be used in case of gastro-esophogeal reflux disease because it may exacerbate the condition. Peppermint oil antagonizes the spasmogenic action of barium chloride, pilocarpine, and physostigmine. It also acts competitively with nifedipine and blocks Ca 2^+ exciting stimuli, thereby inhibiting muscle contractions. A recent study reported that 89.5% of patients with irritable bowel syndrome showed significant improvement in abdominal symptoms after being treated with enteric-coated peppermint oil capsules. The enteric coating allows the peppermint oil to reach the intestines without being absorbed into the stomach. In the intestines, the oil is believed to inhibit the hypercontractility of intestinal smooth muscle and restore proper muscle tone.

  In vitro studies show that peppermint oil can inhibit and destroy influenza A viruses, herpes simplex, mumps virus, *Streptococcus pyogenes*, *Staphylococcus aureus*, *Pseudomonas aeruginosa*, and *Candida albicans*. The menthol and related terpenes found in peppermint oil have been shown by several studies to dissolve gallstones by lowering bile cholesterol levels while raising bile acid and lecithin levels in the gallbladder.

  Peppermint works as an external analgesic by blocking muscle contractions caused by serotonin and substance P, but it also stimulates cold receptors on the skin, which may influence the spinal cord's pain transmissions. The oil also relaxes the pericranial muscles and increases blood flow to the capillaries, making it an effective treatment for headaches.

Dosage Ranges and Duration of Administration

- For digestion and upset stomach, peppermint tea (infusion), 1 to 2 tsp. of dried leaves per 8 oz. of water, 3 to 4 cups daily between meals; peppermint glycente for children, 1 to 2 ml daily
- For gallstones and irritable bowel syndrome, 1 to 2 enteric-coated capsules tid between meals
- As an external analgesic, menthol in a cream or ointment form no more than tid to qid
- For upset stomach or vomiting, 3 to 6 g of leaf, or 5 to 15 drops of tincture
- For tension headaches, tincture of peppermint oil. Apply light coating to entire forehead with fingertips or small sponge. If there is occipital pain, apply to back of neck as well. Allow to evaporate.

Cautions

- **Adverse Effects/Toxicology**
  When taken as a tea, peppermint is usually considered safe, although hypersensitivity reactions have been reported. Rare negative reactions to enteric-coated peppermint oil capsules may include skin rash, heartburn, bradycardia (slowed heartbeat), and muscle tremors. Menthol or peppermint oil applied topically could cause contact dermatitis or rash. Peppermint oil should be diluted and taken in small amounts, as excessive ingestion could cause interstitial nephritis and acute renal failure. An estimated fatal dose of menthol is 2 to 9 g if taken internally. There are no known mutagenic or carcinogenic effects.

- **Warnings/Contraindications/Precautions**
  No contraindications to peppermint as an herb. Peppermint oil is contraindicated by biliary tract obstruction, cholecystitis, and severe liver damage. Infants and small children should not use peppermint tea or oil. Pregnant or nursing mothers should use peppermint tea only in small doses and those with a history of miscarriage should avoid it. Do not mistake oil for tincture preparations.

Interactions

None known.

Regulatory and Compendial Status

On the U.S. FDA's list of herbs, peppermint is generally regarded as safe as a dietary supplement. The German Commission E approves it for internal use as an antispasmodic, carminative, choleretic, and decongestant, and for external use as an analgesic.

References

Blumenthal M, ed. *The Complete German Commission E Monographs.* Boston, Mass: Integrative Medicine Communications; 1998.

Castleman M. *The Healing Herbs.* New York, NY: Bantam Books; 1991.

Dew MJ, Evans BK, Rhodes J. Peppermint oil for the irritable bowel syndrome: a multicentre trial. *Br J Clin Pract.* 1984;(11–12):394, 398.

Duke J. *The Green Pharmacy.* Emmaus, Pa: Rodale Press; 1997.

Feng XZ. Effect of Peppermint oil hot compresses in preventing abdominal distension in postoperative gynecological patients [In Chinese]. *Chung Hua Hu Li Tsa Chih.* 1997; 32:577–578.

Hills J. The mechanism of action of peppermint oil on gastrointestinal smooth muscle. *Gastroenterology.* 1991;101:55–65.

Koch TR. Peppermint oil and irritable bowel syndrome [In Process Citation]. *Am J Gastroenterol.* 1998;93:2304–2305.

Kowalchik C, Hylton W, eds. *Rodale's Illustrated Encyclopedia of Herbs.* Emmaus, Pa: Rodale Press; 1987.

Lawson MJ, Knight, RE, Tran K, Walker G, Robers-Thompson, IC. Failure of enteric-coated peppermint oil in the irritable bowel syndrome: a randomized double-blind crossover study. *J Gastroent Hepatol.* 1988;3:235–238.

Mowrey D. *The Scientific Validation of Herbal Medicine.* New Canaan, Conn: Keats Publishing, Inc; 1986.

Murray MT. *The Healing Power of Herbs.* Rocklin, Calif: Prima Publishing; 1995.

Pittler MH, Ernst E. Peppermint oil for irritable bowel syndrome: a critical review and metaanalysis. *Am J Gastroenterol.* 1998;93:1131–1135.

Rees W. Treating irritable bowel syndrome with peppermint oil. *Br Med J.* 1979;II:835–836.

Schulz V, Hnsel R, Tyler V. *Rational Phytotherapy.* Berlin, Germany: Springer; 1998.

Tyler V. *Herbs of Choice: The Therapeutic Use of Phytomedicinals.* New York, NY: Pharmaceutical Products Press; 1994.

© *Copyright Integrative Medicine Communications*

Rosemary

Names

- **English**
  Rosemary

- **Botanical**
  Rosmarinus officinalis

- **Plant Family**
  Lamiaceae

- **Pharmacopeial**
  Rosmarini

Overview

Native to Portugal and the Mediterranean area, rosemary is widely cultivated in several parts of the world, especially Morocco, Spain, Tunisia, and France. Rosemary takes it name from *ros marinus,* a Latin term which means "sea dew." Well known to the ancients, this plant was touted as a remedy for improving memory.

Rosemary today is used more frequently as a household spice and a food flavoring than a medicinal agent. However, it has traditionally been employed as a diuretic, emmenagogue, and antispasmodic remedy. The oil is a skin irritant in humans, and when administered externally, it increases blood supply. During the 19th century, rosemary leaf and its essential oil were used as a tonic for hypotension and other circulatory ailments. However, the evidence for the effectiveness of rosemary given orally in treating chronic circulatory weakness is controversial.

Rosemary oil is often unsafe for internal consumption since a large amount of it is required for therapeutic benefits. Ingesting excessive quantities of rosemary can irritate the stomach, intestines, and kidneys.

Macro Description

Rosmarinus officinalis is an erect evergreen shrub that grows to a height of two meters. It thrives in somewhat dry soil and a light, warm environment. The woody rootstock bears rigid branches with fissured bark. The long, linear, needle-like leaves are dark green above and white beneath. Both the fresh and dried leaves are pungently aromatic with a slight camphor-like scent. The small, labiate flowers are pale-blue. Volatile oil is found in the leaves and calyces of the flowers.

Part Used/Pharmaceutical Designation

- Leaves
- Twigs

Constituents/Composition

- Volatile oil (1.0% to 2.5%); chief components are monoterpene hydrocarbons, camphene and limonene, 1,8-cineole (20% to 50%), alpha-pinene (15% to 25%), camphor (10% to 25%); other compounds include cineole, linalool, verbinol, camphene, borneol, isobutyl acetate, beta-caryophyllene, p-cymene, myrcene, terpineol, 3-octonone, isobornyl acetate)
- Terpenoids: carnosol (diterpene, bitter), carnosolic acid (picrosalvin), oleanolic acid (10%), ursolic acid (5%) (triterpenes), isorosmanol, rosmadial, rosmaridiphenol, rosmariquinone
- Phenols: caffeic acid derivatives (e.g., rosmarinic, neochlorogenic, cholorogenic, and labiatic acids)
- Flavonoids: cirsimarin, diosmetin, diosmin, hesperidin, luteolin and derivatives, hispidulin, apigenin, homoplantiginin, phegopolin
- Tannins: oligomeric proanthocyanidins (15%)

Commercial Preparations

Commercial preparations of rosemary are available as powdered herb, dry extract, and other preparations derived from fresh or dried leaves. Infusions for internal and external use are made with cut or ground dried leaf material collected during flowering. Rosemary herb generally contains a minimum of 1.2% (v/w) volatile oil, and is often added to remedies for dyspeptic and rheumatic conditions. Plant material grown in southern regions such as Dalmatia is especially valued for medicinal preparations because of its more pungent aroma.

Medicinal Uses/Indications

Traditional internal uses: dyspepsia (gastrointestinal ailments), headache, spasmolytic, sedative, diuretic, antimicrobial, diaphoretic (perspiration-promoting), emmenagogues (menstrual-flow stimulating), abortifacients

Traditional external uses: poultice for wound healing, eczema; topically for myalgia, sciatica, intercostal neuralgia, rubefacient, mild analgesic, parasiticidal; balneotherapy; supportive therapy (adjuvant) for circulatory disorders, rheumatic conditions

Conditions: digestive (dyspepsia), circulatory, pain, neuralgia, spasm nervousness, diuretic, wounds, eczema, myalgia, sciatica, rheumatism, parasites

Clinical applications: loss of appetite, blood pressure problems, liver and gallbladder complaints, rheumatism

Pharmacology

Numerous studies have shown that rosemary has a wide array of pharmacological properties. Rosemary oil exhibited antibacterial and anti fungal activities in vitro. Two of its constituents, carnosol and ursolic acid, had antioxidant effects against spoilage microbes. The oil and several of its active principles produced spasmolytic effects in smooth muscle (gallbladder and small intestines) and, to a lesser extent, in cardiac muscle. A calcium antagonistic action of rosemary may be responsible for the antispasmolytic activity.

In an in vivo study, rosemary extract added to the diet produced a significant (47%) decline in mammary tumor incidence compared to controls. Topical preparations of both carnosol and ursolic acid inhibited tumor promotion. In other research, carnosol inhibited the initiation of carcinogenesis by increasing detoxification of a procarcinogen in human bronchial epithelial cells.

Recent evidence suggests that rosmarinic acid, one of the major constituents of the leaves, has anticomplement and antioxidant properties, thus making rosemary a potential prophylactic for endotoxin shock and adult respiratory distress syndrome. In another investigation, ethanol extracts of young sprouts from rosemary produced significant dose-related choleretic effects while aqueous extracts of young sprouts showed significant hepatoprotective activity.

In an animal study evaluating the abortive effects of rosemary, an extract elicited an anti-implantation effect during the pre-implantation period. However, rosemary did not interfere with the normal development of conception following implantation.

Rosemary oil administered orally or by inhalation enhanced locomotion activity in animals. Other constituents isolated from rosemary reduced capillary permeability.

Dosage Ranges and Duration of Administration

Internal:

- Tincture (1:5): 2 to 4 ml tid
- Infusion: 2 to 4 g tid
- Fluid extract (1:1 in 45% alcohol): 1 to 2 ml tid
- Essential oil (traditional preparation): 2 to 4 drops (however, Germany's Commission E advises against internal use of essential oil)
- Rosemary wine: 20 g herb is added to 1 liter of wine and allowed to stand for five days, shake occasionally

External:

- Essential oil (6% to 10%): 2 drops semisolid or liquid in 1 tablespoon base oil
- Infusion: 50 g herb in 1 liter hot water is added to bath water

Cautions

Adverse Effects/Toxicology

Rosemary oil is generally non-irritating and non-sensitizing when used topically in humans. However, erythema and dermatitis can occur in hypersensitive individuals, and photosensitivity has been reported. The toxicity of rosmarinic acid in mice is low (LD_{50}, 561 mg/kg IV), and this compound is readily removed from the circulation. Doses above 50 mg/kg IV can exacerbate transient cardiovascular actions.

Warnings/Contraindications/Precautions

Rosemary is generally considered safe and devoid of adverse side effects when administered in recommended therapeutic dosages. However, there have been occasional reports of contact allergies.

Large quantities of rosemary leaves, particularly rosemary oil, can cause adverse side effects of coma, spasm, vomiting, gastroenteritis, uterine bleeding, kidney irritation, and in some cases, concomitant pulmonary edema fatal to humans. Rosemary should not be used during pregnancy or lactation.

Topical preparations containing rosemary oil are potentially harmful to hypersensitive individuals who may be allergic to camphor. Excessive quantities of rosemary oil (10% to 20% camphor) taken orally can trigger epileptiform convulsions. Epileptic patients should thus exercise caution in using rosemary and never ingest quantities larger than those used in foodstuffs.

Interactions

None reported.

Regulatory and Compendial Status

In the United Kingdom, rosemary is listed in the General Sale List (GSL). Both the herb and oil are listed in category N2 as a source of natural food flavoring by the Council of Europe. Herbs in this category can be added to foodstuffs in small quantities.

References

Aqel MB. Relaxant effect of the volatile oil of *Rosmarinus officinalis* on tracheal smooth muscle. *J Ethnopharmacol.* 1991;33(1–2):57–62.

Blumenthal M, ed. *The Complete German Commission E Monographs.* Boston, Mass: Integrative Medicine Communications; 1998:197.

Dorland's Illustrated Medical Dictionary. 25th ed. Philadelphia, Pa: WB. Saunders; 1974.

Grieve M. *A Modern Herbal.* Vol. II. New York, NY: Dover; 1971:681–683.

Gruenwald J, Brendler T, Jaenicke C. *PDR for Herbal Medicines.* Montvale, NJ: Medical Economics Company; 1998:1101–1103.

Hoefler C, Fleurentin J, Mortier F, Pelt JM, Guillemain J. Comparative choleretic and hepatoprotective properties of young sprouts and total plant extracts of *Rosmarinus officinalis* in rats. *J Ethnopharmacol.* 1987;19(2):133–143.

Huang MT, Ho CT, Wang ZY, et al. Inhibition of skin tumorigenesis by rosemary and its constituents carnosol and ursolic acid. *Cancer Res.* 1994;54(ISS 3):701–708.

Lemonica IP, Damasceno DC, di-Stasi LC. Study of the embryotoxic effects of an extract of rosemary (*Rosmarinus officinalis* L.) *Braz Med Biol Res.* 1996;19(2):223–227.

Newall C, Anderson L, Phillipson J. *Herbal Medicines: A Guide for Health-care Professionals.* London, England: Pharmaceutical Press; 1996: 229–230.

Offord EA, Mac K, Ruffieux C, Malne A, Pfeifer AM. Rosemary components inhibit benzo[a]pyrene-induced genotoxicity in human bronchial cells. *Carcinogenesis.* 1995;16(ISS 9):2057–2062.

Schulz V, Hansel R, Tyler V. *Rational Phytotherapy: A Physicians' Guide to Herbal Medicine.* 3rd ed. Berlin, Germany: Springer; 1998:105.

Singletary KW, Nelshoppen JM. Inhibition of 7,12-dimethylbenz[a]anthracene (DMBA)-induced mammary umorigenesis and of in vivo formation of mammary DMBA-DNA adducts by rosemary extract. *Cancer Lett.* 1991;10(6):169–175.

Thomson WA. *Medicines from the Earth: A Guide to Healing Plants.* Maidenhead, England: McGraw-Hill Book Company; 1978:95.

Tyler V. *Herbs of Choice: The Therapeutic Use of Phytomedicinals.* Binghamton, NY: Pharmaceutical Products Press; 1994:111.

Tyler V. *The Honest Herbal: A Sensible Guide to the Use of Herbs and Related Remedies.* 3rd ed. New York: Pharmaceutical Products Press; 1993:265–266.

© Copyright Integrative Medicine Communications

Saw Palmetto

Names

■ **English**
Saw Palmetto Berry

■ **Botanical**
Serenoa repens/Sabal serrulata

■ **Plant Family**
Aracaceae

■ **Pharmacopeial**
Sabal fructus

Overview

Saw palmetto is a leading treatment for benign prostatic hyperplasia (BPH) in Germany and Austria, and is among the top five dietary supplements sold in the United States. It relieves bladder and urinary disturbances associated with stage I and II BPH. Stage I symptoms include frequent urination, nocturea, delayed urination, low urinary force, and post-void dribbling; stage II symptoms herald bladder function debility and include urgency and incomplete emptying of the bladder. Sexual dysfunction has also been reported. The majority of men over 60 are considered to have urinary symptoms attributable to BPH. The condition may progress to prostate cancer, bladder infections, and damaged kidneys if left untreated.

First used in the treatment of BPH late in the nineteenth century, saw palmetto has been the subject of at least 20 laboratory studies and 18 clinical studies. These experiments demonstrated saw palmetto's antiestrogenic and antiandrogenic effects and confirmed that the berry extract reduces 5-alpha-reductase. These are considered significant interventions in the treatment of BPH.

Most recently, researchers assessed the results of 18 controlled trials and concluded that saw palmetto can be as effective as finasteride in improving BPH-affected urine flow and urgency. Compared to placebo, saw palmetto relieved nocturia by 25%, urinary tract symptoms by 28%, increased peak urine flow by 28%, and decreased residual volume by 43%. Finasteride does shrink the prostate, however, and saw palmetto does not.

Saw palmetto berries provided food and medicine for Native Americans for centuries. Aside from their nutritional value, the berries were considered expectorant, sedative, and diuretic by traditional folk healers. It was used to reduce inflammation in genitourinary catarrh and to treat breast disorders in women. Some herbalists claim that saw palmetto can increase breast size, and that it is an aphrodisiac. These claims are unsubstantiated, however.

From 1906 to 1916, saw palmetto berries were listed in the U.S. Pharmacopoeia and were described as effective remedies for chronic and subacute cystitis, chronic bronchitis, laryngitis, catarrh that accompanies asthma, and enlarged prostate glands. It was also in the National Formulary from 1926 to 1950.

Macro Description

The saw palmetto shrub is a fan palm that grows from 6 to 10 feet in warm climates, from South Carolina to Mississippi and throughout Florida. Lush palmate leaves have lance-shaped leaflets and are supported by spiny stems. Flowers are white and develop yellow olive-like berries, which become bluish-black when ripe and have an oily sheen attributable to their fatty acid content.

Part Used/Pharmaceutical Designations

- Berries

■ **Constituents/Composition**
Saturated and unsaturated, mostly free fatty acids (capric, caprylic, caproic, lauric, palmitic, and oleic acids); free and conjugated sterols; fruits also contain high-molecular weight polysaccharides and flavonoids. Fat-soluble extracts are standardized to contain 85% to 95% fatty acids and sterols.

■ **Commercial Preparations**
Crude dried berries, tea, powdered encapsulations, tablets, tinctures, and liposterolic extracts standardized to contain 85% to 95% fatty acids and sterols.

Medicinal Uses/Indications

Saw palmetto was historically used as an expectorant and to treat general debility, respiratory catarrh, and muscle wasting due to age or menopause.

Traditional herbal actions: Tonic for both female and male reproductive systems and urinary tracts, nourishing tonic, anti-inflammatory, urinary antiseptic, relaxant, diuretic.

Clinical applications: Used for the relief of symptoms of stage I and II BPH. Future research may lead to the treatment of female androgen excess disorders, such as hirsutism and polycystic ovary disease. Increases milk flow in nursing mothers, used to treat infections of the genito-urinary system, such as cystitis, urethritis, and salpingitis.

■ **Pharmacology**
Liposterolic extracts act at the cytosolic, androgenic receptor of prostate tissue in vitro to inhibit 5-alpha-reductase, block adrenergic receptors, and inhibit DHT-producing enzymes. Inhibition of dihydrotestosterone (DHT) and 5-alpha-reductase may have a positive effect in the treatment of BPH. Finasteride inhibits 5-alpha-reductase, which in turn blocks testosterone from transforming into DHT, and DHT may be responsible for the hyperproliferation of prostate cells involved in the etiology of BPH.

Despite evidence of estrogenic activity, liposterolic extracts also significantly stimulate antiestrogenic effects; it blocked nuclear estrogen receptors in prostatic tissue samples of patients with BPH. After a 90-day treatment period, researchers analyzed the function of androgen, estrogen, and progesterone receptor tissues in 35 study participants. The group given saw palmetto extract had lower cellular and nuclear estrogen and progesterone receptor values than the placebo group. Cellular androgen levels remained the same, but nuclear androgen levels declined. Estrogen may promote BPH due to inhibition of hydroxylation and elimination of DHT. Some investigators feel that estrogen's role in BPH is more significant than that of DHT.

Dosage Ranges and Duration of Administration

To reduce symptoms associated with stages I and II BPH: 160 mg liposterolic extract, standardized to contain 85% to 95% fatty acids and sterols, or equivalent, bid.

- Tincture (1:4): 2 to 4 ml tid
- Fluid extract of dried berry pulp (1:1): 1 to 2 ml tid
- Capsules: 1,000 mg tid
- Tea: 2 tsp. dried berry with 24 oz. water, simmer slowly until liquid is reduced by half, take 4 oz. tid. The tea tastes vile but is effective.

Cautions

■ **Adverse Effects/Toxicology**
Adverse effects are very rare and include mild stomach upset. The American Herbal Products Association gives saw palmetto a class 1 safety rating, indicating that it is safe with appropriate use.

■ **Warnings/Contraindications/Precautions**
Before self-medicating with saw palmetto, patients should get a firm diagnosis of BPH. Although saw palmetto relieves symptoms, it does not shrink the prostate; therefore, the condition should be closely monitored by a health care provider.

Saw palmetto has hormonal effects and should not be used during pregnancy or lactation until specific studies prove otherwise.

Interactions

Saw palmetto may interfere with hormonal therapies such as contraceptive pills and patches and hormone-replacement therapy.

Regulatory and Compendial Status

Dietary supplement in the U.S., saw palmetto is approved for use in the treatment of stage I and II BPH by Germany's Commission E, and is on the General Sales List (GSL) in England.

References

Blumenthal M, ed. *The Complete German Commission E Monographs: Therapeutic Guide to Herbal Medicine.* Boston, Mass: Integrative Medicine Communications; 1998.

Braeckman J. The extract of *Serenoa repens* in the treatment of benign prostatic hyperplasia: A multicenter open study. *Curr Therapeut Res* 1994;55:776–785.

Saw Palmetto — Herbals

Carilla E, Briley M, Fauran F, et al. Binding of Permixon, a new treatment for prostatic benign hyperplasia, to the cytosolic androgen receptor in the rat prostate. *J Steroid Biochem* 1984;20:521–523.

Carraro JC, et al. Comparison of phytotherapy (Permixon) with finasteride in the treatment of benign prostate hyperplasia: a randomized international study of 1,098 patients. *The Prostate.* 1996;29(4):231–240.

Di Silverio F, D'Eramo G, Lubrano C, et al. Evidence that *Serenoa repens* extract displays an antiestrogenic activity in prostatic tissue of benign prostatic hypertrophy patients. *Eur Uro.* 1992;21:309–314.

el-Sheikh M, Dakkak MR, Saddique A. The effect of permixon on androgen receptors. *Acta Obstet Gynecol Scand.* 1988;67:397–399.

Hutchens AR. *Indian Herbalogy of North America.* Boston, Mass: Shambhala Publications; 1973:243–244.

Leung A, Foster S. *Encyclopedia of Common Natural Ingredients Used in Food, Drugs, and Cosmetics.* 2nd ed. New York, NY: John Wiley & Sons; 1996:467–468.

McGuffin M, Hobbs C, Upton R, Goldberg A. *American Herbal Products Association's Botanical Safety Handbook.* Boca Raton, Fla: CRC Press; 1996.

Murray MT. *The Healing Power of Herbs: Tthe Enlightened Person's Guide to the Wonders of Medicinal Plants.* Rocklin, Calif: Prima Publishing; 1995.

Newall CA, Anderson LA, Phillipson JD. *Herbal Medicines: A Guide for Health-Care Professionals.* London, England: The Pharmaceutical Press; 1996.

Schulz V, Hnsel R, Tyler VE. *Rational Phytotherapy: A Physicians' Guide to Herbal Medicine.* Berlin, Germany: Springer-Verlag; 1998.

Skeland J, Albrecht J. A combination of *Sabal* and *Urtica* extracts vs. finasteride in BHP (stage I to II acc. to Alken): A comparison of therapeutic efficacy in a one-year double-blind study. *Urologe A.* 1997;36:327–333.

Mandressi A, et al. Treatment of uncomplicated benign prostatic hypertrophy BPH by an extract of *Serenoa Repens* clinical results. *J Endocrinol Invest* 1987;10(suppl 2):49.

Wilt TJ, Ishani A, Stark G, et al. Saw palmetto extracts for treatment of benign prostatic hyperplasia: a systematic review. *JAMA.* 1998;280:1604–1609.

Wood HC, Osol A. *United States Dispensatory.* 23rd ed. Philadelphia, Pa: J.B. Lippincott; 1943;971–972.

Champault G, Patel JC, Bonnard AM. A double-blind trial of an extract of the plant *Serenoa repens* in benign prostatic hyperplasia. *Br J Clin Pharmacol.* 1984;18:461–462.

© *Copyright Integrative Medicine Communications*

Skullcap

Names

- **English**
  Skullcap

- **Botanical**
  Scutellaria lateriflora

- **Plant Family**
  Labiatae

- **Pharmacopeial**
  Scutellariae herba

Overview

Scutellaria lateriflora is one of 90 species in the genus *Scutellaria* distributed throughout temperate and tropical regions. Most *Scutellaria* species thrive in garden soils (particularly soils with sunny, open borders) and generally die off after two or three years. Many of the closely related species in this genus are found in the United States. Although *Scutellaria lateriflora* is native to North America, it is now widely cultivated in Europe. This particular species is also called mad-dog skullcap because of its traditional use in treating hydrophobia.

Scutellaria lateriflora is slightly astringent and widely touted as a nervine. Its tonic, sedative, and antispasmodic activities are reportedly so pronounced that it has long been hailed as an effective therapy for hysteria, convulsions, hydrophobia, and epilepsy. Among its other varied uses are as a treatment for rickets, neuralgia, pain, hiccough, nervous headaches, and headaches associated with incessant coughing.

Despite these popular uses, precise structure-activity relationships have not been determined for skullcap. Even though flavonoids are presumably responsible for many of its purported pharmacological effects, therapeutic claims for *Scutellaria lateriflora* have not been fully substantiated scientifically.

Skullcap has in the past been frequently adulterated with *Teucrium* species, a group of plants known to contain potential liver toxins. Because of its possibility for causing serious adverse side effects, including hepatotoxicity and hepatitis, skullcap should not be used unless taken under the direct supervision of a qualified health care practitioner knowledgeable about this plant, and care should be taken to buy the herb from a reliable source.

Macro Description

Scutellaria lateriflora is a slender, perennial, herbaceous plant that grows to a height of 60 cm. Although its erect stem is heavily branched, it is rarely shrubby. Skullcap is distinguished by a thick cover of simple and glandular hairs. Its leaves are typically ovate to lanceolate and petioled, with either complete or scalloped margins.

Skullcap blooms in July, giving rise to barely conspicuous blue and sometimes pink flowers that take the form of short lateral false spikes. The fluffy calyx (sepals) is flattened with two rounded, complete lips. The upper and lower sides of the calyx have different appearances. The flowers have four ascending stamens, each with a pair of cilated anthers. The fruit consists of a warty nut that is globular to flattened-ovoid in shape.

Part Used/Pharmaceutical Designations

- Herb (1 to 2 year-old plant harvested in early summer).

- **Constituents/Composition**
  Flavonoids (apigenin, hispidulin, luteolin, scutellarein, scutellarin [bitter glycoside]); catalpol; volatile oils (limonen, terpineol [monoterpenes], d-cadinene, caryophyllene, trans-B-farnesene, B-humulene [sesquiterpenes]); other constituents (lignin, resin, tannin).
  Note: Published findings on the constituents of *Scutellaria lateriflora* are quite limited.

- **Commercial Preparations**
  Available for internal use as a powder or liquid extract made from the pulverized herb.

Medicinal Use/Indications

Traditional uses: epilepsy, chorea, hysteria, nervous tension, convulsions, hydrophobia, grand mal or St. Vitus's dance (epileptic seizure), nervous headaches, neuralgia, pain, hiccough, rickets, headache arising from incessant coughing.

Uses of *Scutellaria baicalensis* roots in Traditional Chinese Medicine: inflammation, suppurative dermatitis, allergic diseases, hyperlipidemia, atherosclerosis.

Conditions: historically used to treat hysteria, nervous tension, epilepsy, chorea, and other nervous disorders; also once used as bitter tonic and febrifuge (for fever).

Clinical applications: nervousness, anxiety, muscle spasm, nervous tics, restless legs syndrome, and mild Tourette's syndrome

- **Pharmacology**

Scutellaria latiflora reportedly possesses sedative, antispasmodic, and anti-inflammatory activities as well as inhibitory effects against lipid peroxidation. However, relatively little research has been conducted on *Scutellaria lateriflora*, and no in vivo data have been located for this species.

Pharmacological studies have been conducted on the root of a related species, *Scutellaria baicalensis*. Flavonoid compounds in *Scutellaria baicalensis* are responsible for several in vitro effects, including blockage of mast cell histamine release comparable to that of disodium cromoglycate; inhibition of lipid peroxidation; and inactivation of lipoxygenase and cyclo-oxygenase pathways.

Flavonoids may also account for certain in vivo activities of *Scutellaria baicalensis* such as hypocholesterolemia in rats. This latter activity has been associated with flavonoid-induced in vitro prevention of experimentally-induced hyperlipidemia and lipolysis, as well as flavonoid-induced in vitro lipogenesis in adipose tissues.

In certain animal investigations, *Scutellaria baicalensis* did not elicit a marked effect on blood pressure in cats and rabbits. Nor did it exert CNS depressant or antispasmodic action on test animals. However, *Scutellaria baicalensis* did exhibit antibacterial effects against several strains of Gram-positive bacteria. It is not clear, however, if these findings are relevant to the pharmacological effects of *Scutellaria lateriflora*.

In clinical trials conducted in China, scutellarin, the active constituent in several *Scutellaria* species, was administered i.m., i.v., or p.o. to over 600 patients diagnosed with cerebral thrombosis, cerebral embolism, and paralysis. An overall rate of efficacy of 88% was reported for this treatment.

Dosage Ranges and Duration of Administration

- Dried herb: 1 to 2 g or by infusion tid
- Fluid extract (1:1 in 25% alcohol): 2 to 4 ml tid
- Tincture (1:2 in 35% alcohol): 2 to 5 ml tid

Cautions

- **Adverse Effects/Toxicology**
  According to some authorities, skullcap is devoid of side effects when taken in recommended therapeutic dosages. However, other experts warn that because of the possibility of adulteration, skullcap should be used with caution.

- **Warnings/Contraindications/Precautions**
  Overdosage of skullcap tincture produces symptoms of giddiness, stupor, mental confusion, seizure, twitching of the limbs, intermission of the pulse, and epileptic-related manifestations. Oral intake of skullcap may be associated with hepatotoxic reactions, probably attributable to adulteration with *Teucrium* species, for example, *Teucrium chamaedrys* (germander).
  Skullcap should be avoided under all circumstances during pregnancy and lactation due to potential adulteration and subsequent liver toxicity.

Interactions

None reported

Regulatory and Compendial Status

Skullcap is an entry on the General Sales List in Great Britain. In the USA, the FDA designates skullcap as herb of undefined safety. This plant is not used in food products.

References

Grieve M. *A Modern Herbal. Vol. II.* New York: Dover; 1971: 724–725.

Gruenwald J, Brendler T, Christof J. *PDR for Herbal Medicines.* Montvale, NJ: Medical Economics Company; 1998: 1128–1129.

Newall C, Anderson L, Phillipson J. *Herbal Medicines: A Guide for Health-care Professionals.* London: Pharmaceutical Press; 1996: 239–240.

Peigen X, Keji C. Recent advances in clinical studies of Chinese medicinal herbs. I. Drugs affecting the cardiovascular system. *Phytotherapy Res.* 1987; 1: 53–57.

Kimura Y, et al. Studies on Scutellariae radix. IV. Effects on lipid peroxidation in rat liver. *Chem Pharm Bull.* 1981; 29: 2610–2617.

Kimura Y, et al. Studies on Scutellariae radix. VI. Effects of flavone compounds on lipid peroxidation in rat liver. *Chem Pharm Bull.* 1982; 30(5): 1792–1795.

Kimura Y, et al. Studies on Scutellariae radix. IX. New component inhibiting lipid peroxidation in rat liver. *Planta Med.* 1984; 50:290–295.

Kubo M, et al Scutellariae radix. X. Inhibitory effects of various flavonoids on histamine release from rat peritoneal mast cells in vitro. *Chem Pharm Bull.* 1984; 32: 5051–5054.

Kurnakov BA. Pharmacology of skullcap. *Farmakol i Toksikol.* 1957; 20: 79–80.

Larrey D, et al. Hepatitis after germander (*Teucrium chamaedrys*) administration: another instance of herbal medicine toxicity. *Ann Coll Physicians.* 1992; 117: 129–132.

© *Copyright Integrative Medicine Communications*

Slippery Elm

Names

- **English**
  Slippery Elm

- **Botanical**
  Ulmus fulva

- **Plant Family**
  Ulmaceae

- **Pharmacopeial**
  Ulmi rubrae

Overview

The inner bark of the slippery elm tree has been used as an herbal remedy in the United States for centuries. The mucilaginous texture of the bark is responsible for the medicinal properties of this plant. In fact, the mucilage is so effective in treating sore throats and coughs that the U.S. Food and Drug Administration has proclaimed slippery elm a safe and effective remedy for soothing throat and respiratory irritation. Slippery elm is an official drug of the U.S. Pharmacopoeia.

Native Americans traditionally employed slippery elm in healing salves for wounds, boils, ulcers, burns, and skin inflammation. Antiseptic poultices made from the mucilage were applied to gangrenous wounds. Legend has it that a drink made from the bark was used to treat typhoid fever. And a pinch of the powder inserted into a painful hollow tooth was said to be effective into preventing decay and discomfort.

Slippery elm is also considered a wholesome nutritional food. Because the mucilage does not dissolve but instead swells in water, it can be prepared as a gruel similar to oatmeal. Consumed three times per day, unsweetened "elm food" provides a sustaining source of nutrients for infants and invalids. It is gentle and easily assimilated, and thus well-tolerated by patients with gastritis and other forms of intestinal inflammation such as gastric catarrh, mucous colitis (inflammation of the colon), and enteritis (inflammation of the small intestine).

Today, the popularity of slippery elm continues to soar, dramatically increasing the demand for it. To further complicate matters, the wood of the slippery elm tree has no commercial value, and the trees are left to die after their bark has been harvested. Overutilization of this species has become such a problem that the National Center for the Preservation of Medicinal Herbs recently launched an effort aimed at promoting sustainable cultivation of slippery elm.

Macro Description

Slippery elm is a small- to medium-size tree native to North America. It can reach a height of 20 m tall and is topped by spreading branches that form an open crown. The red-brown or orange branches grow in a downward direction, and the stalkless flowers are arranged in dense, sessile-like clusters. Slippery elm is characterized by long, obovate to oblong green leaves that darken during the fall.

The bark has deep fissures, a mucilaginous texture, and a slight but distinct odor. The inner bark, or bast, is traditionally sold for medicinal purposes in long flat pieces about 2 to 3 feet long, between 1/8 to 1/16 of an inch in thickness.

Part Used/Pharmaceutical Designation

- Inner bark

- **Constituents/Composition**
  Mucilage (polysaccharides) is composed of hexoses, pentoses, methylpentoses, polyuronides, and one hexosan; after hydrolysis the mucilage yields galactose, glucose, galacturonic acid, *l*-rhamnose, *d*-galactose, trace amount of fructose. It also contains 3.0% to 6.5% tannins (unspecified), starch, minerals, phytosterols, sesquiterpenes, calcium oxalate, cholesterol.

- **Commercial Preparations**
  Commercial preparations are made from the inner bark and wood of slippery elm. Both finely powdered bark for mucilaginous drinks (infusions and decoctions) and coarsely powdered bark for poultices are available. Bark should be about 10 years old to ensure optimal medicinal benefits.

Medicinal Uses/Indications

Traditional uses: inflammation and ulcerations of gastrointestinal tract, demulcent (soother) of alimentary canal and other inflamed areas, emollient (skin softener and soother), nutrient, antitussive (cough preventative), and dumulcent

Internal uses: gastritis, gastric and duodenal ulcers, colitis, diarrhea, esophagitis, diverticulitis, dysentery, enteritis, inflammation of the mouth and throat, diarrhea (simultaneously soothes and astringes), convalescent or digestive food

External uses: poultice to treat wounds, burns, abscesses, boils, scalds, carbuncles (boil-like clusters), inflamed wounds, abrasions, ulcers, and other skin conditions; vaginitis, hemorrhoids, anal fissures, varicose ulcers

Clinical applications: inflammation and ulcerations of gastrointestinal tract; convalescence

- **Pharmacology**
  Only a small amount of scientific information has been published on the pharmacology of slippery elm. The demulcent and emollient properties of this plant presumably derive from mucilages, the main constituent of the bark. Mucilages are known to have beneficial effects on burns, wounds, ulcers, external and internal inflammations and irritations, diarrhea, and dysentery effects. Laboratory research has shown that mucilaginous medicinal plants are capable of decreasing local irritation in acute gastritis. In addition, mucilages from plants suppress coughing by providing a protective coating on the respiratory mucosa.

Dosage Ranges and Duration of Administration

Internal use:

- Decoction (1:8) made from powdered bark, 4 to 16 ml tid; or 5 to 20 ml (1:10) taken as often as needed (can be added to juice or oatmeal)
- Capsules: 2 to 4 g tid in 500 mg capsules
- Infusions: 4 g powdered bark in 500 ml boiling water tid as nutritional supplement

External use:
Coarse powdered bark (with adequate mucilage for viscosity, or mass consistency) is mixed with boiling water for poultices.

Cautions

- **Adverse Effects/Toxicology**
  There is inadequate information to determine the potential toxicity of slippery elm. There are no reports of toxicity and slippery elm is considered by most to be nontoxic, since none of its main constituents are known to produce adverse side effects. Although the Council of Europe lists this plant as a natural food flavoring, the Food Additives and Contaminants Committee (FACC) recommends that it not be used as a food additive.

- **Warnings/Contraindications/Precautions**
  No known side effects or health hazards have been reported for slippery elm when it is properly administered in recommended therapeutic doses.

Interactions

No adverse interactions with other substances have been reported.

Regulatory and Compendial Status

The powdered bark is listed as a licensed product in Schedule 1, Table A in the General Sale List (GSL) in the UK. Unpowdered or whole bark has restricted regulatory status for pharmacy use only. Slippery elm is an official entry in the U.S. Pharmacopoeia, and the U.S. FDA states that slippery elm is a safe and effective throat and respiratory soother.

References

Beveridge RJ, Szarek WA, Jones JK. Isolation of three oligosaccharides from the mucilage from the bark of *Ulmus fulva* (slippery elm mucilage). Synthesis of O-(3-)-Methyl-B-D-galactopyranosyl) (1-4)-L-rhamnose. *Carbohydr Res.* 1971;19:107–116.

Beveridge RJ, Stoddart JP, Szarek WA, Jones JK. Some structural features of the mucilage from the bark of *Ulmus fulva* (slippery elm mucilage). *Carbohydr Res.* 1969;9:429–439.

Blakley T. Slippery elm: Comparative study of the effects of plant spacing on plant development and yield. Research Farm Proposal No. 6088. Collaborating Team, The National Center for the Preservation of Medicinal Herbs. Project Period 1998–2008. Available at: www.ncpmh.org/6088.html.

British Herbal Pharmacopoeia. 4th ed. Great Britain:Biddles Ltd, Guildford and King's Lynn; 1996.

Duke JA. *The Green Pharmacy.* New York: St Martin's Press; 1977: 170, 209, 490 1997

Duke JA. Chemicals and their Biological Activities in: *Ulmus rubra* MUHLENB. (Ulmaceae)—Red Elm, Slippery Elm. Dr. Duke's Phytochemical and Ethnobotanical Databases. Agricultural Research Service (ARS), Phytochemical Database, USDA - ARS - NGRL, Beltsville Agricultural Research Center, Beltsville, Maryland. Available at: www.ars-grin.gov/cgi-bin/duke/farmacy2.pl.

Grieve M. *A Modern Herbal.* Vol. II. New York, NY: Dover; 1971.

Gruenwald J, Brendler T, Jaenicke C. *PDR for Herbal Medicines.* Montvale, NJ: Medical Economics Company; 1998.

Gysling E. *Leitfaden zur Pharmakotherpie.* Vienna: Huber, Bern Stuttgart; 1976:86.

Hahn HL. 1987 Husten: Mechanismen, pathophysiologie und therapie. *Disch Apoth A* 127. 1987;(suppl 5): 3–26.

Hoffman D. Slippery elm, 1995. Available at: www.healthy.net/hwlibrarybooks/hoffman/materiamedica/slippery.htm.

Kurz H. 1989 Antitussiva und Expektoranzien. *Wissenschaftliche.* Verlagsgesellschaft Stuggart; 1989.

Morton JF. Mucilaginous plants and their uses in medicine. *Biol Pharm Bull.* 1993;16: 735–739.

© *Copyright Integrative Medicine Communications*

Stinging Nettle

Names

■ **English**
Stinging nettle herb/stinging nettle leaf/stinging nettle root

■ **Botanical**
Urtica dioica/Urtica urens

■ **Plant Family**
Urticaceae

■ **Pharmacopeial**
Uticae herba/Urticae folium/Urticae radix

Overview

Stinging nettle usually refers to *Urtica dioica*, but it can also include a closely related species, *Urtica urens*, known as garden nettle, and hybrids of these two species. *Urtica dioica* is an annual native to the temperate regions of Eurasia, now found throughout the world.

Healers from many cultures use nettle branches as part of a whipping technique called flagellation or urtification. Whipping paralyzed limbs and other afflicted or painful body parts supposedly activates the muscles and stimulates the organs. Hot leaf poultices and pounded leaves made from nettle were traditionally used as topical treatments for rheumatic pain. The herb was also historically used to treat uterine hemorrhage (particularly after childbirth) and as a snuff for nosebleeds. Today, nettle root is an effective therapy for treating the symptoms of benign prostatic hyperplasia (BPH).

Macro Description

Stinging nettle *(Urica dioica)*, or common nettle, is an herbaceous shrub that reaches a height of nearly 3 feet. It prefers nitrogen-rich soil and blooms between June and September. The heart-shaped, finely toothed, tapered leaves are alternate and elliptical. The small green flowers are incomplete, and multiple types of flowers are often found on a single plant. The entire plant, especially the leaves and stem, is sparsely covered with stinging hairs that are painful when touched.

The stings are glandular hairs, or sharp, polished spines. Each hair contains an acrid fluid filled with histamine and formic acid. These chemical substances are released whenever the plant is forcefully applied to the skin, and they immediately irritate and inflame the skin. Histamine is probably responsible for the initial stinging sensation. However, nettle stings can have a therapeutic effect by acting as counter-irritants. Ironically, nettle juice can also be used as an antidote to painful nettle stings.

Part Used/Pharmaceutical Designations

- Seeds
- Leaves
- Roots (rhizome) and underground parts (fresh and dried)

■ **Constituents/Composition**
Flavonoids (in flowers) include glycosides of quercetins (isoquercitin, rutin), kaempferol, isohamnetin; amines (in stinging hairs) consist of small quantities of histamine, choline, acetylcholine, serotonin); chlorophylls; vitamins; triterpenes; sterols; carboxylic acids; minerals (high potassium and calcium salt content, silicic acid).

■ **Commercial Preparations**
Commercial preparations are made from fresh or dried aerial parts of *Urtica dioica, Urtica urens*, hybrids gathered during the flowering season, or from dried root/rhizome. Tinctures and tea products are available, as are capsules made from dried or freeze-dried herb.

Medicinal Uses/Indications

Traditional herbal actions: nutritive, alterative, circulatory stimulant, galactogogue, hypo-glycemic, topical rubefacient (fresh leaves, only with caution), anti-histaminic and antidote to stings (fresh juice)

Clinical applications: supportive treatments (internal and external) for rheumatic ailments; irrigation therapy for inflammatory diseases of lower urinary tract; prevention and treatment of kidney gravel. Diuretic effect if taken with sufficient fluid. Treatment of seasonal allergies, non-insulin-dependent diabetes. Root is used to treat micturition (urinary) disorders in BPH stages 1 and 2, while the leaf is used for urinary tract infections, kidney and bladder stones, and rheumatism. It is also used as a topical compress or cream for arthritic joints, gout, sprains and strains, neuralgia, sciatica, tendonitis, burns, hemorrhoids, and insect bites. Fresh expressed juice is used for anemia and cardiac insufficiency with edema.

■ **Pharmacology**

Open, observational, and placebo-controlled double-blind studies confirm that nettle root extract is efficacious for several conditions, including BPH. In vivo studies have shown that nettle herb has diuretic activity, presumably due to the presence of flavonoids and high potassium content. An aqueous root extract exhibited mild anti-inflammatory effects in a carrageenan-induced animal edema model.

In other animal studies, nettle had CNS-depressant, analgesic, hypoglycemic, and hyperglycemic effects. Urticin has been identified as the hypoglycemic principle responsible for lowering blood sugar levels in rabbits. Nettle herb extracts showed uterine activity in both pregnant and nonpregnant mice. The uteroactive effect was attributed to betaine and serotonin.

Stinging nettle root has a favorable effect on BPH by increasing urinary volume and maximum urinary flow while reducing residual urine. Although nettle root extract lessens the symptoms of enlarged prostate, it does not actually decrease the enlargement.

Prostate enlargement has been linked to elevated testosterone levels, specifically to increased activity of enzymes involved in testosterone production. An active principle in nettle is thought to either lower the amount of free testosterone or inhibit a crucial enzyme, such as aromase, required for testosterone production.

Nettle root extract interferes with testosterone synthesis by competitively displacing sex-hormone-binding globulin (SHBG). However, the effective concentration needed for competitive displacement may be much greater than the concentration available in therapeutic doses.

The active constituent responsible for the anti-BPH effect has not been unequivocally determined, but it may consist of an agglutinin (a protein mixture called UDA) and several polysaccharides isolated from nettle root. Lectin induces interferon production by human lymphocytes and triggers nonspecific agglutination of erythrocytes. In an in vitro study, a component of UDA from nettle inhibited virus-induced cell damage caused by HIV-1, HIV-2, CMV, RSV, and influenza A.

In human clinical trials, nettle herb juice produced marked diuresis in patients with myocardial and chronic venous insufficiency, and showed hemostatic activity. And in a double-blind investigation, nettle herb was mildly efficacious in the treatment of allergic rhinitis.

Dosage Ranges and Duration of Administration

- Seeds Dried herb: 2 to 4 g tid as infusion
- Seeds Fluid extract (1:1): 2 to 4 ml tid
- Seeds Tincture (1:5): 4 to 8 ml tid
- Seeds Fresh leaf infusion: 8 to 12 g fresh plant and ample liquid (at least 2 liters/day or equivalent)
- Seeds Root tincture/spiritus (1:10), for external use: 4 to 6 g/day or equivalent preparations (may be difficult to acquire in the U.S. except in blends)
- Seeds Topical compress, for external use: 4 to 6 g of herb in infusion

Cautions

■ **Adverse Effects/Toxicology**
No major side effects. Skin exposure to Urtica dioica can cause a stinging sensation (contact urticaria). Nettle root tea taken orally can cause mild gastrointestinal complaints, gastric irritation, burning sensation of the skin, edema, and oliguria (decreased urine output in relation to fluid intake). Allergic reactions (edema, skin afflictions) to leaf preparations have been reported in rare cases.

■ **Warnings/Contraindications/Precautions**
Irrigation therapy should not be used if edema is present. The massive amounts of fluids required for irrigation therapy can cause fluid retention due

to reduced cardiac or renal activity. Nettle has abortifacient activity, and it can alter the menstrual cycle. Pregnant women should not use nettle, and lactating women should avoid excessive use of this herb.

Interactions

Excessive use of nettle may interfere with the actions of hypoglycemic, hyperglycemic, antidiabetic, and CNS depressive drugs.

Regulatory and Compendial Status

The U.S. FDA classifies stinging nettle as a dietary supplement. It is listed on the General Sale List (GSL) in Britain. In Germany, nettle root is used as a therapy for urinary complaints during early stages of BPH. Stinging nettle is approved by the German Commission E.

References

Balzarini J, Neyts J, Schols D, Hosoya M, Van Damme E, Peumans W, De Clercq E. The mannose-specific plant lectins from Cymbidium hybrid and Epipactis helleborine and the (N-acetylglucosamine) n-specific plant lectin from *Urtica dioica* are potent and selective inhibitors of human immunodeficiency virus and cytomegalovirus replication in vitro. *Antiviral Research.* 1992;18:191–207.

Belaiche P, Lievoux O. Clinical Studies on the Palliative Treatment of Prostatic Adenoma with Extract of Urtica Root. *Phytotherapy Research.* 1991;5:267–269.

Blumenthal M, ed. *The Complete German Commission E Monographs. Therapeutic Guide to Herbal Medicines.* Boston, Mass: Integrative Medicine Communications; 1998:47, 132.

Bradley P, ed. *British Herbal Compendium.* Dorset, England: British Herbal Medicine Association; 1992;1:166–167.

Chrubasik S, Enderlein W, Bauer R, Grabner W. Evidence for antirheumatic effectiveness of Herba *Urticae dioica* in acute arthritis: A pilot study. Phytomedicine. 1997;4:105–108.

Grieve M. A Modern Herbal. New York, NY: Dover; 1971;2:574–579.

Gruenwald J, Brendler T; Christof J. *PDR for Herbal Medicines.* Montvale, NJ: Medical Economics Company; 1998:1197–1199.

Hutchens A. *Indian Herbalogy of North America.* Boston, Mass: Shambhala; 1991:204–206.

Krzeski T, Kazon M, Borkowski A, Witeska A, Kuczera J. Combined extracts of *Urtica dioica* and *Pygeum africanum* in the treatment of benign prostatic hyperplasia: double-blind comparison of two doses. *Clin Ther.* 1993;15:1011–1020.

Millspaugh C. *American Medicinal Plants.* New York, NY: Dover; 1974:611–614.

Newall C, Anderson L, Phillipson J. *Herbal Medicines: A Guide for Health-Care Professionals.* London, England: Pharmaceutical Press; 1996:201–202.

Oliver F, Amon E, Breathnach A, Francis D, Sarathchandra P, Black A, Greaves M. Contact urticaria due to the common stinging nettle *(Urtica dioica*—histological, ultrastructural and pharmacological studies.*) Clin Exp Dermatology.* 1991;267:1–7.

Schneider H, Honold E, Masuhr T. Treatment of benign prostatic hyperplasia. Results of a treatment study with the phytogenic combination of Sabal extract WS 1473 and Urtica extract WS 1031 in urologic specialty practices. *Fortschr Med.* 1995;267:37–40.

Schulz V, Hnsel R, Tyler VE. *Rational Phytotherapy: A Physician's Guide to Herbal Medicine. 3rd* ed. Berlin, Germany: Springer-Verlag; 1998:228–238.

Schottner M, Gansser D, Spiteller G. Lignans from the roots of *Urtica dioica* and their metabolites bind to human sex hormone binding globulin (SHBG). *Planta Med.* 1997;63(6):529–32.

Tyler VE. *Herbs of Choice: The Therapeutic Use of Phytomedicinals.* Binghamton, NY: Haworth; 1994:84–85.

Wylie G, et al. A comparative study of Tenidap, a cytokine-modulating anti-rheumatic drug, and diclofenac in rheumatoid arthritis: a 24 week analysis of a 1-year clinical trial. *Br J Rheumatol.* 1995;34:554–563.

© *Copyright Integrative Medicine Communications*

St. John's Wort

Names

■ **English**
St. John's wort

■ **Botanical**
Hypericum perforatum

■ **Plant Family**
Hypericaceae

■ **Pharmacopeial**
Hyperici herba

Overview

Medicinal use of St. John's wort dates back to ancient Greece. The renowned physicians Dioscorides and Hippocrates used it to treat various illnesses, and it was long believed to rid the body of evil spirits. Belief in the herb's powers continued through the Middle Ages, but by the end of the 19th century, interest in it—and most other medicinal plants—had waned. Recent research on St. John's wort has focused attention on the herb, and it has become extremely popular with health product consumers in the United States. In Europe, where St. John's wort has a longer history of use, it is used to treat wounds, gastritis, kidney and lung problems, insomnia, and depression.

Most clinical studies of St. John's wort have focused on its use in treating mild to moderate depression. In a 1996 meta-analysis, researchers examined 23 randomized trials of St. John's wort in 1,757 patients with mild to moderate depression. Acknowledging the limitations of using pooled data from studies that used different dosages and preparations, experimental designs and patient populations, the researchers still concluded that St. John's wort is better than placebo in treating some types of depression. However, they could not draw firm conclusions about whether St. John's wort is as effective as standard antidepressants. The analysis did find that St. John's wort causes fewer side effects than standard antidepressants.

The National Institute of Mental Health (NIMH) does not currently recommend the use of St. John's wort for treatment of depression and has called for more rigorous research on the herb. Along with two other branches of the National Institutes of Health—the Office of Alternative Medicine and the Office of Dietary Supplements—NIMH has funded a three-year controlled clinical study of the herb in clinically depressed patients.

In at least one controlled trial, patients with seasonal affective disorder (SAD) responded well to treatment with St. John's wort, and the herb seems to be even more effective when used in combination with light therapy.

The antiretroviral activity of St. John's wort has raised hopes for using it to treat acquired immunodeficiency syndrome (AIDS). Results of small pilot studies have been promising, with patients showing stable or increased helper T cell counts, improved helper-to-suppressor T cell ratios, and low incidence of opportunistic infection, but larger and longer-term studies are still needed.

Topical preparations of St. John's wort have shown antibacterial and wound-healing activity and have been used to treat burns, muscle pain, and hemorrhoids. Topical preparations also have been used to reduce pain, inflammation, and to promote nerve-tissue regeneration. Interestingly, debate continues over the most active ingredient in St. John's wart, although its therapeutic effects are widely accepted and acknowledged.

Macro Description

St. John's wort is a shrubby perennial with flat-topped clusters of bright yellow flowers. The plant is native to Britain and Europe but now grows wild in many other parts of the world, including the United States. It grows best in sunny sites with dry, gravelly, or chalky soil.

Part Used/Pharmaceutical Designations

- Leaves
- Flowering tops

■ **Constituents/Composition**
The best-studied active components are hypericin and pseudohypericin, found in both the leaves and flowers. There has been recent research to suggest that these best-studied components may not be the most active in the plant, with significant debate ensuing within the industry. Other components include flavonoids, xanthones, phenolic carboxylic acids, essential oils, carotenoids, alkanes, phloroglucinol derivatives, phytosterols, and medium-chain fatty acid alcohols.

■ **Commercial Preparations**
St. John's wort is available in various forms, including dried herb (chopped or powdered), capsule, liquid extract, tincture, infused oil, and tea infusion.

The recommended preparation of St. John's wort currently accepted by the industry is an extract standardized to contain 0.3% hypericin.

Medicinal Uses/Indications

- Reduces symptoms of anxiety, depression, apathy, anorexia, and feelings of worthlessness
- Relieves insomnia and hypersomnia
- In topical form, promotes healing of wounds and burns; antimicrobial; reduces swelling
- Shows promise as adjuvant therapy for viral infections such as herpes simplex, influenza, mononucleosis, AIDS, M.S., Fibromyalgia, and neuro-muscular inflammations

■ **Pharmacology**

- Antidepressant activity. Initial research suggested that hypericin acts as a monoamine oxidase (MAO) inhibitor, but more recent work shows that xanthones and flavonoids may be responsible for this activity. The most recent studies indicate that hypertorin, a phoraglucinal, is partly responsible for the anti-depressant activity.
- Antibacterial activity. Extracts show broad-spectrum antimicrobial activity against such organisms as Escherichia coli, Staphylococcus aureus, Streptococcus mutans, Pseudomonas aeruginosa, and Proteus vulgaris in-vitro.
- Antiviral activity. Active components hypericin and pseudohypericin show antiviral activity against herpes simplex virus types 1 and 2, Epstein-Barr virus, influenza types A and B, and vesicular stomatitis virus in vitro. These components have also been shown to be active against a number of retroviruses, including the human immunodeficiency virus (HIV).

Dosage Ranges and Duration of Administration

As an antidepressant, RDA is 300 to 500 mg of a 0.3% standardized extract, tid with meals, for a minimum of four to six weeks.

Cautions

■ **Adverse Effects/Toxicology**
St. John's wort causes severe photosensitivity in grazing animals that eat large amounts of the plant. Such reactions are rare in humans and have been seen only in people taking very large doses for HIV infection. However, as a precaution, people with fair skin and people who take St. John's wort in large doses or over long periods should use a sunscreen with a skin protection factor (SPF) of at least 15 and should not use sun-lamps or tanning beds or booths while taking the herb.

Other side effects are usually mild. They may include:

- Abdominal pain, bloating, constipation
- Nausea, vomiting
- Dizziness
- Dry mouth
- Itching, hives, skin rash
- Sleep problems
- Elevated blood pressure
- Unusual tiredness

■ **Warnings/Contraindications/Precautions**

- Take with food to reduce chances of gastric upset.
- Do not take during pregnancy or while breast-feeding.

Interactions

- Using St. John's wort (*Hypericum perforatum*) with antiviral agents like indinavir and other protease inhibitors is not recommended. There is the

possibility of an interaction between this herb and these medications that could undermine the effectiveness of the antiviral medications.
- There have also been reports of breakthrough bleeding in women taking St. John's wort (*Hypericum perforatum*) with birth control medications. The interaction between St. John's wort and birth control medications may result in decreased effectiveness of these medications.
- May interact with L-dopa, 5-hydroxytryptophan
- Should be taken cautiously with MAO inhibitors such as furazolidone (Furoxone®), isocarboxazid (Marplan®), moclobemide (Manerex®), phenelzine (Nardil®), procarbazine (Matulane®), selegiline (Eldepryl®) or tranylcypromine (Parnate®)
- Can be effective complement to selective serotonin reuptake inhibitors (SSRIs) such as fluoxetine (Prozac®), paroxetine (Paxil®) or sertraline (Zoloft®). Debate exists whether they may be taken in combination if under careful observation.

Regulatory and Compendial Status

St. John's wort is labeled as a dietary supplement by the U.S. Food and Drug Administration.

References

Bombardelli E, Morazzoni P. Hypericum perforatum. *Fitoterapia*. 1995;LXVI:43–68.

Degar S, et al. Inactivation of the human immunodeficiency virus by hypericin: Evidence for phytochemical alterations of p24 and a block in uncoating. *AIDS Res Hum Retroviruses*. 1992;8:1929–1936.

De Smet P, Peter AGM, Nolen WA. St. John's wort as an antidepressant. *Br Med J*. 1996;313:241–247.

Furner V, Bek M, Gold JA. A phase I/II unblinded dose ranging study of hypericin in HIV-positive subjects. *Int Conf AIDS*. 1991;7:199.

Cott JM. In vitro receptor binding and enzyme inhibition by *Hypericum perforatum* extract. *Pharmacopsychiatry*. 1997;30(suppl 2):108–112.

Gulick R, et al. Human hypericism: A photosensitivity reaction to hypericin (St. John's wort). *Int Conf AIDS*. 1992; 8:B90.

Lavie G, et al. Studies of the human mechanism of action of the antiviral agents hypericin and pseudohypericin. *Proc Natl Acad Sci USA*. 1989;86:5963–5967.

Linde K, Ramirez G, Mulrow CD, et al. St. John's wort for depression: an overview and meta-analysis of randomised clinical trials. *BMJ*. 1996;313:253–257.

Martinez B, Kasper S, Ruhrmann S, Moller HJ. Hypericum in the treatment of seasonal affective disorders. *J Geriatr Psychiatry Neurol*. 1994;7(Suppl 1):S29–33.

Meruelo D, Lavie G, Lavie D. Therapeutic agents with dramatic antiretroviral activity and little toxicity at effective doses: Aromatic polycyclic diones hypericin and pseudohypericin. *Proc Natl Acad Sci USA*. 1988;85:5230–5234.

Muller WE, Rolli M, Schafer C, Hafner, U. Effects of *hypericum* extract (LI 160) in biochemical models of antidepressant activity. *Pharmacopsychiatry*. 1997;30(suppl):102–107.

Murray MT. *The Healing Power of Herbs: The Enlightened Person's Guide to the Wonders of Medicinal Plants*. Rocklin, Calif: Prima Publishing; 1995.

Piscitelli S, Burstein AH, Chaitt D, et al. Indinavir concentrations and St. John's wort [letter]. *Lancet*. 2000;355:547–548.

Rasmussen P. St. John's wort: a review of its use in depression. *Australian Journal of Medical Herbalism*. 1998;10:8–13.

Tyler VE. *The Honest Herbal: A Sensible Guide to the Use of Herbs and Related Remedies*. Binghamton, NY: Pharmaceutical Products Press; 1993.

Yue Q, Bergquist C, Gerden B. Safety of St. John's wort (*Hypericum perforatum*) [letter]. *Lancet*. 2000;355:576–577.

© *Copyright Integrative Medicine Communications*

Turmeric

Names

- **English**
  Turmeric

- **Botanical**
  Curcuma longa

- **Plant Family**
  Zingiberaceae

- **Pharmacopeial**
  Curcumae longae rhizoma

Overview

Turmeric is indigenous to the tropical regions of southern Asia. It is widely used as a yellow food color and spice, including an ingredient in curry powder, throughout India, China, and Indonesia. It is also popular in Asian traditional medicine, even though there is no known basis for all of its many varied uses in folk healing.

However, both in vitro and in vivo pharmacological studies show that turmeric and its active constituents have antioxidant, antitumor, anti-inflammatory, and antimicrobial effects. In in vivo research, turmeric extracts displayed antitumor activity against skin cancer, breast cancer, and oral cancer cell lines. Turmeric extracts thus may be clinically beneficial in treating a range of carcinomas in humans.

Turmeric is also a cholagogue, an agent that stimulates the flow of bile from the duodenum. It has choleretic actions that enhance bile secretion by the liver as well as cholecystokinetic properties that promote gallbladder contraction. It is also an antihepatotoxic agent.

Macro Description

Turmeric is an erect, perennial plant distinguished by its oblong tubers and by its large, petioled leaves that are tapered at each end. The dull, yellowish white or yellow flowers radiate from a stem encased in a sheathing petiole. The cone-shaped, tubular infloresences are about four to six inches long with a three-lobed calyx.

The palate tubers have a characteristically yellowish-brown exterior and a deep orange or reddish-brown interior. Each tuber gives rise to multiple, secondary, finger-shaped, tuber-like rhizomes that bear no offshoots of their own. Turmeric has a noticeable fragrance, and its bitter, mildly acrid taste is reminiscent of ginger. The dried rhizomes have a transversely ringed appearance.

Part Used/Pharmaceutical Designations

- Tubers
- Dried rhizome

- **Constituents/Composition**
  Volatile oil (4 to 14%, 60% sesquiterpene ketones, or tumerones, including alpha-tumerone, beta-tumerone, artumerone, alpha-atlantone, gamma-atlantone, curlone, zingiberene, curcumol); curcuminoids (curcumin [diferuloylmethane], bidemethoxycurcumin, demethoxycurcumin); 1,5-diaryl-penta-1,4-dien-3-on-derivatives; sugars.

- **Commercial Preparations**
  Turmeric is typically available as hydroalcoholic fluid extracts, tinctures, and encapsulated powders. Decoctions are rarely employed since both the volatile oil and curcuminoids are not particularly water soluble. All turmeric products should be protected from light when stored.

Medicinal Use/Indications

Internal: liver obstruction, jaundice, intestinal worms, fever, diarrhea, bronchitis, leprosy, headache, arthritis, menstrual complaints, toothache, hemorrhage, stomach tonic, blood purifier, antifertility agent, insect repellent.
External: ulcers, inflammation, wounds, bruises, eye infections, leech bites.
Conditions: liver and gallbladder disorders; loss of appetite, dyspepsia.

Clinical applications: dyspeptic complaints, liver toxicity, hyperlipidemia inflammation, tumors; antioxidant, anti-inflammatory, and antimicrobial agent.

- **Pharmacology**
In in vitro studies, both turmeric extracts and curcumin exhibited significant antioxidant and free radical scavenging activity at least comparable to that of vitamins C and E. Turmeric inhibited oxidative insults in vivo and in vitro by interrupting oxidative chain reactions caused by free radicals. The volatile oil and alcohol extracts suppressed microbial growth of numerous bacterial and fungal pathogens in vitro.

Aqueous turmeric extracts produced antimutagenic action against several mutagens in test animals. In clinical studies, smokers administered oral doses of 1 to 5 g turmeric daily for 30 days showed significantly lower levels of mutagens in their urine when compared to nonsmokers given placebo.

Turmeric also has cardiovascular, hepatic, and gastrointestinal actions. Curcumin and turmeric, even in small doses, reduced cholesterol levels and inhibited platelet aggregation in vivo. Curcumin decreased cholesterol levels by several mechanisms: disrupting cholesterol uptake from the intestines, increasing the transformation of cholesterol into bile acids, and promoting choleretic action leading to increased excretion of bile acid.

The volatile oil is responsible for the choleretic action, while the curcuminoids account for the anti-inflammatory and cholekinetic properties of turmeric. Curcumins presumably block platelet aggregation by suppressing the formation of thromboxanes and simultaneously elevating prostacyclin levels.

Turmeric decreased symptoms of skin cancers and reduced the incidence of chemically caused breast cancer in laboratory animals. Curcumins exhibit anticancer activity during the tumor initiation, promotion, and progression stages of development.

Combinations of curcumin and genistein, an isoflavone derived from soy, may help to combat breast cancer. In an in vitro experiment, curcumin/genistein mixtures had a synergistic effect on inhibiting the pesticide-induced proliferation of estrogen-positive cells. In another study, curcumin administered i.p. to female rats suppressed DMBA-induced mammary tumorigenesis in the test animals.

The volatile oil fraction of turmeric showed anti-inflammatory properties in several studies. Curcumin was comparable to either cortisone or phenylbutazone in eliciting anti-inflammatory effects without adverse side effects in in vivo models of acute inflammation, but only 50% as effective in chronic inflammation.

Dosage Ranges and Duration of Administration

- Standardized powder (curcumin): 400 to 600 mg tid (1.5 to 3.0 g daily)
- Tincture (1:2): 3 to 5 ml tid

Note: Curcumin should be taken on an empty stomach 20 minutes before meals or between meals. Oral doses of curcumin are not readily absorbed; 40 to 85% of the compounds may never be absorbed in the gastrointestinal tract. Combinations of curcumin and bromelain may increase the absorption of curcumin.

Cautions

- **Adverse Effects/Toxicology**
Turmeric and curcumin are safe when taken in recommended doses. However, extended oral use of curcumin occasionally produces gastrointestinal upset and, in extreme cases, ulcers.

- **Warnings/Contraindications/Precautions**
Excessive dosing of standardized curcumin products may lead to gastric complaints and possibly ulcers. Patients diagnosed with either gallstones or obstruction of bile passages should consult a qualified health care practitioner before using turmeric products.

Interactions

None reported.

Regulatory and Compendial Status

Commission E classifies turmeric as an approved drug for use as a cholagogue and digestive aid.

References

Arora R, et al. Anti-inflammatory studies on *Curcuma longa* (turmeric). *Indian J of Med Res.* 1971; 59: 1289–1295.

Azuine MA, Bhide SV. Chemopreventive effect of turmeric against stomach and skin tumors induced by chemical carcinogens in Swiss mice. *Nutr Cancer,* 1992; 17(1): 77–83.

Blumenthal M, ed. *The Complete German Commission E Monographs. Therapeutic Guide to Herbal Medicines.* Boston: Integrative Medicine Communications; 1998: 222.

Dorland's Illustrated Medical Dictionary. 25th ed. Philadelphia: W.B. Saunders; 1974.

Grieve M. *A Modern Herbal. Vol.* II. New York: Dover; 1971:822–823.

Gruenwald J, Brendler T, Christof J. *PDR for Herbal Medicines.* Montvale, NJ: Medical Economics Company; 1998: 786–788.

Murray M. *The Healing Power of Herbs: The Enlightened Person's Guide to the Wonders of Medicinal Plants.* 2nd ed. Rocklin, CA: Prima Publishing; 1995: 327–335.

Nadkarni AK *Indian Materia Medica.* Bombey: Popular Prakashan; 1976: 414–418.

Nagabhushan N, Bhide SV. Curcumin as an inhibitor of cancer. *J Am Coll Nutr.* 1992; 11: 192–198.

Polasa K, et al. Effect of turmeric on urinary mutagens in smokers. *Mutagenesis.* 1992; 7: 107–109.

Piper JT, Singhal SS, Salameh MS, Torman RT, Awasthi YC, Awasthi S. Mechanisms of anticarcinogenic properties of curcumin: the effect of curcumin on glutathione linked detoxification enzymes in rat liver. *Int J Biochem Cell Biol.* 1998; 30(4): 445–456.

Singletary K, MacDonald C, Iovinelli M, Fisher C, Wallig M. Effect of the beta-diketones diferuloylmethane (curcumin) and dibenzoylmethane on rat mammary DNA adducts and tumors induced by 7,12-dimethylbenz[a]anthracene. *Carcinogenesis.* June 1998; 433(3):1039–1043.

Srinivasan K, Samaiah K. The effect of spices on cholesterol 7 alpha-hydroxylase activity and on serum and hepatic cholesterol levels in the rat. *Int J Vitam Nutr Res.* 1991; 61: 364–369.

Tyler V. *Herbs of Choice: The Therapeutic Use of Phytomedicinals.* Binghamton, NY: Haworth; 1994: 61–62.

Verma SP, Salamone E, Goldin B. Curcumin and genistein, plant natural products, show synergistic inhibitory effects on the growth of human breast cancer MCF-7 cells induced by estrogenic pesticides. *Biochem Biophys Res Commun.* 1997; 233(3): 692–696.

© *Copyright Integrative Medicine Communications*

Valerian

Names

■ **English**
Valerian root

■ **Botanical**
Valeriana officinalis

■ **Plant Family**
Valerianaceae

■ **Pharmacopeial**
Valerianae radix

Overview

Valerian root relieves anxiety and nervousness-related chronic and periodic insomnia. Herbalists have understood the mildly sedating, sleep-enhancing properties of valerian for centuries, and also recommend its use for mild stomach pains, headaches, and menstrual pain. Currently, the FDA is considering the approval of valerian root as an OTC sleep aid.

Macro Description

This three-to-five-foot herbaceous perennial has erect grooved, hollow stems that are hairy at the base and branch out toward the top. Dark green leaves grow in four to eight pairs from each stem; simple, pinnately lobed, and opposite, with hairy leaf veins on underside. Small fragrant flowers are white, lavender, or pink with three stamens and bloom in June in four-inch-wide panicles. Ornamental and medicinal, this perennial grows wild in damp, elevated locations.

Rhizomes, roots, and occasional stolons are sources of the crude drug. Superior preparations are light brown with a faint scent; darker, more pungent scents are considered inferior. The rhizome is one to two inches tall, ovoid, cylindrical, and light grayish-brown; with a "dirty sock" smell when dried. Darker offshoots of multiple joints with coarse longitudinal wrinkles grow from the rhizome. Stolons are gnarled and also light grayish-brown. Fresh root tastes sweet, spicy, and bitter. Soils rich in minerals grow healthier roots and provide stronger tinctures. These roots have sweeter taste and reduced "dirty sock" smell.

Part Used/Pharmaceutical Designations

- Roots

■ **Constituents/Composition**

The rhizome contains 0.8% to 1% iridoid valepotriates, 80% to 90% of which occur as valtrates (didrovaltrate, isovaltrate) and other iridoids. Many of these preparations no longer contain all of these constituents.

Rhizome hypodermis contains 0.3% to 0.8% volatile oil, which consists of monoterpenes and sesquiterpenes, which occur mostly as esters, including 0.1% to .03% valerenic (sometimes called valeric) as well as acetoxyvalerenic acids in medicinal valerian, as well as bornyl isovalerate, bornyl acetate, and bornyl formate. Valerian also contains alkaloids—including actinidine, valerine, and valerianine—and polyphenolic acids (caffeic and chlorogenic acids), tannins, gum, and resin.

■ **Commercial Preparations**

Aqueous, aqueous-alcohol, and glycerite extracts, which are standardized to contain 0.8% valerenic acid content, are available in liquid, tablet, or capsule form. Non-standardized dried-root material is available cut and sifted (for tea) or in capsules. *Valeriana officinalis* is the species most frequently used in the United States, often compounded with other sedative herbs (passionflower, hops, lemon balm, kava) to enhance relaxation and provide mild sedation.

Medicinal Uses/Indications

Traditional: sedative, mild hypnotic, carminative, antispasmodic, bactericide, anodyne (pain relief), nervine

Conditions: insomnia, nervousness, stress-related anxiety, migraine, stomach or intestinal cramps, hysteria, exhaustion, and abdominal, pelvic, or menstrual cramps

Clinical applications: insomnia, anxiety, stress, fever, convulsions, neuralgia, spastic muscles, night leg cramps

■ **Pharmacology**

The whole root drug is mildly sedating and reduces smooth muscle spasms. Actions may be due to increased concentrations of GABA (gamma-aminobutyric acid) in the synaptic cleft; increased GABA concentrations may decrease CNS activity, result in sedation, and reduce anxiety. Components in valerian extracts apparently decrease GABA catabolism, inhibit GABA uptake and release (secondary to a reversal of the NA(+) and Ca(2+)-independent GABA carrier release of [3H]GABA), and trigger peripheral nervous system spasmolytic effects.

Individual components of volatile oil and iridoids depress the central nervous system, reduce smooth muscle spasms in laboratory animals, with positive inotropic/negative chronotropic effects on coronary smooth muscle, and reduce arrhythmia and convulsion.

In human studies, valerian enhances sleep, reduces nighttime sleep disturbances, and improves overall sleep quality (in geriatric sleep-disturbed patients, nonelderly chronic insomniacs, and periodic insomniacs) and mood.

Although clinical trials are not yet conclusive, early results suggest that valerian can be as effective as benzodiazepines for sleep disorders, without benzodiazepine "hangover" or addiction risk.

Dosage Ranges and Duration of Administration

To reduce nervousness, anxiety, or headache or menstrual pain, any of the following forms and dosages may be used. Dosages repeated three times a day will also reduce sleeplessness. To relieve insomnia, patients must take a dosage at least 30 to 45 minutes before bedtime. For chronic insomnia, allow two weeks of continued use to achieve optimum therapeutic effect, then continue use for another two to four weeks.

- 2 to 3 g dried root in tea, up to several times daily
- $^1/_4$ to $^1/_2$ tsp. (1 to 3 ml) tincture, up to several times daily
- $^1/_4$ tsp. (1 to 2 ml) fluid extract (1:1)
- 150 to 300 mg valerian extract, dried or liquid, standardized to contain 0.8% valerenic acid, 1% to 1.5% valtrates

Cautions

■ **Adverse Effects/Toxicology**

Valerian is a safe, mild, herbal medicine. The German Commission E lists no side effects. The American Herbal Products Association (AHPA) rates valerian class 1 (safe when used appropriately). Mild gastrointestinal upset infrequently reported. Reports that chronic use (longer than two to four months) causes insomnia are controversial. Some individuals develop a "paradoxical reaction" of nervousness and excitability with valerian (rare).

■ **Warnings/Contraindications/Precautions**

Valerian has not posed risks to fetuses or breast-fed newborns, but all pregnant and lactating women should consult with a professional when considering taking any herb.

Valepotriates, valtrate, didrovaltrate, dihydrovaltrate, and isovaltrate have cytotoxic and mutagenic properties in vitro on specific cultured tumor cells and strains of bacteria. In humans, the degradation of these substances into baldrinals and possible polymers are believed to form nonmutagenic metabolites. Although the specific risks to human stomach, liver, and intestines have not been proven, species with high valepotriate content (e.g., Mexican and Indian valerian) are not recommended, and valerenic acid preparations, such as *V. officinalis*, are advised.

Interactions

Valerian may interfere with anxiolytics, hypnotics, analgesics, and antiepileptics, and may enhance effects of kava, passionflower, lemon balm, hops, poppy, and skullcap.

Regulatory and Compendial Status

Valerian is considered a dietary supplement and GRAS (generally recognized as safe) as a food additive in the United States. It is awaiting FDA approval as an over-the-counter sleep aid. Valerian is approved in Germany by the German Commission E to treat nervous restlessness and sleeping disorders and in Canada as a sedative and spasmolytic.

References

Balderer G, Borbely AA. Effect of valerian on human sleep. *Psychopharmacol.* 1985;87:406–409.

Blumenthal M, ed. *The Complete German Commission E Monographs.* Boston, Mass: Integrative Medicine Communications; 1998.

Blumenthal M, Riggins C. *Popular Herbs in the U.S. Market: Therapeutic Monographs.* Austin, Tex: The American Botanical Council; 1997.

Brown D. *Herbal Prescriptions for Better Health.* Rocklin, Calif: Prima Publishing; 1996.

DeSmet PAGM, ed. *Adverse Effects of Herbal Drugs.* New York, NY: Springer-Verlag; 1997:3.

Diefenbach K, et al. Valerian effects on microstructure of sleep in insomniacs. (2nd Congress of the European Assoc. for Clinical Pharmacology and Therapeutics, Berlin, Germany, Sept. 17–20.) *Eur J Clin Pharmacol.* 1997;52 (suppl):A169.

Hobbs C. *The Herbal Prescriber.* Santa Cruz, Calif. Botanica Press; 1995.

Kowalchik C, Hylton W, eds. *Rodale's Illustrated Encyclopedia of Herbs.* Emmaus, Pa: Rodale Press; 1998:495–496.

Leathwood PD. Aqueous extract of valerian root *Valeriana officinalis* L.) improves sleep quality in man. *Pharmacol Biochem Behav.* 1982;17:65–71.

Leung A, Foster S. *Encyclopedia of Common Natural Ingredients Used in Food, Drugs, and Cosmetics.* 2nd ed. New York, NY: John Wiley and Sons; 1996.

Lindahl O, Lindwall L. Double-blind study of a valerian preparation. *Pharmacol Biochem Behav.* 1989;32:1065–1066.

Lindahl O, Lindwall L. Double-blind study of valopotriates by hairy root cultures of *Valeriana officinalis* var. sambucifolia. Planta Med. 1992;58:A614.

McGuffin M, Hobbs C, Upton R, Goldberg A. *American Herbal Products Association's Botanical Safety Handbook.* Boca Raton, Fla: CRC Press; 1997:120.

Murray, MT. *The Healing Power of Herbs: The Enlightened Person's Guide to the Wonders of Medicinal Plants.* Rocklin, Calif: Prima Publishing; 1995.

Newall CA, Phillipson JD. Interactions of Herbs with Other Medicines. Kings Centre for Pharmacognosy, the School of Pharmacy, University of London. *The European Phytojournal.* 1998; 1. Available at: www.ex.ac.uk/phytonet/phytojournal.

Petkov V. Plants with hypotensive, antiatheromatous and coronarodilating actions. *Am J Chin Med.* 1979;7:197–236.

Samuelsson G. *Drugs of Natural Origin: A Textbook of Pharmacognosy.* Stockholm, Sweden: The Swedish Pharmaceutical Press; 1992.

Santos MS. Synaptosomal GABA release as influenced by valerian root extract—involvement of the GABA carrier. *Arch Int Pharmacodyn Ther.* 1994; 327:220–231.

Schultz V, Hansel R, Tyler V. *Rational Phytotherapy: A Physician's Guide to Herbal Medicine.* New York, NY: Springer-Verlag; 1998.

Seifert T. Therapeutic effects of valerian in nervous disorders: a field study. *Therapeutikon.* 1988;2(94).

Schultz H, Stolz C, Muller J. The effect of valerian extract on sleep polygraph in poor sleepers: a pilot study. *Pharmacopsychiatry.* 1994;27:147–151.

Wagner et al. Comparative studies on the sedative action of valeriana extracts, valepotriates, and their degradation products. *Planta Med.* 1980;39:358–365.

© *Copyright Integrative Medicine Communications*

Wild Yam

Names

- **English**
  Wild Yam

- **Botanical**
  Dioscorea villosa

- **Plant Family**
  Dioscoreaceae

- **Pharmacopeial**
  Dioscoreae villosae rhizoma

Overview

Dioscorea villosa, commonly known as wild yam, is native to Canada and the southern United States. It is one of an estimated 600 species of yam in the genus, *Dioscorea*, found in warm tropical habitats. Many of these are wild species that flourish in damp woodlands and thickets.

Yams are important cultigens, and some yam species are major food staples in tropical countries. The potato-like tubers of yam plants are grown as both edible and ceremonial plants throughout the world, even in subtropical and temperate regions. The formation and morphology of the tubers can vary from species to species. The tubers of *Dioscorea villosa*, for example, arise as fleshy rhizomes.

The tubers of wild yam and certain related species contain saponin compounds, including steroid-like constituents that are used as starting material for the synthesis of hormones. Wild yam tubers contain diosgenin, a steroid precursor that can be converted into the female hormone progesterone in the laboratory.

The discovery of diosgenin revolutionized the pharmaceutical industry several decades ago. It paved the way for synthesizing hormones and developing oral contraceptives. Today, diosgenin is still used as an active industrial agent in the half-synthesis of steroidal hormones. This chemical compound was traditionally obtained from Mexican yam *(Dioscorea mexicana)*, but it is also present in wild yam *(Dioscorea villosa)*. Wild species of yam tend to contain higher concentrations of diosgenin than do cultivated, edible species.

A closely related species of wild yam, *Dioscorea alata*, is used in the Amazon as a treatment for fever, gonorrhea, leprosy, piles, and tumors. Amazonian medicinal plant remedies made from other *Dioscorea* species are administered for skin inflammation, stomachache, boils, cancer, dysentery, goiter, and syphilis. In Belize, a "wild yam" species *(Dioscorea belizensis)* is a popular treatment for urinary tract infections, cold, bilious colic, rheumatism, arthritis, and diabetes.

Both cultivated and uncultivated yam species are employed in folk medicine for a wide variety of ailments. Diosgenin is conceivably responsible for pharmacological activities such as the purported anti-inflammatory effects of wild yam. The tubers of *Dioscorea villosa* and other wild yam species have a long history of use in traditional herbalism, but their importance will forever be linked to modern medicine. The synthesis of hormones and the birth control pill from diosgenin marks one of the major advances in plant drug medicine this century. This discovery helped to legitimize ethnopharmacology—the search for pharmaceutical drugs from natural products, particularly natural products from the plant kingdom.

Macro Description

Wild yam is a perennial, twining vine with pale brown, knotty, woody, cylindrical rootstocks, or tubers. The rootstocks are crooked and bear lateral branches of long creeping runners. The thin reddish-brown stems grow to a length of 5 to 12 meters. The tubers have no characteristic odor. The roots initially taste starchy, but soon thereafter become bitter and acrid to the tongue.

The wild yam plant has clusters of small green-white to green-yellow single flowers that are sessile-like. The heart-shaped leaves are broadly ovate and long-stemmed, with prominent longitudinal veins. The leaves are glabrous on the upper surface and pubescent on the underside.

Part Used/Pharmaceutical Designation

- Dried rhizome with roots

- **Constituents/Composition**
  Dioscorea villosa roots contain saponins (e.g., dioscin, an aglycone diosgenin), isoquinuclidine alkaloids (e.g., dioscorin)

- **Commercial Preparations**
  Commercial preparations of wild yam are available as liquid extracts and powdered tuber products. Raw plant material for commercial use is typically harvested from the eastern and central United States, and supplied to commercial outlets in the form of cut or broken tubers.

Medicinal Uses/Indications

Traditional uses: used as anti-inflammatory, cholagogue (stimulates flow of bile to duodenum), antispasmodic, carminative, sudorific, mild diaphoretic (perspiration-promoting agent), anodyne (analgesic), emetic (vomit-causing agent), expectorant; used for rheumatic conditions, gallbladder colic, dysmenorrhea, cramps, asthma, diuretic, dyspepsia, liver ailments, parturition, uterotonic, pain and inflammation of diverticulai, bilous colic, nausea associated with pregnancy, cramps, neuralgia, spasmodic hiccup, spasmodic asthma, women's reproductive health (e.g., salve made from inner root applied topically for breast inflammation and postmenopausal vaginal dryness).

Conditions: inflammation, spasm, rheumatic conditions, cramps; mild diaphoretic.

Clinical applications: anti-inflammatory, cholagogue, antispasmodic, mild diaphoretic, rheumatic conditions, gallbladder colic, dysmenorrhea, cramps, biliousness, nausea, intestinal colic.

- **Pharmacology**
  Although various species of *Dioscorea* have been investigated extensively for their pharmacological properties, relatively few published studies were located on *Dioscorea villosa*. Various preparations of wild yam reportedly have exhibited anti-inflammatory, antitumor, estrogenic, hemolytic, hypocholesterolemic, amebicidal, mastogenic (pertaining to breasts), pesticidal, and piscicidal effects. However these claims have not necessarily been confirmed by laboratory research. Similarly, the putative antifatigue, antistress, and antigliomic (antitumor against cancers of brain and nervous tissue) effects of wild yam await further scientific verification.

  However, studies on other species of *Dioscorea* clearly show that a related species of wild yam has antidiabetic activity. In one investigation, the effects of hydroalcoholic extracts of *Dioscorea dumetorum* tubers were evaluated on either fasting normal mice or rabbits, and on fasting alloxan-diabetic rabbits. Both the whole extract and the steroidal fractions, especially the glycosidic portion, produced significant hypoglycemic action in normal test animals and in fasting alloxan-diabetic rabbits. A fraction containing alkaloids actually elevated blood sugar in the fasting normal mice. This suggests that the active constituent responsible for the hypoglycemic effect is probably a steroidal derivative. Nigerian researchers have also reported that *Dioscorea dumetorum* tubers possess antidiabetic properties.

Dosage Ranges and Duration of Administration

- Dried herb: 1 to 2 tsp tid
- Tincture: 2 to 4 ml tid

Cautions

- **Adverse Effects/Toxicology**
  No adverse side effects have been reported for wild yam preparations when taken in recommended therapeutic dosages.

- **Warnings/Contraindications/Precautions**
  Overdosing can be potentially poisonous because dioscorin, one of the active constituents, can have picrotoxin-like effects.

Regulatory and Compendial Status

Wild Yam is listed in the *British Herbal Pharmacopeia*.

References

Aikman L. *Nature's Healing Arts: From Folk Medicine to Modern Drugs*. Washington, DC: National Geographic Society; 1977:186–189, 196.

Arvigo R, Balick M. *Rainforest Remedies:One Hundred Healing Herbs of Belize*. Twin Lakes, Wis: Lotus Press; 1993: 194–195.

British Herbal Pharmacopoeia. 4th ed. Great Britain: Biddles Ltd, Guildford and King's Lynn; 1996:187.

Dorland's Illustrated Medical Dictionary. 25th ed. Philadelphia, Pa: W.B. Saunders; 1974.

Duke JA. *The Green Pharmacy.* New York, NY:St Martin's Press; 1997:111, 209–210, 352

Duke JA. Phytochemical Database, USDA–ARS–NGRL, Beltsville Agricultural Research Center, Md. Available at: www.ars-grin.gov/cgi-bin/duke/farmacy2.pl

Duke J, Vasquez R. *Amazonian Ethnobotanical Dictionary.* Boca Raton, Fla: CRC Press; 1994:66–67.

Etkin N, ed. *Plants in Indigenous Medicine and Diet: Biobehavioral Approaches.* Bedford Hills, NY: Redgrave Publishing; 1986: 131–150.

Grieve M. *A Modern Herbal.* Vol. II. New York, NY: Dover; 1971:863.

Gruenwald J, Brendler T, Jaenicke C. *PDR for Herbal Medicines.* Montvale, NJ: Medical Economics Company; 1998:809–810.

Mabberley DJ. *The Plant-Book: A Portable Dictionary of the Higher Plants.* England: Cambridge University Press; 1987: 185.

Thomson WA, ed. *Medicines from the Earth: A Guide to Healing Plants.* Maidenhead, England: McGraw-Hill Book Company; 1978:61.

Vasiukova N, Paseshnichenko V, Davydova M, Chalenko G. Pharmacological evaluation of *Dioscorea dumetorum* tuber used in traditional antidiabetic therapy. *J Ethnopharmacol.* 1986;15(ISS 2):133–144.

© *Copyright Integrative Medicine Communications*

Yarrow

Names

■ **English**
Yarrow Flower/Yarrow Herb

■ **Botanical**
Achillea millefolium

■ **Plant Family**
Asteraceae

■ **Pharmacopeial**
Millefolii flos/Millefolii herba

Overview

Yarrow is the name given to a number of subspecies of *Achillea millefolium* that have a virtually identical appearance but different numbers of chromosomes. The taxonomy of *Achillea millefolium* is inconsistent, and subspecies as well as related species are variously categorized as *Achillea millefolium*. Subspecies of yarrow are found in many regions, particularly in eastern, southeastern, and central Europe.

Legend has it that the botanical grouping, or genus, of yarrow was named *Achillea* because Achilles, the Greek mythical figure, used yarrow to staunch the bleeding wounds of his soldiers. Popular in European folk medicine, yarrow has traditionally been used to treat menstrual ailments and bleeding hemorrhoids. This plant is a distant botanical relative of German (or Hungarian) chamomile and English chamomile, and it has some of the same chemical constituents found in the two chamomiles. As in the case of chamomile, yarrow is a common herbal remedy for bloating, flatulence, and mild gastrointestinal cramping.

Chamomile and yarrow belong to the Asteraceae, or daisy, family. Plants in this family contain a bluish-colored essential oil that owes its color to the presence of intensely blue azulene derivatives. The azulene constituents and other active principles in the volatile oil of yarrow have anti-inflammatory effects.

While the chemistry of various subspecies of yarrow has not been fully elucidated, some of the therapeutic claims for this plant have been documented. Pharmacological studies indicate that yarrow has diaphoretic (perspiration-promoting), antipyretic, hypotensive, astringent, diuretic, and urinary antiseptic activity.

Macro Description

Yarrow grows as a simple, erect, and hairy stem that reaches a height of 0.1 to 1.5 m. It flourishes in a sunny and warm habitat, and is frequently found along meadows and roadsides, as well as on dry, sunny slopes. The entire plant (with the exception of the fruit) is draped in white, silky appressed hairs, which gives it a white hairy-like appearance. Growing from underground runners are tough, angular, horizontal stems that bear flowers.

Yarrow blooms between June and September. The flowers are typically white, but either pink or pale purple inforesences are common in species found in mountain areas. The flowers are composite and densely arranged in flattened, umbel-like clusters. The leaves are alternate, lanceolate, and multi-pinnate with a feathery appearance.

Part Used/Pharmaceutical Designation

- Flowers (flowerhead)
- Whole herb
- Above-ground parts

■ **Constituents/Composition**
Volatile oil (0.2% to 1.0%, components are variable depending on strain/subspecies; e.g., chamazulene [blue, 6% to 19%, maximum 40%], camphor, beta-pinene, 1,8-cineole, carophyllene, alpha-thujone). Sesquiterpene lactones (primarily guaianolides, e.g., achillicin, achillin, millefin, millefolide; sesquiterpenes may be converted to chamazulene [proazulenes] through steam distillation); flavonoids, acids, alkaloids/bases (e.g., betonicine, stachydrine [pyrrolidine]), polyynes, alkamids, tannins, unknown cyanogenetic compound, sugars.

■ **Commercial Preparations**
Commercial preparations are made from both the herb (fresh or dried above-ground parts) and dried yarrow flowers of *Achillea millefolium*. Plant material is harvested during the flowering season and then dried. Essential oil preparations should not be stored in synthetic containers. Yarrow drug contains volatile oil which must be protected from light and moisture. Yarrow is a component in multi-herbal formulations of two gastrointestinal teas listed in the German Standard Registration of phytopharmaceutical products.

Medicinal Uses/Indications

Traditional uses:

- Internal: cold, fever, measles, essential hypertension, cerebral and coronary thromboses, amenorrhea, dysentery, diarrhea; whole plant decoction used for bleeding piles, kidney disorders
- External: wound healing, skin inflammations; sitz (partial) bath for pain and cramps in lower female pelvis, liver ailments

Conditions: used as diaphoretic, antipyretic, anti-inflammatory, spasmolytic, hemostatic, hypotensive, emmenagogue (induces menstruation), choleretic (stimulates production of bile by the liver), cholagogue (stimulates flow of bile to duodenum), antibacterial astringent, antispasmodic, gallbladder therapeutic
Clinical applications: loss of appetite, dyspeptic (digestive) complaints, liver and gallbladder complaints, hypertension, menorrhagia, irritable bowel disease, influenza

■ **Pharmacology**
In in vitro experiments, ethanolic extracts of yarrow showed moderate antibacterial activity, with the sesquiterpene lactone fraction also exhibiting antibacterial properties. In in vivo studies, an aqueous extract of true yarrow produced anti-inflammatory activity in paw edema models of mouse and rat, and had topical anti-inflammatory activity in rabbits. In general, anti-inflammatory properties have been associated with azulenes, the major component of the essential oil.

Yarrow extract administered to mice at a dose over twice that needed for anti-inflammatory effect showed diuretic activity. The diuretic action has been attributed to terpinen-4-ol. The essential oil also yielded CNS depressant activity by reducing spontaneous activity of mice and by lowering body temperature of rats. In test animals, the volatile oil from yarrow prolonged barbiturate-induced sleep and inhibited pentetrazole-induced convulsions.

Another chief constituent, achilleine (0.5 g/kg IV) displayed hemostatic effects by reducing blood-clotting time by 32% in rabbits for 45 minutes and was devoid of observable toxic side effects. Azulene compounds in the flavonoid-containing fraction of yarrow may account for the antispasmodic activity of this plant on isolated rabbit intestine. Other research suggests that azulene-related constituents such as chamazulene and prochamazulenes also have anti-inflammatory properties. Additional investigations reveal that the basic fraction of yarrow extracts (containing alkaloid/base) exhibited antipyretic and hypotensive effects, while the sesquiterpene lactone fraction elicited cytotoxic action.

Dosage Ranges and Duration of Administration

- Dried herb: 1 to 4 g tid as infusion or capsules
- Extract (1:1, 25% ethanol): 1 to 4 ml tid
- Tincture (1:5, 40% ethanol): 2 to 4 ml tid
- Yarrow flowers, or equivalent preparations: 3 g per day as infusion
- Sitz baths: 100 g yarrow per 20 liters (5 gal) of water.

Cautions

■ **Adverse Effects/Toxicology**
Although yarrow is described as nontoxic, it can cause allergic reactions in sensitized individuals.

■ **Warnings/Contraindications/Precautions**
While yarrow is reportedly free of adverse side effects when administered in designated therapeutic dosages, some individuals have allergic reactions to this plant. Yarrow has a potential for sensitization.

Yarrow should be avoided during pregnancy since it has abortifacient properties and affects the menstrual cycle. Lactating women should avoid excessive use.

Interactions

While some sources report no interactions between yarrow and other therapeutics, excessive dosing may interfere with the pharmacological actions of anticoagulant, hypotensive, and hypertensive medications taken concurrently with yarrow. Any interactions could potentially produce sedative and diuretic effects.

Regulatory and Compendial Status

Yarrow is listed in the General Sale List (GSL) of approved therapeutic agents in the United Kingdom. It is listed as an approved herb by the German Commission E, and accepted in Belgium and France for specific indications. The Council of Europe approves yarrow as a natural source of food flavoring (category N2) but prohibits certain concentrations of alpha and beta thujone in foods and alcoholic beverages. In the United States, yarrow is not approved as a food additive, and alcoholic beverages containing yarrow must be thujoid-free.

References

Blumenthal M, ed. *The Complete German Commission E Monographs.* Boston, Mass: Integrative Medicine Communications; 1998:223–224.

Bradley P, ed. *British Herbal Compendium.* Vol. I. Dorset, Great Britain: British Herbal Medicine Association; 1992:227–229.

Chandler RF, Hooper SN, Harvey MJ. Ethnobotany and phytochemistry of yarrow, *Achillea millefolium,* Compositae. *Econ Botany.* 1982;36:203–223.

Goldberg AS, Mueller EC, Eigen E, Desalva S. Isolation of anti-inflammatory principles from *Achillea millefolium* (Compositae). *J Pharm Sci.* 1969;58:938–941.

Grieve M. A Modern Herbal. Vol. II. New York, NY: Dover; 1971:863–865.

Gruenwald J, Brendler T, Jaenicke C. *PDR for Herbal Medicines.* Montvale, NJ: Medical Economics Company; 1998:604–606.

Kudrzycka-Bicloszabska FW, Glowniak K. Pharmacodynamic properties of *oleum chamomillae* and oleum millefolii. Diss Pharm Phamacol. 1966;18:449–454.

Moskalenko SA. Preliminary screening of far-Eastern ethnomedicinal plant for antibacterial activity. *J Ethnopharmacol.* 1986;15:231–259.

Newall C, Anderson L, Phillipson J. *Herbal Medicines: A Guide for Health-care Professionals.* London: Pharmaceutical Press; 1996:271–273.

Schulz V, Hansel R, Tyler V. *Rational Phytotherapy: A Physicians' Guide to Herbal Medicine.* 3rd ed. Berlin, Germany: Springer; 1998:182–183, 239

Shipochliev T, Fournadjiev G. Spectrum of the antiinflammatory effect of *Arctostaphylos uva ursi* and *Achillea millefolium.Probl Vutr Med.* 1984;12:99–107.

Thomson WA. *Medicines from the Earth: A Guide to Healing Plants.* Maidenhead, England: McGraw-Hill Book Company; 1978:61.

Tyler V. *The Honest Herbal: A Sensible Guide to the Use of Herbs and Related Remedies.* 3rd ed. Binghampton, NY: Pharmaceutical Products Press; 1993:83–85.

© *Copyright Integrative Medicine Communications*

SUPPLEMENTS 101

Alpha-Linolenic Acid ALA

Overview

The fatty acid alpha-linolenic acid (ALA) is an essential nutrient. It is the 18-carbon polyunsaturated fatty acid (PUFA) in the omega-3 series found in unhydrogenated oils derived from plants. ALA is found primarily in margarines as well as as rapeseed (canola), flaxseed, and soybean oils.

ALA is a "parent" fatty acid. Our bodies convert it into the longer-chain omega-3 fatty acids (such as docosahexaenoic acid [DHA] and eicosapentaenoic acid [EPA]), which are found primarily in fish oils. Scientists studying DHA and EPA have shown that omega-3 oils have several beneficial effects. Because these fatty acids are produced by ALA, this research can be applied to ALA as well.

The beneficial effects of omega-3 series oils include: lowering cholesterol and triglyceride levels, reducing the risk of heart disease, lowering blood pressure, improving rheumatoid arthritis, and protecting myelin formation and function. Omega-3 oils may also be helpful in treating multiple sclerosis and diabetes, and in preventing cancer.

ALA may help prevent coronary heart disease, and inhibit atherosclerosis. In one small study, 15 obese persons took 20 g of ALA from margarine products based on flax oil daily. As a result, the subjects showed improvement in arterial compliance, and thus had a decreased risk of cardiovascular disease, despite a rise in LDL oxidizability. At the same time, insulin sensitivity and HDL cholesterol diminished. Another study found that ALA supplements from vegetable oil and EPA and DHA supplements from a fish source have largely parallel effects on hemostatic factors. Other research has indicated that ALA acts equivalently to n-6 fatty acids with respect to lipid and lipoprotein effects. However, very large amounts of ALA, which is plant-based, were needed to reduce tricylglycerol concentrations, which is the hallmark effect of the fish-based omega-3 fatty acids. The study concluded that plant-derived ALA is not equivalent to fish-based acids in its effect on lipoprotein metabolism. Scientists agree that the relationship among the fatty acids and the ratio of ALA to linoleic acid in the diet is an important area for further study.

Scientists are also investigating other uses for ALA. The anti-inflammatory and immunoregulatory effects of ALA, and its successor fatty acids, have been demonstrated. Successful treatment of migraines and alleviation of depression with ALA have been reported. Topical application of ALA inhibits melanin production and accelerates turnover of the stratum corneum, thus aiding in the removal of melanin pigment from the epidermis.

Sources

■ **Dietary Sources**

- Flax seeds
- Flaxseed oil
- Linseed oil
- Canola (rapeseed) oil
- Soybean oil
- Margarine, if based on canola or soybean oil
- Pumpkin
- Walnuts

■ **Constituents/Composition**

Alpha-linolenic acid is a long-chain polyunsaturated fatty acid with 18 carbon atoms. It is the parent fatty acid in the omega-3 series. It is converted to eicosapentaenoic acid (EPA), then to decosahexaenoic acid (DHA), then to the prostaglandin E_3 series (PGE_3). Some fish products (e.g., mackerel and salmon) can introduce EPA and DHA directly into the body.

The essential fatty acids, including ALA, are known as vitamin F. The Food and Drug Administration prohibits the use of the term "vitamin F" in advertising, because foods like french fries could be advertised as being "vitamin enriched" because they were fried in oil containing these fatty acids.

■ **Commercial Preparations**

ALA is commercially prepared in two ways.

- Cooking oils (canola oil, soybean oil, margarines made from these oils). Hydrogenated products are not preferred.
- Medicinal oil (flaxseed oil, gelatin capsules of flaxseed oil)

Several manufacturing methods can destroy the nutritional value of the products. Some preferred manuafacturers use proprietary names for their packaging processes. Bio-Electron Process (Barlean's Organic Oils), Spectra-Vac (Spectrum Naturals), or Omegaflo (Omega Nutrition) are some examples. Generally, a high quality oil will be certified as organic by a reputable third party, is packaged in light-resistant containers, may be refrigerated, and will be dated.

Therapeutic Uses

The primary uses of ALA and other omega-3 oils include the following.

- Cardiovascular disease: reducing cholesterol levels and blood pressure
- Allergic and inflammatory conditions: e.g., for treatment of psoriasis and eczema
- Autoimmune diseases: e.g., for treatment of multiple sclerosis, lupus, and cancer

Dosage Ranges and Duration of Administration

There is no recommended dietary allowance of ALA.

A healthy person eating a normal diet should consume fewer saturated fats and more polyunsaturated essential fatty acids.

Cautions

■ **Adverse Effects/Toxicology**
N/A

■ **Warnings/Contraindications/Precautions**
Total fat intake should be considered.
The ratio of ALA to other essential fatty acids may be important in treating some conditions.

Interactions

ALA interacts with other fatty acids.

References

Ando H, Ryu A, Hashimot A, Oka M, Ichihashi M. Linoleic acid and alpha-linolenic acid lightens ultraviolet-induced hyperpigmentation of the skin. *Arch Dermatol Res.* 1998;290:375–381.

Billeaud C, Bougle D, Sarda P, et al.. Effects of preterm infant formula supplementation with alpha-linolenic acid with a linoleate/alpha-linoleate ration of 6. *Eur J Clin Nutr.* August 1997;51:520–527.

DeDeckere EA, Korver O, Verschuren PM, Katan MB. Health aspects of fish and n-3 polyunsaturated fatty acids from plant and marine origin. *Eur J Clin Nutr.* 1998;52:749–753.

Edwards R, Peet M, Shay J, Horrobin D. Omega-3 polyunsaturated fatty acid levels in the diet and in red blood cell membranes of depressed patients. *J Affect Disord.* 1998;48:149–155.

Ensminger AH, Ensminger ME, Konlande JE, Robson JRK. *Foods & Nutrition Encyclopedia.* 2nd ed. Baton Rouge, Fla: CRC Press, Inc; 1994:1:684–708.

Ferretti A, Flanagan VP. Antithromboxane activity of dietary alpha-linolenic acid. *Prostaglandins Leukot Essent Fatty Acids.* 1996;54:451–455.

Freese R, Mutanen M. Alpha-linolenic acid and marine long-chain n-3 fatty acids differ only slightly in their effects on hemostatic factors in healthy subjects. *Am J Clin Nutr.* 1997;66:591–598.

Garrison Jr RH, Somer E. *The Nutrition Desk Reference.* 3rd ed. New Canaan, Conn: Keats Publishing, Inc; 1995:23–64.

Haas EM. *Staying Healthy with Nutrition.* Berkley, Calif: Celestial Arts Publishing; 1992:65–79.

Harris WS. N-3 fatty acids and serum lipoproteins: human studies. *Am J Clin Nutr.* 1997;65:1645S (10).

de Lorgeril M, Renaud S, Mamelle N, et al. Mediterranean alpha-linolenic acid-rich diet in secondary prevention of coronary heart disease. *Lancet.* 1994;343:1454–1459.

Mantzioris E., James MJ, Gibson RA, Cleland LG. Dietary subsitutions with an alpha-linolenic acid-rich vegetable oil increases eicosapentaenoic acid concentrations in tissues. *Am J Clin Nutr.* 1994;59:1304–1309.

Murray MT. Encyclopedia of Nutritional Supplements. Rocklin, Calif: Prima Publishing; 1996:239–278.

Nestel PJ, Pomeroy SE, Sasahara T, et al. Arterial compliance in obese subjects is improved with dietary plant n-3 fatty acid from flaxseed oil despite increased LDL oxidizability. *Arterioscler Thromb Vasc Biol.* 1997;17:1163–1170.

Newstrom H. *Nutrients Catalog.* Jefferson, NC: McFarland & Co, Inc; 1993:103–105.

Simon JA, Fong J, Bernert JT Jr, Browner WS. Serum fatty acids and the risk of stroke. *Stroke.* 1995;26:778–782.

Shils ME, Olson JA, Shike M, Ross AC. *Modern Nutrition in Health and Disease.* 9th ed. Baltimore, Md: Williams & Wilkins; 1999:90–92, 1377–1378.

Voskuil DW, Feskens EJM, Katan MB, Kromhout D. Intake and sources of alpha-linolenic acid in Dutch elderly men. *Eur J Clin Nutr.* 1996;50:784–787.

Wapnir RA. Copper absorption and bioavailability. *Am J Clin Nutr.* 1998;67:1054s.

Wagner W, Nootbaar-Wagner U. Prophylactic treatment of migraine with gamma-linolenic and alpha-linolenic acids. *Cephalalgia.* April 1997:17:127–130.

Werbach MR. *Nutritional Influences on Illness.* 2nd ed. Tarzana, Calif: Third Line Press;1993:13–22;655–671.

Yehuda S, Rabinovitz S, Carasso RL, Mostofsky DI. Fatty acids and brain peptides. *Peptides.* 1998;19:407–419.

© *Copyright Integrative Medicine Communications*

Alpha-Lipoic Acid

Overview

In recent years, increasing attention has been paid to the group of vitamins, minerals, and enzymes known as antioxidants. Some of the better known antioxidants are vitamins A, C and E, beta-carotene, selenium, and melatonin. Antioxidants play an important role in preventing aging-related degenerative conditions through their actions in fighting free radicals. Free radicals are wastes generated by the regular metabolic processes in the cells. Free radicals are normally present in the body and actually serve useful purposes, such as aiding in the production of hormones and activating enzymes. However, when there is an excess of free radicals in the body, they become destructive.

In addition to being by-products of normal metabolic processes, free radicals also can result from exposure to radiation, toxic chemicals (such as those contained in cigarette smoke, automobile exhaust, and other environmental pollutants), and from overexposure to the sun's rays. Free radicals are atoms or molecules that contain unpaired electrons. They tend to bind to other molecules, causing chemical reactions that can be destructive to the body. They can damage cells, interfere with the immune system, and contribute to degenerative diseases such as cancer and cardiovascular disease. In fact, free radical damage may be the basis for the aging process. Antioxidants bind with these reactive molecules to counteract their harmful effect.

The antioxidant alpha-lipoic acid (also called thioctic acid) is made by the body and directly supports detoxifying abilities of the liver. It enhances the antioxidant functions of vitamins C and E and glutathione. Alpha-lipoic acid (ALA) has growth-stimulating properties, prevents cell damage, regulates blood sugar, and chelates toxic metals out of the blood. In animal studies, it has been shown to enhance cognitive function as well. It is also involved in the production of muscular energy and directs calories toward energy production. Because it is both water- and fat-soluble, ALA is able to function in almost any part of the body, including the brain.

Sources

■ Dietary Sources
Dietary sources of alpha-lipoic acid include the following:

- Spinach
- Broccoli
- Beef
- Yeast
- Kidney
- Heart

■ Constituents/Composition
Alpha-lipoic acid, along with glutathione, is one of the thiol antioxidants. It is a carboxy acid with two sulfur atoms in its molecule, and occurs as an amide in plant and animal tissues.

■ Commercial Preparations
Alpha-lipoic acid is available commercially in capsule form.

Therapeutic Uses

Because alpha-lipoic acid relieves stress on the liver and directly supports its detoxifying functions, it has been used in the treatment of chronic hepatitis and Amanita (a particularly toxic mushroom) poisoning. It is able to bind to toxic metals and is used for heavy metal detoxification. Alpha-lipoic acid can help eliminate toxic effects of anasthesia, analgesics, or other drugs used in the course of surgery, and to ease subsequent pain. A recommended dose is two 100-mg capsules tid one week before surgery and two weeks postoperatively.

The thiols are central to antioxidant defense in the brain. Alpha-lipoic acid has a low molecular weight; it is readily absorbed from nutritional sources and crosses the blood-brain barrier. Current research indicates that alpha-lipoic acid and its metabolite dihydrolipoate have protective effects on brain and neural tissue. Preliminary human studies support conclusions of animal and in vitro studies showing a role for ALA in the treatment of stroke and other brain disorders involving free radical damage. In an animal study, treatment with ALA was associated with a four-fold increase in stroke survival.

Alpha-lipoic acid has shown great promise in the treatment of nerve dysfunction in diabetics. Diabetes mellitus is associated with free radicals; studies with diabetics have revealed oxidative stress loads. In more than one study, treatment with alpha-lipoic acid has significantly reduced the pain, burning, paresthesia, and numbness associated with diabetic neuropathy. Alpha-lipoic acid has also been shown to increase glucose transport in diabetics, and to lead to improved heart rate variability.

Dosage Ranges and Duration of Administration

Currently, no recommended dosages have been established for ALA. ALA manufacturers suggest one or two 50-mg capsules daily as a dietary supplement.

Cautions

■ Adverse Effects/Toxicology
Studies investigating the effects of alpha-lipoic acid on nerve damage related to diabetes found no side effects at the dosage levels they were testing.

■ Warnings/Contraindications/Precautions
Diabetics should take ALA with caution as it can cause hypoglycemia.

Interactions

Alpha-lipoic acid enhances the functions of antioxidant vitamins C and E, and of glutathione (another thiol produced by the body). While there have been claims of alpha-lipoic acid's ability to regenerate vitamin E, this has not been supported by animal studies.

References

Hocking GM. *A Dictionary of Natural Products.* Medford, NJ: Plexus Publishing; 1997:39;449,797.

Mindell E, Hopkins V. *Prescription Alternatives.* New Canaan, Conn: Keats Publishing; 1998:55–56.

Packer J, Tritschler HJ, Wessel K. Neuroprotection by the metabolic antioxidant alpha-linoic acis. *Free Radic Biol Med.* 1997;22:359–378.

Walker LP, Brown E. *The Alternative Pharmacy.* Paramus, NJ: Prentice Hall; 1998:36, 78, 216, 326, 362, 375.

Ziegler D, Gries FA. Alpha-lipoic acid in the treatment of diabetic peripheral and cardiac autonomic neuropathy. *Diabetes.* 1997;46 (suppl 2):S62–66.

© *Copyright Integrative Medicine Communications*

Betaine

Overview

Betaine, also known as trimethylglycine, or oxyneurine, is involved in methylation reactions that play a critical role in the health of the cardiovascular system. Homocysteine (Hcy) has been shown to be a major independent risk factor for coronary artery disease (CAD). Betaine is formed through oxidation of choline. Once formed, it can donate a methyl group to homocysteine, thereby producing dimethylglycine and methionine. The end result is a reduction in potentially toxic homocysteine levels. It is believed that accumulation of homocysteine, over time, can damage the endothelial cells and predispose individuals to premature atherosclerosis. Mild hyperhomocysteinemia is common in patients with premature vascular disease. Mild hyperhomocysteinemia, significant enough to cause vascular problems, is also relatively common in the general population, and may account for a substantial proportion of vascular disease in the United States. Some researchers estimate that 10% of the populations's CAD risk is attributable to Hcy.

S-adenosylmethionine (SAM) is synthesized from methionine, a byproduct of homocysteine methylation. Oral administration of betaine to laboratory rats has been shown to cause an increase in S-adenosylmethionine levels. This has lead researchers to conclude that betaine may be a possible alternative to expensive SAM in the treatment of liver disease and other disorders.

Folic acid, vitamin B_{12} and vitamin B_6 are also involved in methylation reactions that convert homocysteine to methionine. The Third National Health and Nutrition Examination Survey, conducted by the U.S. Department of Health & Human Services Center for Disease Control, found that Americans are consuming inadequate amounts of these three vitamins. Furthermore, Americans typically consume inadequate amounts of fruits and vegetables, which may limit their dietary intake of betaine. These statistics indicate that Americans may significantly benefit by increasing intake of these nutrients, either by diet or supplementation. Supplementation is necessary to achieve the high levels of betaine (6 grams per day) required to treat hypercysteinemia in premature vascular disease or genetic homocystinuria.

Sources

■ Dietary Sources

Betaine is widely distributed in plants and animals. Broccoli, spinach, and beets are rich sources of betaine.

■ Constituents/Composition

Anhydrous betaine, betaine monohydrate

Note: Betaine-HCL is a stomach acidifier that is *not* the same as trimethylglycine (betaine).

■ Commercial Preparations

Betaine supplements are a byproduct of sugar beet processing.

- Powder
- Tablets (500, 750, 1000 mg)
- Capsules (500, 750, 1000 mg)

Therapeutic Uses

Cardiovascular disease: Betaine (0.84 g twice daily for one week) was shown to significantly reduce homocysteine levels in patients with premature vascular disease, comparable to choline, pyridoxine, or folic acid treatment. In a similar study, 6 g of betaine per day was shown to reduce homocysteine levels in the majority of patients tested.

Liver disease: It is hypothesized that betaine may be a promising therapeutic agent in the treatment of liver disease. Oral administration of betaine has been shown to increase SAM levels sufficiently enough to protect against the early stages of alcoholic liver injury in rats.

Homocystinuria: Homocystinuria is an inherited disease caused by a deficiency in 5–10-methylenetetrahydrofolate reductase or cystathionine beta-synthase activity, or a defect in cobalamin metabolism. Betaine treatment (6 g per day) has been shown to correct metabolic abnormalities in patients with homocystinuria caused by methylenetetrahydrofolate reductase, and cystathione beta-synthase, deficiency.

In some forms of homocystinuria, betaine may be more efficacious than vitamin B_6, B_{12}, or folate. In one study, treatment with betaine monohydrate caused a significant improvement in symptoms in an adolescent with 5–10-methylenetetrahydrofolate reductase defiency, while the B vitamins caused no response. SAM levels were significantly elevated in the cerebrospinal fluid after treatment with betaine.

Dosage Ranges and Duration of Administration

- Most experts recommend that patients with homocystinuria or premature vascular disease be kept on a methylation regimen (folic, B_6, B_{12}, and/or betaine) indefinitely.
- General cardiovascular health: 500 to 1000 mg/day
- Inherited homocystinuria: 6 g/day
- Premature vascular disease: 6 g/day

Cautions

■ Adverse Effects/Toxicology

No side effects were observed at a dosage of 6 grams betaine, daily.

■ Warnings/Contraindications/Precautions

None.

Interactions

Folic acid (vitamin B_9), pyridoxine (vitamin B_6), and cobalamin (vitamin B_{12}) are involved in methylation reactions that convert homocysteine to methionine. For best results, these vitamins should be taken in combination with betaine.

References

Barak AJ, et al. S-adenosylmethionine generation and prevention of alcoholic fatty liver by betaine. *Alcohol*. Nov-Dec 1994; 11(6): 501–503.

Barak AJ, et al. Betaine, ethanol, and the liver: a review. *Alcohol*. Jul-Aug 1996; 13(4): 395–398.

Berkow R, et al, eds. *The Merck Manual of Diagnosis and Therapy*. 15th ed. Rahway: Merck Sharp & Dohme Research Laboratories; 1987: 556.

Boushey CJ, et al. A quantitative assessment of plasma homocysteine as a risk factor for vascular disease. Probable benefits of increasing folic acid intakes. *JAMA*. Oct 4, 1995; 274(13): 1049–1057.

Budavari S, O'Neil MJ, Heckelman PE, Kinneary JF, eds. *The Merck Index*. 12th ed. Whitehouse Station: Merck & Co., Inc.; 1996: 198.

Dudman NPB, et al. Disorderd Methionine/Homocysteine Metabolism in Premature Vascular Disease. *Arteriosc and Thromb*. 1993; 13(9): 1253–1260.

Franken DG, et al. Treatment of mild hyperhomocysteinemia in vascular disease patients. *Arterioscler and Thromb*. March 1994;14 (3): 465–470.

Holme E, et al. Betaine for treatment of homocystinuria caused by methylenetetrahydrofolate reducatase deficiency. *Arch Dis Child*. 1989; 64: 1061–1064.

Kishi T, et al. Effect of betaine on S-adenosylmethionine levels in the cerebrospinal fluid in a patient with methylenetetrahydrofolate reductase deficiency and peripheral neuropathy. *J Inherit Metab Dis*. 1994; 17(5): 560–565.

Shils M, Olson J, Shike M, eds. *Modern Nutrition in Health and Disease Vol 1*. 8th ed. Media: Williams & Wilkins; 1994: 452.

Shils M, Olson J, Shike M, eds. *Modern Nutrition in Health and Disease*. 7th ed. Media: Williams & Wilkins; 1988: 1363–1365.

Stampfer MJ, Malinow MR. Can lowering homocysteine levels reduce cardiovascular disease *N Engl J Med*. Feb. 2, 1995; 332: 328–329.

Steinmetz CA, et al. Vegetables, fruit, and cancer prevention: A review. *Am Diet Assoc*. 1996: 1027–1039.

The Third National Health and Nutrition Examination Survey. Phase 1, 1989–91. The National Center for Health Statistics. Accessed at: www.cdc.gov/nchs/faq/hanesii1.htm. on November 3, 1999.

Wilcken DE, et al. Homocystinuria due to cystathione beta-synthase deficiency–the effects of betaine treatment in pyridoxine-responsive patients. *Metab*. Dec 1985; 34(12): 1115–1121.

© *Copyright Integrative Medicine Communications*

Brewer's Yeast

Overview

Brewer's yeast, which is often called nutritional yeast, was originally a by-product of the brewing of beer. While still used for brewing, it is also now produced for its nutritional value. Nutritional yeast is not exactly the same as brewer's yeast. Brewer's yeast was originally used as a nutritional supplement, then other yeasts were made available for this purpose. Brewer's yeast differs from live baker's yeast in that its live yeast cells have been destroyed, leaving the nutrients behind. Live yeast cells can actually deplete the body of B vitamins and other nutrients.

Nutritional yeast contains high levels of many important nutrients, including all of the B vitamins (except for B_{12}), 16 out of 20 amino acids, and 14 different minerals. The amino acids in yeast are protein components which help the body repair tissue and fight disease. Brewer's yeast has a high protein content, with one tbsp. providing 4.6 g, making it a rich source of protein for vegetarians. It is also high in phosphorus.

Because yeast is such a rich source of the B vitamin family, it enhances the roles these vitamins play in the body. The B-complex vitamins support and optimize carbohydrate, fat, and protein metabolism. They also support the nervous system and maintain tonicity in gastrointestinal muscles. Different B vitamins play different roles, particularly in their support of the nervous system. They relieve stress, depression, irritability, and fatigue, and also help protect against aging. When under the pressures of stress or infection, the body needs higher supplies of these important vitamins. The body does not store excess B vitamins, so they must be continually replenished. B vitamins can also help deter morning sickness.

Biotin, one of the B vitamins that brewer's yeast supplies, has been shown to strengthen brittle nails and improve the health of hair. It also improves the metabolism of scalp oils, which make it an important treatment for seborrheic dermatitis, a condition seen most often in infants ("cradle cap") and the elderly. Biotin is also used to treat diabetes, since it enhances insulin sensitivity, increases glucokinase activity, and is helpful for treating diabetic neuropathy.

Brewer's yeast is also an important source of chromium. There is no official RDA for chromium, but the U.S. FDA recommends 120 mcg daily. However, 90% of Americans are deficient in this important mineral. Chromium has the ability to significantly lower low density lipoprotein (LDL) levels in the blood and raise high density lipoprotein (HDL) levels. Studies have shown that cardiac patients can have 40% lower blood levels of chromium than those without coronary artery disease. Some research has suggested that brewer's yeast also contains other hypocholesterolemic factors beyond its rich chromium content.

Chromium is also an important supplement for those with Type II (adult onset) diabetes. It can significantly lower blood glucose levels by aiding transmission of insulin into the cells. Researchers have been able to lower some glucose levels in diabetics to almost normal levels with daily chromium doses of 1,000 mcg. Chromium supplementation should be considered as an adjunct to started medications.

Even if blood glucose levels are normal, skin glucose tolerance appears to be impaired in cases of acne. Several studies have tested the use of chromium for acne treatment, with good results. Chromium's ability to increase the effectiveness of insulin's activity in the body has also led to its use as a weight loss aid. Chromium can be difficult for the body to absorb, but brewer's yeast is one of most absorbable ways to take it.

Sources

■ Constituents/Composition
Chromium, thiamine, nicotinic acid, riboflavine, pyridoxine, pantothenic acid, biotin, folic acid, cyanocobalamin, aminobenzoic acid, and inositol.

■ Commercial Preparations
Brewer's yeast comes in powder, flake, tablet, and liquid form.

Therapeutic Uses

- As a source of chromium: to reduce blood sugar levels in Type II diabetics, to lower blood cholesterol levels, to aid in weight loss, and to aid in the treatment of acne
- As a source of B vitamins: to relieve stress, depression, irritability, and fatigue
- As a source of biotin: to strengthen hair and nails and treat seborrheic dermatitis and diabetes

Dosage Ranges and Duration of Administration

Can be taken in juice or water. Four tbsp. per day are recommended. If the body's diet is low in B vitamins, this amount may cause gas. It is best to begin with 1 tsp. in a glass of juice and work slowly up to 4 tbsp. Nutritional yeast may be taken as a source of chromium to assist weight loss and treat impaired glucose tolerance, or of biotin to promote strong nails and healthy hair and treat cradle cap, diabetes, and diabetic neuropathy.

Cautions

■ Adverse Effects/Toxicology
Brewer's yeast has no known side effects.

■ Warnings/Contraindications/Precautions
Be cautious with yeast products if you have an overgrowth of intestinal yeast (*Candida albicans* or *rhodotorula* yeast). People with osteoporosis should avoid yeast because of its high levels of phosphorus. If taking a yeast supplement, also take extra calcium.

Interactions
None reported

References

Balch J, Balch P. *Prescription for Nutritional Healing*. Garden Park City, NY: Avery Publishing Group; 1997.

Bentley JP, Hunt TK, Weiss JB, et al. Peptides from live yeast cell derivative stimulate wound healing. *Arch Surg*. 1990;125:641–646.

Chromium necessary to regulate blood sugar. *Conscious Choice: The Journal of Ecology and Natural Living*. June 1998;11:33.

Hegoczki J, Suhajda A, Janzso B, Vereczkey G. Preparation of chromium enriched yeasts. *Acta Alimentaria*. 1997;26:345–358.

Li Y-C. Effects of brewer's yeast on glucose tolerance and serum lipids in Chinese adults. *Biol Trace Elem Res*. 1994;41:341–347.

McCarty MF. Insulin resistance in Mexican Americans: a precursor to obesity and diabetes? *Med Hypotheses*. 1993;41:308–315.

Murray M. Biotin: An overlooked essential B vitamin. *The America Journal of Natural Medicine*. May 1996;3:5–6.

Murray M. The chromium connection. *Health Counselor*. March 1997;9:48–59.

Rabinowitz MB, Gonick HC, Levin SR, Davidson MB. Effects of chromium and yeast supplements on carbohydrate and lipid metabolism in diabetic men. *Diabetes Care*. 1983;6:319–327.

© Copyright Integrative Medicine Communications

Bromelain

Overview

Bromelain is a proteolytic digestive enzyme that is extracted from the stem and the fruit of the pineapple plant *(Ananas comosus)*. It is best known as a digestive aid and for its anti-inflammatory effects in soft tissue injury and edema. However, bromelain has been used successfully to treat a number of disorders including cardiovascular disease, joint disease, upper respiratory tract infection, and Peyronie's disease. Bromelain has also been used successfully to debride wounds and to potentiate the actions of antibiotics and chemotherapeutic agents.

Sources

■ Dietary Sources

Bromelain is one of the simple digestive enzymes that is extracted from tropical fruits, in this case pineapples.

■ Constituents/Composition

Bromelain A and B, the proteolytic enzymes of pineapples, constitute bromelain. Bromelain also consists of peroxidase, acid phosphatase, protease inhibitors, and calcium.

■ Commercial Preparations

Bromelain is available in tablet (500 mg) or capsule form for oral use.

Therapeutic Uses

- Traumatic injuries and surgery. Bromelain's anti-inflammatory effects reduce the pain, bruising, and swelling from trauma (e.g., sports injuries) or surgery and speed the healing process. (The pain reduction is probably due to decreased tissue inflammation rather than to a direct analgesic effect.)
- Digestive aid. Bromelain has been used as a digestive enzyme, especially in patients with pancreatic insufficiency. It has been known to relieve gastrointestinal upset in humans and to heal ulcers in experiments in animals.
- Cardiovascular disease. Bromelain can relieve the symptoms of angina pectoris, inhibit platelet aggregation and clot formation, and break down arterial plaques by promoting fibrolysis; thus, it can be used to treat angina, thrombosis, thromophlebitis, varicose veins, and atherosclerosis.
- Joint inflammation. Because bromelain's anti-inflammatory effects reduce joint inflammation, it can be used for rheumatoid arthritis, osteoarthritis, sciatica, bursitis, tendinitis, and scleroderma.
- Potentiation of antibiotics and chemotherapeutic agents. By increasing absorption and tissue penetration, bromelain may potentiate the actions of chemotherapeutic agents and antibiotics. It has been shown to result in tumor regression when used in combination with selected chemotherapeutic agents.
- AIDS. Bromelain is a natural protease inhibitor (a protein-digesting enzyme) that may prove useful in the treatment of AIDS patients to control the replication of HIV. It is less expensive and is associated with fewer side effects than the protease inhibitors that are currently used for this function. More study is needed on bromelain's clinical usefulness in treating persons with HIV and AIDS.
- Upper respiratory tract infections. Bromelain has demonstrated effectiveness in suppressing mucolytic cough and decreasing bronchial secretions, resulting in increased lung function in patients with upper respiratory tract infections. It has also proved effective in patients with sinusitis.
- Peyronie's disease. The deposition of fibrin, which is responsible for the thickening of the fibrous connective tissue in the penis, can be prevented with bromelain.
- Wound debridement. Bromelain as a topical agent can accelerate the healing of burns.
- Anti-metastatic. Several studies suggest use as an anti-metastatic agent with chemotherapy.

Dosage Ranges and Duration of Administration

For use as a digestive aid, 500 mg with meals are recommended. For other uses, the following dosages are recommended.

- Traumatic injuries—500 mg qid on an empty stomach
- Cardiovascular disease—500 to 750 mg tid on an empty stomach
- Joint inflammation—500 to 2,000 mg/day in two doses
- Antitumor activity—1,000 mg/day

The standard duration of administration is 8 to 10 days, but longer periods are tolerated.

Cautions

■ Adverse Effects/Toxicology

Bromelain may cause nausea, vomiting, diarrhea, metrorrhagia, and hypermenorrhea, but no serious side effects have been reported in humans. Experiments in animals have not shown bromelain to cause cancer or birth defects.

■ Warnings/Contraindications/Precautions

- Allergic reactions, including skin reactions and asthma, may occur if the patient is allergic to pineapples.
- Caution must be used in patients with coagulation disorders and liver or kidney disease.
- Caution must be used in patients with hypertension.
- No data are available for use during pregnancy.

Interactions

- Increased bleeding may result if given simultaneously with anticoagulants.
- Bromelain can potentiate the blood levels of tetracyclines.
- Tachycardia may result when given to patients with hypertension.

References

Bromelain. *Alternative Medicine Review.* August 1998;3:302–305.

Desser L, Rehberger A, Kokron E, Paukovits W. Cytokine synthesis in human peripheral blood mononuclear cells after oral administration of polyenzyme preparations. *Oncology.* 1993;50:403–407.

Haas EM. *Staying Healthy with Nutrition: The Complete Guide to Diet and Nutritional Medicine.* Berkeley, Calif: Celestial Arts; 1992:257–258.

Harborne J, Baxter H, eds. *Phytochemical Dictionary: A Handbook of Bioactive Compounds from Plants.* London, England: Taylor & Francis; 1993:376.

Masson M. Bromelain in blunt injuries of the locomotor system. A study of observed applications in general practice. *Fortschr Med.* 1995;113:303–306.

Murray MT. *Encyclopedia of Nutritional Supplements: The Essential Guide for Improving Your Health Naturally.* Rocklin, Calif: Prima Publishing; 1996:429.

Murray MT, Pizzorno JE. *Encyclopedia of Natural Medicine.* 2nd ed. Rocklin, Calif: Prima Publishing; 1998:208,297–298,568,807,829–830.

Reynolds JEF, ed. *Martindale: The Extra Pharmacopoeia.* 31st ed. London, England: Royal Pharmaceutical Society; 1996:1681.

Taussig SJ, Batkin S. Bromelain, the enzyme complex of pineapple (Ananas comosus) and its clinical application. An update. *J Ethnopharmacol.* 1998;22:191–203.

Uhlig G, Seifert J. The effect of proteolytic enzymes (traumanase) on posttraumatic edema. *Fortschr Med.* 1981;99:554–556.

Walker JA, Cerny FJ, Cotter JR, Burton HW. Attenuation of contraction-induced skeletal muscle injury by bromelain. *Med Sci Sports Exerc.* 1992;24:20–25.

Werbach MR. *Nutritional Influences on Illness: A Sourcebook of Clinical Research.* New Canaan, Conn: Keats Publishing; 1987:64–65,268–269,386.

© Copyright Integrative Medicine Communications

Carnitine

L-Carnitine

Overview

Carnitine, in the form of L-carnitine, is a trimethylated amino acid that is essential for the transformation of fatty acids into energy for muscular activity. This transformation occurs in the mitochondria, producing coenzyme A.

A typical daily diet contains from 5 to 100 mg of carnitine. Most of the carnitine in the human body is synthesized from the essential amino acid lysine with the aid of methionine, another essential amino acid. The normal rate of carnitine synthesis in humans is approximately 1.2 micromoles per kg body weight per day.

Deficiency or depletion can occur secondary to various genetic and acquired disorders and conditions that impair the efficiency of carnitine reabsorption or increase the rate of excretion. Primary carnitine deficiency usually results from genetic disorders in carnitine transport. Such deficiency usually presents before age 5, and may be manifested by progressive cardiomyopathy, skeletal muscle weakness, and episodes of fasting hypoglycemia. Dietary deficiencies are rare, but occur most often in vegetarians, preterm infants, and during pregnancy or lactation. However, as vegetarians often have low-fat diets, they often have less risk of cardiovascular disease. Deficiencies may increase symptoms of fatigue, angina, muscle weakness, or confusion.

For supplementation, the L-carnitine form, alone or bound either to acetic or propionic acid, should be used. The D-carnitine form has produced undesirable side effects and should not be used.

Sources

■ Dietary Sources

The primary dietary sources of L-carnitine are red meats. Secondary sources include other animal-based food products such as fish, poultry, and milk products. Lesser sources include tempeh (fermented soybeans), wheat, and avocados.

■ Constituents/Composition

Carnitine is a zwitterionic quaternary amine with a molecular weight of 161.2 g/mol. The chemical name is beta-hydroxy-gamma-N,N,N-trimethylaminobutyric acid. The body produces carnitine, primarily in the liver and kidneys, from lysine with the help of vitamin C, pyridoxine, niacin, iron, and methionine. It is stored primarily in the skeletal muscles and heart; it is also concentrated in sperm and in the brain.

■ Commercial Preparations

- Carnitine is available in several commercial preparations. The L-carnitine form is most often recommended. It is available alone, or linked with acetic acid or propionic acid.
- L-carnitine (LC) is the most widely available form, is least expensive, and has been studied the most.
- L-acetylcarnitine (LAC) appears to be best for Alzheimer's disease and brain defects.
- L-propionylcarnitine (LPC) may be best for angina and other cardiac problems.

Therapeutic Uses

- Prevention of cardiovascular diseases: Carnitine facilitates oxidation of glucose in working hearts by relieving inhibition of pyruvate dehydrogenase by fatty acids.
- Congestive heart failure: L-propionylcarnitine (LPC) improves cardiac function.
- Early administration in patients with heart attacks has been found to reduce heart damage.
- Reduction of pain of angina; may be an effective alternative to other antianginal agents.
- One study has suggested that carnitine may be as beneficial as quinidine in treating cardiac arrhythmia without depressing blood pressure.
- Reduction of blood triglycerides and cholesterol levels; increase in HDL levels.
- AIDS: Reduced levels of carnitine are associated with AIDS; carnitine prevents toxicity of the drug AZT on the muscle cells, thereby reducing muscle fatigue and pain.
- Alcoholism: May inhibit alcohol-induced fatty liver.
- Alzheimer's disease: L-acetylcarnitine (LAC) may delay progression of the disease; also may be beneficial in treating senile depression and age-related memory defect.
- Anorexia: Supplementation may be beneficial.
- Diabetes mellitus: Supplementation with carnitine assists in glucose tolerance, stimulating immune defenses, and reducing the risk and severity of some secondary complications.
- Down syndrome: Treatment with L-acetylcarnitine (LAC) improves visual memory and attention.
- Epilepsy (childhood): intravenous L-carnitine is indicated for valproate (VPA)-induced hepatotoxicity and overdose. Oral supplementation is suggested for VPA-associated hyperammonemia or renal-associated symptoms in infants and young children, and for individuals with epilepsy using the ketogenic diet who have hypocarnitinemia.
- Chronic fatigue syndrome: L-carnitine supplementation is beneficial in the treatment of CFS.
- Hemodialysis: Relatively low doses of L-carnitine supplementation may be beneficial for hypertriglyceridemic hemodialysis patients.
- Immune system response: Even at low concentration levels, L-carnitine has been shown to neutralize lipid-induced immunosuppression; it has also been shown to increase the proliferative response of human lymphocytes following mitogenic stimulation.
- Infertility, male: In one study, supplementation was shown to increase sperm count and motility in 80% of men with abnormal sperm mobility.
- Weight loss: In addition to aiding in weight loss, or perhaps as a consequence of weight loss, carnitine has been linked to improvement of exercise capacities and endurance.

Dosage Ranges and Duration of Administration

- To improve fat metabolism and muscular performance, supplementation levels of 1,000 to 2,000 mg per day, usually divided into two doses
- For treatment of ischemic heart disease and hyperlipid states (specifically, Type IV hyperlipidemia): doses of 600 to 1,200 mg tid or 750 mg bid
- For AIDS patients being treated with AZT: 6 g/day
- For treatment of alcoholic fatty liver: 300 mg tid
- For treatment of male infertility: 300 to 1,000 mg tid

Cautions

■ Adverse Effects/Toxicology

Supplements in large quantities (approximately 5 g/day by an adult) may cause diarrhea or fish odor syndrome.

■ Warnings/Contraindications/Precautions

- Not recommended for individuals with active liver or kidney disease.
- Supplementation for improvement of fat metabolism and muscular performance should probably be stopped one week each month.
- Additional research into long-term safety as a supplement is needed.

Interactions

- Coenzyme Q10 appears to enhance the effects of carnitine.
- Pantethine appears to enhance the effects of carnitine.
- Choline appears to conserve carnitine.
- Antibiotics containing pivalic acid and valproic acid may reduce circulating carnitine in humans.
- Vitamin C may increase urinary excretion.

References

Brass EP, Hiatt WR. The role of carnitine and carnitine supplementation during exercise in man and in individuals with special needs. *J Am Coll Nutr.* 1998;17:207–215.

De Vivo DC, Bohan TP, Coulter DL, et al. L-Carnitine supplementation in childhood epilepsy: current perspectives. *Epilepsia.* 1998;39:1216–1225.

Elisaf M, Bairaaktari E, Katopodis K, et al. Effect of L-Carnitine supplementation on lipid parameters in hemodialysis patients. *Am J Nephrol.* 1998;18:416–421.

Haas EM. *Staying Healthy with Nutrition* Berkley, California: Celestial Arts Publishing; 1992:65–79.

Kelly GS. L-Carnitine: therapeutic applications of a conditionally-essential amino acid. *Alt Med Rev.* 1998;3:345–60.

Murray MT. *Encyclopedia of Nutritional Supplements*. Rocklin, Calif: Prima Publishing; 1996:283–295.

Murray MT, Pizzorno JE. *Encyclopedia of Natural Medicine*. 2nd ed. Rocklin, Calif: Prima Publishing; 1996:206, 216, 246–247, 424, 505–506, 584.

Newstrom H: *Nutrients Catalog*. Jefferson, NC: McFarland & Co., Inc.; 1993:103–105.

Plioplys AV, Plioplys S. Amantadine and L-carnitine treatment of chronic fatigue syndrome. *Neuropsychobiology*. 1997;35(1):16–23.

Shils ME, Olson JA, Shike M, Ross AC. *Modern Nutrition in Health and Disease*. 9th ed. Baltimore, Md: Williams & Wilkins; 1999: 90–92; 1377–1378.

Werbach MR. *Nutritional Influences on Illness*. 2nd ed. Tarzana, Calif: Third Line Press; 1993:13–22, 655–671.

© *Copyright Integrative Medicine Communications*

Cartilage

Overview

Cartilage is elastic, translucent connective tissue found in animals and man. Most cartilage is converted to bone as an animal matures, but some remains in such sites as the nose, ears, knees, and other joints. Cartilage extracts and supplements are made from cows (bovine cartilage), whose bodies contain both cartilage and bone, and sharks (shark cartilage), whose bodies contain cartilage and no bone.

Cartilage supplements are said to shrink tumors; to cure, or at least slow the development of, cancers; to reverse bone diseases such as osteoporosis; and to treat other conditions, such as macular degeneration and psoriasis, in which overgrowth of blood vessels causes disease symptoms.

The notion of using cartilage medicinally began in 1954, when bovine tracheal cartilage was found to promote wound healing. Since then, clinical trials have shown this substance to be effective against a broad range of conditions ranging arthritis to cancers. In studies at the Comprehensive Medical Clinic in Southern California, patients reported pain relief in as little as three weeks, though patients should be cautioned against expecting rapid relief. Early reports claimed that sharks do not get cancer, which proved to be untrue, although it is true that the incidence of cancer in sharks is low.

Shark cartilage that has been dried and pulverized into fine powder for use as a supplement contains many active components. Among the most important is an angiogenesis inhibitor (a protein that, at least in laboratory research, suppresses the development of new blood vessels). In cancer, this angiogenesis inhibitor deprives tumors of nutrients by blocking their ability to develop new blood vessels. In macular degeneration, it prevents blindness by blocking the uncontrolled growth of blood vessels in the eye. These effects have been demonstrated in the laboratory but have not yet been proven in human trials. Phase III clinical trials began in December 1998 on a liquid antiangiogenesis drug called Neovastat, which is made from shark cartilage. The 550 patients with small-cell lung cancer who participated were given chemotherapy; half were also given Neovastat, the other half a placebo. The joint studies are being conducted by the U. S. National Cancer Institute and a biotechnology company.

Bovine cartilage that has been cleaned, dried, and powdered to be used as a supplement helps to accelerate wound healing and reduce inflammation. Bovine tracheal cartilage was initially called catrix (from the Latin *cicatrix*, which refers to a healed wound). Today it is recognized as one of the few substances that speed wound healing. Both shark and bovine cartilage are beneficial for psoriasis, rheumatoid arthritis, and ulcerative colitis.

Sources

■ Dietary Sources

Commercially prepared supplements of bovine or shark cartilage.

■ Constituents/Composition

Shark cartilage contains angiogenesis inhibitor proteins; approximately 16% calcium and 8% phosphorus, which are absorbed as nutrients; and immune system-stimulating mucopolysaccharides, carbohydrates that form chemical bonds with water.

Bovine cartilage is believed to inhibit tumor growth, and the polysaccharides it contains are believed to combat cancer by stimulating the immune system.

■ Commercial Preparations

Neither shark nor bovine cartilage is U.S. FDA-approved for safety or effectiveness. (Shark cartilage was under study by the National Cancer Institute when it was discovered that every one of the cartilage supplements provided for the study had been contaminated. The trials were stopped.)

Both shark and bovine cartilage may be obtained at health stores or by mail-order as nutritional supplements. They maybe purchased in powder or capsule form under a variety of brand names, typically in capsules of 750 mg.

Therapeutic Uses

Shark and/or bovine cartilage is used to:

- Treat or prevent cancer by stopping the growth of blood vessels upon which tumors depend for nutrients
- Arrest the growth of new blood vessels in macular degeneration
- Treat arthritis
- Treat psoriasis
- Treat regional enteritis
- Relieve or reduce pain, inflammation, and joint damage associated with osteoarthritis and rheumatoid arthritis

Dosage Ranges and Duration of Administration

When using shark or bovine cartilage as a dietary supplement, 3 to 4 capsules per day.

When using shark or bovine cartilage to treat cancer, the normal supplement dose may increase by 3 fold.

Cautions

■ Adverse Effects/Toxicology

Some shark cartilage products have a strong fish odor and flavor that may be unpleasant. Taken in large doses, shark cartilage has a very unpleasant taste and often causes nausea.

■ Warnings/Contraindications/Precautions

With their providers' approval, most people can take shark cartilage safely as an adjunct to conventional treatments for arthritis and cancer; however, cartilage supplements should not be used in place of conventional treatments. Shark cartilage should not be used by:

- Children
- Pregnant women
- Patients who recently underwent surgery
- Patients who recently survived a heart attack

Interactions

Bovine cartilage is not known to interfere with other medications. Shark cartilage is believed to be safe when taken with other medications.

People who ingest large quantities of shark cartilage may also need extra magnesium and potassium supplements to maintain the body's correct mineral balance.

References

Balch J, Balch P. *Prescription for Nutritional Healing.* 2nd ed. Garden City Park, NY: Avery Publishing Group; 1997.

Burton Goldberg Group. *Alternative Medicine: The Definitive Guide.* Puyallup, Wash: Future Medicine Publishing, Inc; 1994.

Cassileth BR. *The Alternative Medicine Handbook.* New York, NY: W. W. Norton & Company; 1998.

Dupont E, Savard PE, Jourdain C, et al. Antiangiogenic properties of a novel shark cartilage extract: potential role in the treatment of psoriasis. *J Cutan Med Surg.* 1998;2:146–152.

Horsman MR, Alsner J, Overgaard J. The effect of shark cartilage extracts on the growth and metastatic spread of the SCCVII carcinoma. *Acta Oncol.* 1998;37:441–445.

Kriegal H, John Prudden and Bovine Tracheal Cartilage Research. *Alternative & Complementary Therapies.* April/May 1995.

Miller DR, Anderson GT, Stark JJ, Granick JL, Richardson D. Phase I/II trial of the safety and efficacy of shark cartilage in the treatment of advanced cancer. *J Clin Oncol.* 1998;16:3649–3655.

Moss R. *Cancer Therapy.* Brooklyn, NY: Equinox Press Inc; 1992.

Murray M. *Encyclopedia of Nutritional Supplements.* Rocklin, Calif: Prima Publishing; 1996.

Prudden JF. The treatment of human cancer with agents prepared from bovine cartilage. *Biol Response Mod.* 1985;4:551–584.

Romano CF, Lipton A, Harvey HA, Simmonds MA, Romano PJ, Imboden SL. A phase II study of Catrix-S in solid tumors. *J Biol Response Mod.* 1985;4:585–589.

Sheu JR, Fu CC, Tsai Ml, Chung WJ. Effect of U-995, a potent shark cartilage-derived angiogenesis inhibitor, on anti-angiogenesis and anti-tumor activities. *Anticancer Res.* 1998;18:4435–4441.

© Copyright Integrative Medicine Communications

Chromium

Overview

Chromium is an essential trace element for humans. Chromium in tissue is highest during infancy and decreases steadily with age. The average adult body contains about 600 mcg of chromium. Absorption occurs primarily in the jejunum and is affected by interactions with other metals, such as zinc, iron, and vanadium, and chelating agents, such as oxalate and phytate. After absorption, transferrin binds trivalent chromium and transports it to body tissues. Absorbed chromium is excreted primarily in the urine, with small amounts lost in hair, perspiration, and bile. Unabsorbed chromium (>99%) is lost in the feces.

Chromium must be converted to a biologically active form for physiological function. Glucose tolerance factor (GTF), a biologically active form isolated from brewer's yeast, contains chromium (III), nicotinic acid, and the amino acids glycine, glutamic acid, and cysteine. GTF potentiates insulin's actions and therefore influences carbohydrate, lipid, and protein metabolism. It works with insulin to facilitate glucose uptake, regulate blood sugar levels, and stimulate protein synthesis. The exact nature of the chromium-insulin interaction is unknown. Chromium may potentiate insulin action through direct action on insulin or its receptor, or it may regulate the synthesis of a molecule that potentiates insulin action. In clinical studies, GTF chromium has been shown to potentiate the effects of insulin and decrease serum cholesterol and triglycerides.

It is estimated that as many as 90% of all American diets are low in chromium. Individuals often consume less than the suggested minimum intake for chromium. The trend toward consuming highly processed foods may be a major contributing factor to this problem; appreciable losses of chromium occur in the refining of foods. Children with protein-calorie malnutrition, diabetics, and older individuals may be especially susceptible to chromium deficiency. Stressors such as elevated simple sugars, strenuous physical exercise or work, infection, and physical trauma may increase the loss of chromium, thereby increasing the need for chromium. Symptoms of chromium deficiency include glucose intolerance, elevated circulating insulin, glycosuria, fasting hyperglycemia, impaired growth, decreased longevity, elevated serum cholesterol and triglycerides, increased incidence of aortic plaques, peripheral neuropathy, brain disorders, decreased fertility and sperm count, negative nitrogen balance, and decreased respiratory quotient.

Sources

■ Dietary Sources

- Brewer's yeast (best dietary source when grown on chromium-rich medium)
- Lean meats (especially processed meats)
- Cheeses
- Pork kidney
- Whole-grain breads and cereals
- Molasses
- Spices
- Some bran cereals

Vegetables, fruits, and most refined and processed foods (except for some processed meats, which contain high amounts of chromium) contain low amounts of chromium. Hard tap water can supply 1% to 70% of one's daily intake. Cooking in stainless steel cookware increases the chromium content of food.

■ Constituents/Composition

Chromium is a white, hard, brittle metal that occurs in any oxidation state from -2 to $+6$. Trivalent chromium is the most stable and biologically active oxidation state and forms compounds with other organic compounds.

■ Commercial Preparations

Chromium is available commercially in several forms, including chromium polynicotinate, chromium picolinate, chromium-enriched yeast, and chromium chloride. Chromium is available in multivitamins and alone in tablet and capsule forms. Daily preparation doses are typically between 15 and 200 mcg chromium in multivitamins.

Therapeutic Uses

Diabetes. Chromium supplementation may improve glucose tolerance in healthy individuals and Type II diabetics with low chromium levels, and older individuals with abnormal glucose tolerance. Not all healthy individuals show a response to chromium supplementation. Individuals with low chromium levels appear to benefit the most from supplementation.

Poor dietary intake of chromium results in impaired glucose tolerance and symptoms similar to those of Type II diabetes mellitus. Individuals with marginally elevated blood glucose concentrations may benefit from chromium supplementation. One study assessed the effects of chromium supplementation (200 mcg chromium chloride per day) on 20 normal subjects with marginally impaired glucose tolerance. By the end of the three-month trial, 18 of the 20 subjects exhibited significant improvement in glucose tolerance.

Supplementation with chromium has also been shown to improve glucose tolerance in some diabetic patients. There is some indication that Type II diabetics may have an increased requirement for chromium. In one study, diabetic patients with severe complications, such as retinopathy and nephropathy, showed lower blood concentrations of chromium.

Older individuals are more susceptible to low tissue chromium levels, abnormal glucose tolerance, and increased incidence of diabetes and cardiovascular disease. Several studies have examined the correlation between low chromium levels and impaired glucose tolerance. In one clinical study, chromium supplementation improved glucose tolerance in 50% of older subjects (> age 70) tested. Older individuals with mild abnormalities in glucose metabolism appear to benefit more from supplementation than those with extreme diabetic-like abnormalities in glucose intolerance.

Chromium is also used to treat the following conditions.

- Hypoglycemia. Chromium deficiency may be an underlying contributing factor of hypoglycemia in some individuals. Supplementation with 200 mcg of chromium improves the symptoms of hypoglycemia in some individuals.
- Cardiovascular disease. A low amount of chromium in the diet is associated with increased blood cholesterol and increased risk of developing cardiovascular disease. Supplementation with chromium has been shown to increase HDL cholesterol and lower triglyceride and total cholesterol levels in diabetics and in individuals with impaired glucose tolerance.
- Glaucoma. Chromium affects insulin receptors in the eye. There is a strong association between chromium deficiency and increased risk of glaucoma.
- Obesity. Preliminary evidence suggests that chromium supplementation may help reduce body fat and increase lean body mass in some individuals. Chromium's ability to increase insulin sensitivity may explain these effects.
- Osteoporosis. Chromium picolinate has been shown to decrease urinary excretion of calcium and hydroxy-proline in women, and may help preserve bone density in postmenopausal women.

Dosage Ranges and Duration of Administration

There are no RDAs established for chromium. The estimated safe and adequate daily dietary intakes of chromium are as follows:

- Infants birth to 6 months: 10 to 40 mcg
- Infants 6 to 12 months: 20 to 60 mcg
- Children 1 to 3 years: 20 to 80 mcg
- Children 4 to 6 years: 30 to 120 mcg
- Children 7 to 10 years: 50 to 200 mcg
- 11+ years: 50 to 200 mcg

Dosage for disease prevention and treatment is typically 200 mcg chromium one to three times a day.

Cautions

■ Adverse Effects/Toxicology

Excess intake or tissue accumulation of chromium can inhibit the effectiveness of insulin.

■ Warnings/Contraindications/Precautions

Hexavalent chromium is more toxic than trivalent. Industrial exposure to high amounts of chromium, usually airborne, can result in toxicity symptoms, including allergic dermatitis, skin ulcers, and bronchogenic carcinoma. Trivalent chromium, the form found in foods, is poorly absorbed; thus, extremely high amounts are necessary to attain toxic levels. Gastric irritation can occur at extremely high doses.

Interactions

Chromium combines with niacin to form glucose tolerance factor (GTF). Calcium carbonate and antacids reduce the absorption of chromium.

References

Anderson RA, Cheng N, Bryden NA, et al. Elevated intakes of supplemental chromium improve glucose and insulin variables in individuals with type 2 diabetes. *Diabetes.* 1997;46:1,786–1,791.

Anderson RA, Polansky MM, Bryden NA, Bhathena SJ, Canary JJ. Effects of supplemental chromium on patients with symptoms of reactive hypoglycemia. *Metabolism.* 1987;36:351–355.

Bahadori B, Wallner S, Schneider H, Wascher TC, Toplak H. Effect of chromium yeast and chromium picolinate on body composition of obese, non-diabetic patients during and after a formula diet. *Acta Med Austriaca.* 1997;24:185–187.

Friedman E, ed. *Biochemistry of the Essential Ultratrace Elements.* New York, NY: Plenum Press; 1984.

Fujimoto S. Studies on the relationships between blood trace metal concentrations and the clinical status of patients with cerebrovascular disease, gastric cancer, and diabetes mellitus. *Hokkaido Igaku Zasshi.* 1987;62:913–932.

Krause MV, Mahan LK. *Food, Nutrition, and Diet Therapy.* 7th ed. Philadelphia, Pa: WB Saunders Co; 1984.

McCarty MF. Anabolic effects of insulin on bone suggests a role for chromium picolinate in preservation of bone density. *Med Hypotheses.* 1995;45:241–246.

Murray MT, Pizzorno JE. *Encyclopedia of Natural Medicine.* 2nd ed. Rocklin, Calif: Prima Publishing; 1998.

Shils ME, Olsen JA, Shike M, eds. *Modern Nutrition in Health and Disease.* 8th ed. Media, Pa: Williams and Wilkins Co; 1994:1.

Somer E. *The Essential Guide to Vitamins & Minerals.* New York, NY: HarperCollins Publishers; 1992

Urberg M, Zemel MB. Evidence for synergism between chromium and nicotinic acid in the control of glucose tolerance in elderly humans. *Metabolism.* 1987;36:896–899.

Wilson BE, Gondy A. Effects of chromium supplementation on fasting insulin levels and lipid parameters in healthy, non-obese young subjects. *Diabetes Res Clin Pract.* 1995;28:179–184.

© *Copyright Integrative Medicine Communications*

Coenzyme Q10

Overview

Coenzyme Q10, also known as ubiquinone, is found in the mitochondria, and it is essential for energy production. It is classified as an antioxidant, although it has been suggested that it should be classified as a fat-soluble vitamin.

An increasing body of research is demonstrating that supplementation with coenzyme Q10 can be beneficial in the treatment of a number of health problems, particularly cardiac conditions and diseases. Studies have suggested that supplementation may be beneficial in the treatment of breast cancer, diabetes mellitus, immune deficiency, muscular dystrophy, and periodontal disease.

Deficiency primarily affects the heart and may lead to heart failure. Deficiency can result from impaired coenzyme Q10 synthesis or increased needs from diseases such as angina, hypertension, and congestive heart failure. Additionally, coenzyme Q10 levels may decrease as part of the aging process.

Sources

■ Dietary Sources

Coenzyme Q10 is found in every plant and animal cell, hence the alternative name, ubiquinone. Primary dietary sources include oily fish, organ meats, and whole grains.

■ Constituents/Composition

Coenzyme Q10 is a component of the mitochondria within each cell. It is a coenzyme and an antioxidant involved in the process of creating ATP, and thus critical to providing useable energy to the body.

■ Commercial Preparations

Coenzyme Q10 is available commercially in many forms including the following.

- Softgel capsules containing coenzyme Q10 suspension in oil (soybean oil); solubilized (Q-Gel) (good bioavailability)
- Powder-filled hardshell capsules
- Powder-based tablets

Therapeutic Uses

- Coenzyme Q10 can reverse or prevent degenerative lesions of the heart associated with angina, hypertension, and congestive heart failure by providing optimal nutrition at the cellular level.
- Congestive heart failure: Coenzyme Q10 as an adjunct to conventional drug therapy has been demonstrated to improve symptoms such as cyanosis, edema, venous congestion, heart palpitations, sweating arrhythmia, vertigo, and insomnia, in patients with moderate to severe CHF. Coenzyme Q10 alone may be sufficient to improve symptoms in patients with mild CHF.
- Hypertension: 39% of patients with hypertension have a coenzyme Q10 deficiency; studies have shown that coenzyme Q10 supplementation lowers HBP after 4 to 12 weeks. Coenzyme Q10 is not a typical antihypertensive drug; it apparently corrects a metabolic abnormality that favorably affects blood pressure.
- Angina: May reduce anginal episodes and improve cardiac function.
- Myocardial infarction: May provide protective effects in patients with acute myocardial infarction if administered within three days of onset of symptoms.
- Arrhythmia: May be beneficial in controlling cardiac arrhythmia.
- Ischemia: Acute intravenous coenzyme Q10 improves function and efficiency and decreases oxidant injury after cardiac ischemia and reperfusion.
- Cardiomyopathy: May be beneficial for cardiomyopathy by increasing cardiac ejection fraction, reducing shortness of breath, and increasing muscle strength.
- Mitral valve prolapse: One study has demonstrated that heart function returns to normal when coenzyme Q10 is taken for at least 8 weeks in doses of 2 mg per kg of body weight. When taken for 18 months or more, relapse rarely occurred; however, when taken for only 12 to 17 months, there were more frequent relapses.
- Cardiac bypass surgery: Pretreatment supplementation with coenzyme Q10 has been shown to reduce oxidative damage and protect the heart during surgery.
- Breast cancer: In Danish studies, coenzyme Q10 in dosages of 390 mg per day, as part of a nutritional protocol, was found to support at least partial remission, tumor reductions, and retarded metastasis.
- Chemotherapy: Coenzyme Q10 reduces the cardiotoxicity of adriamycin.
- Diabetes mellitus: In one study, coenzyme Q10 reduced fasting blood sugar by at least 20% in 14 of 39 patients, and by at least 30% in another 12 of 39 patients; ketone bodies fell by at least 30% in 13 of 22 patients.
- Exercise/weight loss: May be beneficial in improving capacity at submaximal heart rate, maximal work load, maximal oxygen consumption after about four weeks of supplementation. May assist in weight loss by correcting energy consumption and expenditure balance in certain individuals.
- Immune deficiencies: Supplementation with coenzyme Q10 may enhance immune response.
- Mitochondrial and neurodegenerative diseases: Coenzyme Q10 supplementation may improve energy production in muscle cells, thereby improving physical performance.
- Periodontal disease: Coenzyme Q10 deficiency in gingival tissue is present in 60 to 96 percent of patients with periodontal disease. Low levels of coenzyme Q10 may indicate a systemic imbalance, or a response to the periodontitis itself. Oral treatment with coenzyme Q10 reverses the gingival tissue deficiency and appears to accelerate healing by correcting abnormal citrate metabolism and by generally improving energy-dependent healing and repair.

Dosage Ranges and Duration of Administration

General supplementation dose is 25 mg bid.

Experimental doses:

- 100 mg/day in patients with congestive cardiomyopathy
- 60 mg/day for four to eight weeks to enhance athletic performance
- 120 mg/day for 28 days in patients with acute myocardial infarction
- 400 mg per day for potential prevention and treatment of breast cancer, and possibly other forms of cancer

Coenzyme Q10 should be taken with a meal with oil since it is oil soluble. Absorption decreases in the absence of oil.

Cautions

■ Adverse Effects/Toxicology

Coenzyme Q10 appears to be safe with no significant side effects.

■ Warnings/Contraindications/Precautions

Coenzyme Q10 appears to be safe; however, there have been no studies pertaining to safety during pregnancy and lactation.

Interactions

There are no significant adverse interactions noted. Coenzyme Q10 enhances the performance of carnitine and pantethine. Coenzyme Q10 supplementation counteracts the adverse effects of the following.

- Cholesterol-lowering drugs including lovastatin (Mevacor), pravastatin (Pravachol), and simvastatin (Zocor), which can block the manufacture of coenzyme Q10 and other necessary enzymes. (Supplement with 100 mg per day.)
- Beta-blockers: One study suggested supplementation of 60 mg per day for patients taking propranolol, which can inhibit coenzyme Q10-dependent enzymes.
- Psychotropic drugs: Studies suggest that supplementation may reduce cardiac side effects from the use of phenothiazines and tricyclic antidepressants.

References

Chan A, Reichmann H, Kogel A, Beck A, Gold R. Metabolic changes in patients with mitochondrial myopathies and effects of coenzyme Q10 therapy. *J Neurol.* 1998;245:681–685.

Chopra RK, Goldman R, Sinatra ST, Bhagavan HN. Relative bioavailability of coenzyme Q10 formulations in human subjects. *Int J Vitam Nutr Res.* 1998;68:109–113.

Haas EM. *Staying Healthy with Nutrition.* Berkley, Calif: Celestial Arts Publishing; 1992:65–79.

Jolliet P, Simon N, Barre J, et al. Plasma coenzyme Q10 concentrations in breast cancer: prognosis and therapeutic consequences. *Int J Clin Pharmacol Therapeu.* 1998;36:506–509.

Matthews RT, Yang L, Browne S, Baik M, Beal MF. Coenzyme Q10 administration increases brain mitochondrial concentrations and exerts neuroprotective effects. *Proc Natl Acad Sci USA*. July 21, 1998; 95:8892–8897.

Murray MT. *Encyclopedia of Nutritional Supplements*. Rocklin, Calif: Prima Publishing; 1996:296–308.

Murray MT, Pizzorno JE. *Encyclopedia of Natural Medicine*. 2nd ed. Rocklin, Calif: Prima Publishing; 1996.

Niibori K, Yokoyama H, Crestanello JA, Whitman GJ. Acute administration of liposomal coenzyme Q10 increases myocardial tissue levels and improves tolerance to ischemia reperfusion injury. *J Surg Res*. 1998;79:141–145.

Shils ME, Olson JA, Shike M, Ross AC. *Modern Nutrition in Health and Disease*. 9th ed. Baltimore, Md: Williams & Wilkins; 1999:90–92: 1377–1378.

Singh RB, Wander GS, Rastogi A, et al. Randomized, double-blind placebo-controlled trial of coenzyme Q10 in patients with acute myocardial infarction. *Cardiovasc Drugs Ther*. 1998;12:347–353.

Werbach MR. *Nutritional Influences on Illness*. 2nd ed. Tarzana, Calif: Third Line Press; 1993:66, 119, 122, 179, 421.

© *Copyright Integrative Medicine Communications*

Copper

Overview

Copper is an essential nutrient required for hemoglobin formation and many other functions. Copper is involved in producing and releasing energy through enzymes in the cytochrome system of cell respiration. It is essential for the development and maintenance of skeletal structures; specifically, copper helps to form collagen, especially in the bone and connective tissues. In the nervous system, copper conducts electrical impulses and helps maintain the myelin sheath around nerve fibers through the synthesis of phospholipids. In addition, copper has been linked to anti-inflammatory effects through oxygen-free radical metabolism and control of histamine levels. Copper is involved in iron metabolism and may play a role in thermal regulation, glucose metabolism, and blood clotting. Recent evidence suggests it also plays a role in proper functioning of the immune system.

The average daily intake by individuals consuming a typical Western diet has now been established as 1.0 to 1.5 mg. This is lower than the 1.5 to 3.0 mg per day recommended to be safe and adequate. Pregnant women have higher needs, and greater supplementation may be indicated.

Copper deficiency in human beings is considered rare. Anemia resulting from copper deficiency has been found in individuals who have undergone intestinal bypass surgery, in patients receiving parenteral nutrition, in malnourished infants, and in persons ingesting excessive amounts of zinc. Copper deficiency in human beings has been linked to anemia, red blood cell rupture, demyelination and degeneration of the nervous system, pigmentation abnormalities in both skin and hair, abnormalities of the immune system, poor collagen integrity, faulty bone development, reduced activity of the antioxidant selenoglutathione peroxidase, elevated LDL cholesterol and reduced HDL cholesterol, and leukopenia (particularly granulocytopenia). Copper is important for converting T_3 to T_4, so low copper levels may reduce thyroid function. Animal studies indicate that copper deficiency results in central nervous system disturbances similar to Parkinson's disease, including symptoms of ataxia, tremors, and uncontrolled movements.

Wilson's disease, a genetic disorder, affects copper metabolism and leads to low serum and hair copper levels with high liver and brain copper levels. Serious problems, such as irreversible liver, kidney and brain damage, and even death, may result. It is treated with chelating agents; penicillamine is most often used as it binds copper in the gut and carries it out. Copper levels may be reduced through a low-copper diet, combined with more zinc and manganese in the diet and as supplements.

In Menkes disease, a rare problem of copper malabsorption in infants, that can often be fatal, decreased intestinal absorption causes copper to accumulate in the intestinal lining.

Indian childhood cirrhosis, a hereditary disease with accumulating copper in the liver, used to be fatal, but can now be treated with chelators. The incidence of ICC in India has decreased in recent years, but similar diseases have appeared elsewhere.

Sources

■ Dietary Sources

Copper is found in many varied food sources. The best sources include:

- Seafood (especially raw oysters; also squid, whelk, lobster, mussels, crab)
- Organ meats (beef liver, kidneys, heart)
- Nuts (e.g., cashews, filberts, macadamia nuts, pecans, almonds, pistachio nuts)
- Legumes (especially lentils, navy beans, peanuts)
- Chocolate (unsweetened or semisweet baker's chocolate, cocoa)
- Cereals (e.g., bran flakes, shredded wheat, raisin bran)
- Fruits and vegetables (e.g., dried fruits, mushrooms, tomatoes, potatoes, bananas, grapes, avocado)
- Blackstrap molasses
- Black pepper

An additional source is water that flows through copper piping.

■ Constituents/Composition

Copper is the third most abundant essential trace mineral. (Iron and zinc are first and second.) In biologic systems, copper is primarily found as Cu^{2+}, although it can appear as Cu^+ or even Cu^{3+}.

■ Commercial Preparations

Copper is available combined with sulfate, picolinate, gluconate, and amino acids. Data is not available to evaluate one form against another.

Superoxide dismutase (SOD), with copper, has been used to treat arthritis. Stability in the stomach and small intestine is an issue, however, and oral use may be contraindicated. Enteric-coated tablets of active SOD may improve suitability for oral treatment of arthritis and other inflammatory disorders. In a Danish study, arthritis patients who were treated with injections of SOD obtained relief from many of their symptoms, such as joint swelling, pain, and morning stiffness.

Therapeutic Uses

Therapeutic uses for copper include:

- Arthritis: Copper bracelets have been shown to reduce pain and inflammation associated with arthritis, although the exact mechanism is unknown. Recent research suggests that copper salicylate used to treat arthritis reduces symptoms more effectively than either copper or aspirin alone. SOD injections have reportedly provided relief in several European studies.
- Leukopenia and anemia
- Chemical hypersensitivity
- Cardiovascular disease: to prevent aortic aneurysms, treat high cholesterol
- Where copper levels are low, used to treat vitiligo, fatigue, allergies, and stomach ulcers

Dosage Ranges and Duration of Administration

- Daily dietary copper intake recommended by the National Research Council of the United States: 1.5 to 3.0 mg per day for adults. For children 2 to 11 years, 1.5 to 2.5 mg. Not recommended for children under 2.
- A zinc-to-copper ratio in the range of 8:1 to 15:1 is consistently recommended.
- For leukopenia and anemia, daily doses up to 0.1 mg/kg of cupric sulfate orally, or 1 to 2 mg per day added to nutrient solution of nutrients for parenteral administration.

Cautions

■ Adverse Effects/Toxicology

Copper toxicity is rare. Circumstances in which acute copper poisoning has occurred include accidental consumption by children, ingestion of several grams in suicide attempts, application of copper salts to burned skin, drinking water from contaminated water supplies, and consumption of acidic food or beverages stored in copper containers.

Toxicity results in nausea, vomiting, epigastric pain, headache, dizziness, weakness, diarrhea, and a characteristic metallic taste. In severe (but rare) cases, tachycardia, hypertension, jaundice, uremia, coma, or death can result.

■ Warnings/Contraindications/Precautions

Chronic copper toxicosis has been observed in dialysis patients following months of hemodialysis when copper tubing was used and in vineyard workers using copper compounds as pesticides.

Copper is an emetic. As little as 10 mg usually produces nausea, and 60 mg usually produces vomiting. The lethal dose for copper may be as little as 3.5 g. Copper supplements should be kept away from children.

Interactions

Excess copper can interfere with absorption of zinc.
Copper deficiency may be aggravated by:

- Alcohol
- Egg
- Fructose

Excretion losses may be increased by:

- Molybdenum

Copper absorption may be adversely affected by:

- Calcium
- Iron
- Manganese
- Tin

Copper SUPPLEMENTS

- Zinc
- Phytates
- Vitamin B$_6$
- Vitamin C (high levels of supplementation)
- Cysteine
- Antacids in very high amounts

References

Asseth J, Haugen M, et al. Rheumatoid arthritis and metal compounds—perspectives on the role of oxygen radical detoxification. *Analyst.* 1998;123:3–6.

Ensminger AH, Ensminger ME, Konlande JE, Robson JRK. *Foods and Nutrition Encyclopedia.* 2nd ed. Baton Rouge, Fla: CRC Press Inc; 1994;1:476–479.

Garrison Jr RH, Somer E. *The Nutrition Desk Reference.* 3rd ed. New Canaan, Conn: Keats Publishing Inc; 1995:188–192.

Haas EM. *Staying Healthy With Nutrition.* Berkley, Calif: Celestial Arts Publishing; 1992:190–194.

Hardman JG, Gilman AG, Limbird LE, eds. *Goodman and Gilman's Pharmacological Basis of Therapeutics.* 9th ed. New York, NY: McGraw-Hill; 1996:1325–1326.

Heinerman J. *Heinerman's Encyclopedia of Nature's Vitamins and Minerals.* Paramus, NJ: Prentice Hall Inc; 1998:250–255.

Mazzetti I, Grigolo B, Borzai RM, Meliconi R, Facchini A. Serum copper/zinc superoxide dismutase levels in patients with rheumatoid arthritis. *J Clin Lab Res.* 1996;26(4):245–249.

Murray MT. *Encyclopedia of Nutritional Supplements.* Rocklin, Calif: Prima Publishing, 1996:199–203.

Newstrom H. *Nutrients Catalog.* Jefferson, NC: McFarland & Co. Inc; 1993:141–151.

Olivares M, Uauy R. Copper as an essential nutrient. *Am J Clin Nutr.* 1996;63:791S–796S.

Pennington JA, Schoen SA. Total diet study: estimated dietary intakes of nutritional elements. *Int J Vitam Nutr Res.* 1996;66:350–362.

Shils ME, Olson JA, Shike M, Ross AC. *Modern Nutrition in Health and Disease.* 9th ed. Baltimore, Md: Williams & Wilkins; 1999:241–252.

Uauy R, Olivares M, Gonzalez M. Essentiality of copper in humans. *Am J Clin Nutr.* 1998;67(5 suppl):952S–959S.

Wapnir RA. Copper absorption and bioavailability. *Am J Clin Nutri.* May 1998;67;5:1054s.

Werbach MR. *Nutritional Influences on Illness.* 2nd ed. Tarzana, Calif: Third Line Press; 1993:655–680.

© *Copyright Integrative Medicine Communications*

Creatine

Overview

Creatine is an amino acid (a protein building block) which is absorbed into the bloodstream in the small intestine and excreted as the by-product creatinine in the urine. Creatine in the form of creatine phosphate (phosphocreatine) is an important form of high-energy phosphate found in skeletal muscle cells. During high-intensity exercise lasting for a short time (15 to 30 seconds), phosphocreatine is broken down into phosphate and creatine. The energy released is used to regenerate ATP, the primary source of energy. As phosphocreatine becomes depleted, output power drops because ATP cannot be regenerated fast enough. Therefore, more energy is available for use. In short-duration, high-intensity anaerobic sports such as weight lifting or sprinting, it is logical that more creatine phosphate in the muscles would allow greater ATP regeneration to produce more energy and increase performance.

Research has shown that taking creatine monohydrate supplements enhances performance for athletes who participate in high-intensity, short-duration sports. Several studies have been recently conducted to study a variety of sports and various dosages of creatine. The results are generally concurrent. After an initial "loading" phase of about a week, a "maintenance" phase keeps most athletes' muscle concentrations of creatine high enough to see noticeable changes in endurance and strength, and also an increase in lean muscle mass. However, some individuals are genetically predisposed to have high stores of creatine already in their muscles, or have a high efficiency or inefficiency in producing ATP. These people will not see a dramatic ergogenic (energy-producing) effect from creatine monohydrate supplementation.

Sources

■ Dietary Sources

About half of an individual's daily need of creatine is synthesized in the liver, kidneys, and pancreas from the amino acids glycine, arginine, and methionine. The other half is provided from the diet.

Meat or fish are the best natural sources of creatine. There is about 1 g of creatine in a half pound of raw meat. However, for purposes of "loading" the skeletal muscles to gain ergogenic benefits, it is not feasible to get extra creatine from the diet alone. Supplementation is necessary.

■ Constituents/Composition

There are three different forms of creatine. Creatine is primarily stored in the skeletal muscles as free creatine and phosphocreatine. Creatine monohydrate is the form primarily used for supplementation to increase the skeletal muscles' stores of both free creatine and the phosphorylized form used to fuel energy release during the conversion of ATP.

■ Commercial Preparations

Creatine monohydrate is available in a variety of forms. The most common form is a powder which is ingested by mixing with juice or water. Generally, about 1 tsp. provides a 5 g dose of creatine monohydrate. Liquid creatine monohydrate, a more recently marketed preparation, is now competing with the powdered form. Claimed benefits of the liquid form are faster absorption and convenience over the powdered variety. Creatine monohydrate is also available in tablets, capsules, energy "bars," chews, drink mixes, and other preparations. Since combining creatine monohydrate with glucose is reported to be more effective than taking creatine alone, there are many preparations with differing combinations of creatine and glucose or other carbohydrates.

Therapeutic Uses

- Primarily used by athletes as a supplement to "load" muscle stores of creatine to improve strength, endurance, and lean muscle mass for high-intensity, short-duration exercise
- May reduce blood lipids
- May improve glucose metabolism
- Reduces muscle wasting in post-surgical patients
- May benefit heart patients by increasing myocardial metabolism and reducing fibrillation as well as allowing increased exercise capacity
- May provide anti-inflammatory and analgesic activity

Dosage Ranges and Duration of Administration

The typical loading regimen for the average weight athlete consists of taking creatine monohydrate supplements in the dose of 5 g, qid (20 g/day) for seven days, depending on body weight. After that, the maintenance phase consists of 2 to 5 g/day to sustain the stores of creatine in the muscles.

Cautions

■ Adverse Effects/Toxicology

The only well-documented side effect has been weight gain. This is due to water being stored in the muscle cells (volumization), general water weight gain, and also an increase in lean muscle tissue.

Unsubstantiated side effects which have been reported include greater incidence of muscle cramping, strains and pulls; gastrointestinal distress; kidney impairment; and liver damage. However, studies have been done which negate these claims.

■ Warnings/Contraindications/Precautions

Not useful to increase performance in endurance (aerobically oriented) exercise.

Interactions

Caffeine has been proven to negate any of the ergogenic effects of creatine supplementation. Coffee, tea, and soft drinks should be avoided. Creatine monohydrate in combination with glucose seems to be more effective in increasing muscle energy and endurance than just supplementing with creatine monohydrate alone.

References

Bosco C, et al. Effect of oral creatine supplementation on jumping and running performance. *Int J Sports Med.* 1997;18:369–372.

Earnets, C.P., Almada, A.L., Mitchell, T.L. High-performance capillary electrophoresis: pure creatine monohydrate reduces blood lipids in men and women. *Clin Sci.* 1996;91:113–118.

Grindstaff PD, et al. Effects of creatine supplementation on repetitive sprint performance and body composition in competitive swimmers. *Int J Sport Nutr.* 1997;7:330–346.

Juhn, MS, Tarnopolsky M. 1998. Potential side effects of oral creatine supplementation: a critical review. *Clin J Sport Med.* 1998;8:298–304.

Juhn, MS, Tarnopolsky M. Oral creatine supplementation and athletic performance: a critical review. *Clin J Sport Med.* 1994;8:286–297.

Kreider RB, Ferreira M, et al. Effects of creatine supplementation on body composition, strength and sprint performance. *Med Sci Sports Exerc.* 1998;30(1):73–82.

Kreider RB, Rasmussen C, Ransom J, Almada AL. Effects of creatine supplementation during training on the incidence of muscle cramping, injuries and GI distress. Presented at the National Strength and Conditioning Association Convention; June 24–28, 1998; Nashville, Tenn. Accessed at www.eas.com/research/creatine/0698.html on February 21, 1999.

Kreider RB, Ferreira M, Wilson M, et al. Effects of creatine supplementation on body composition, strength, and sprint performance. *Med Sci Sports Exerc.* 1998;30:73–82.

Lawrence SR, et al. The effect of oral creatine supplementation on maximal exercise performance in competitive rowers. *Sports Medicine, Training and Rehabilitation.* 1997;7:243–253.

McNaughton LR, Dalton B, Tarr J. The effects of creatine supplementation on high-intensity exercise performance in elite performers. *Eur J Appl Physiol.* 1998;78:236–240.

Odland LM, et al. Effect of oral creatine supplementation on muscle [PCr] and short-term maximum power output. *Med Sci Sports Exerc.* 1997;29:216–219.

Poortmans JR, et al. Effect of short-term creatine supplementation on renal responses in men. *Eur J Appl Physiol.* 1997;76:566–567.

Prevost MC, Nelson AG, Morris GS. Creatine supplementation enhances intermittent work performance. *Res Q Exerc Sport.* 1997;68:233–240.

Schneider DA, et al. Creatine supplementation and the total work performed during 15-s and 1-min bouts of maximal cycling. *Aust J Sci Med Sport.* 1997;29:65–68.

Smith, J.C., et al. Effect of oral creatine ingestion on paarameters of the work rate-time relationship and time to exhaustion in high-intensity cycling. *Eur J Appl Physiol.* 1998;77:360–365.

Thompson CH, et al. Effect of creatine on aerobic and anaerobic metabolism in skeletal muscles in swimmers. *Br J Sports Med.* 1996;30:222–225.

Vandenberghe K, et al. Caffeine counteracts the ergogenic action of muscle creatine loading. *J Appl Physiol.* 1996;80:452–457.

Vandebuerie F, Vanden Eynde B, Vandenberghe K, Hespel P, et al. Effects of creatine loading on endurance capacity and sprint power in cyclists. *Int J Sports Med.* 1998;19:490–495.

Vandenberghe K, et al. Long-term creatine intake is beneficial to muscle performance during resistance training. *J Appl Physiol.* 1997;83:2055–2063.

Volek JS, et al. Creatine supplementation enhances muscular performance during high-intensity resistance exercise. *J Am Diet Assoc.* 1997;97:765–770.

Werbach MR. *Nutritional Influences on Illness: A Sourcebook of Clinical Research.* New Canaan, Conn: Keats Publishing, Inc; 1988.

© *Copyright Integrative Medicine Communications*

Cysteine

Overview

Cysteine is a sulfur-containing, water-soluble amino acid that is found in many proteins. Cysteine is considered a non-essential amino acid because it is formed from methionine in the body. Cysteine is very unstable and is readily oxidized to the amino acid cystine. Cystine contains two cysteines linked with a disulfide bond. It is thought that both amino acids probably undergo similar reactions in the body. Cysteine may be metabolized by several routes to yield pyruvate, taurine, or sulfide and sulfate. Insulin, CoA, glutathione (GSH), and vasopressin are other important sulfur-containing compounds derived from cysteine and cystine.

Cysteine plays an important role in liver detoxification conjugation reactions. Chemical toxins, such as bromobenzene, chlorobenzene, iodobenzene, naphthalene, benzyl chloride, are converted to mercapturic acids by conjugation with cysteine and acetylation.

The cysteine derivative N-acetyl-L-cysteine (NAC) helps prevent cellular oxidative damage in two ways: first, as an antioxidant capable of scavenging non-peroxyl radicals and, secondly, as a substrate for GSH synthesis. NAC has been used for a number of therapeutic purposes including treating respiratory diseases, acetaminophen poisoning, angina pectoris, and glutathione/antioxidant replenishment in HIV/AIDS. Newer research suggests an additional benefit in helping prevent cardiovascular disease and treating ocular symptoms in Sjogren's syndrome.

There is some controversy over the bioavailability of NAC, and its effectiveness at enhancing endogenous GSH levels. Some experts believe that cysteine is as effective as NAC, and it is less costly.

Sources

■ Dietary Sources

- wheat germ
- granola
- oat flakes
- ricotta
- cottage cheese
- yogurt
- pork, sausage meat
- chicken, turkey, duck
- luncheon meat

■ Constituents/Composition

L-Cysteine, N-Acetylcysteine

■ Commercial Preparations

- NAC aerosol spray (pharmaceutical)
- NAC liquid solution (pharmaceutical)
- L-Cysteine powder
- Cysteine/NAC tablets/capsules: (500, 600, and 1,000 mg)

The following is a list of N-Acetylcysteine Commercial Drug Preparations.

- Airbron
- Broncholysin
- Brunac
- Fabrol
- Fluatox
- Fluimucil
- Fluimucetin
- Fluprowit
- Mucocedyl
- Mucolator
- Mucolyticum
- Mucomyst
- Muco Sanigen
- Mucosolvin
- Mucret
- Neo-Fluimucil
- Parvolex
- Tixair

Therapeutic Uses

Sjogren's syndrome: Preliminary research indicates that N-acetylcysteine may have a therapeutic benefit on ocular symptoms, such as ocular soreness and irritability, associated with Sjogren's syndrome.

Respiratory diseases: Pulmonary dysfunction that occurs in adult respiratory distress syndrome (ARDS) is thought to be the result of neutrophil-mediated oxidant injury. Inflammatory metabolites of membrane phospholipids (leukotrienes, thromboxanes, prostacyclin, and PAF) may also cause oxidant injury in ARDS. NAC, as a substrate for glutathione synthesis, may reduce the oxidative damage and acute lung injury that occurs in ARDS.

Oral and aerosol NAC treatment may improve some of the symptoms associated with chronic bronchitis.

Cardiovascular Disease: NAC may potentiate the vasodilatory effects of nitroglycerin (NTG) in patients with unstable angina pectoris. NAC, administered orally or intravenously with nitroglycerin, has been shown to significantly reduce the incidence of acute myocardial infarctions in patients with angina pectoris. Intravenous administration of NAC has been shown to reduce infarct size and preserve left ventricular function after acute myocardial infarction.

Elevated plasma homocysteine levels are associated with increased risk of CHD. NAC may reduce homocysteine levels in hyperhomocysteinaemic conditions by forming mixed, low molecular weight, NAC-homocysteine disulfides with enhanced renal clearance.

NAC, administered orally, has also been shown to cause a dose-related increase in HDL-cholesterol levels without altering TC, TG, or lipoprotein (a) levels. A 16.2% increase in HDL cholesterol was seen at the highest dose (3,600 mg per day).

HIV: HIV patients have been shown to have a compromised antioxidant defense system and decreased intracellular GSH levels in their circulating T cells. NAC has been proposed as a treatment to replenish depleted GSH and inhibit reactive oxygen intermediates in HIV. However, the ability of NAC to increase GSH levels in white blood cells of AIDS patients is still controversial.

Acetaminophen poisoning: NAC is commonly used in the treatment of acetaminophen (paracetamol) overdosage. NAC (oral and intravenous) mitigates acetaminophen-induced hepatorenal damage if given within 10 hours, but becomes less effective thereafter. NAC may also help combat the enhanced acetaminophen toxicity that is associated with alcohol ingestion.

Corneal damage: Glutathione is found in high concentrations in the cornea and lens of the eye, where it probably functions as an antioxidant, protecting the eyes against cataracts. Animal studies indicate that NAC may help reduce cigarette smoke-induced oxidative damage to corneal cells, possibly by enhancing GSH levels.

Dosage Ranges and Duration of Administration

- Acetaminophen poisoning: The typical oral dosage of NAC is 140 mg/kg body weight, followed four hours later by 70 mg/kg every four hours for an additional 17 doses. Oral treatment must be started within eight hours of an acetaminophen overdose to prevent hepatoxicity. Oral NAC is typically administered for 72 hours; intravenous NAC for 20 to 52 hours. It is recommended to give the intravenous loading dose over 60 minutes, instead of 15 minutes, to reduce the risk of adverse reactions.
- Bronchial disease: 200 mg bid
- HDL cholesterol: 1,200 to 3,600 mg per day
- Antioxidant protection/general health: 500 mg/day to start. Individuals may increase the dose to 3 to 4 g/day as tolerated.

Cautions

■ Adverse Effects/Toxicology

Taking high doses (over 7 g) of cysteine may be harmful and should be avoided.

Oral NAC treatment may cause nausea, vomiting, and diarrhea.

NAC infusion in acetaminophen poisoning may cause anaphylactoid reactions including angioedema, bronchospasm, flushing, hypotension, nausea/vomiting, rash, tachycardia, and respiratory distress.

Intravenous nitroglycerin combined with intravenous NAC may cause symptomatic hypotension.

Fatalities have occurred from intravenous overdosage of NAC.

■ Warnings/Contraindications/Precautions

Oral NAC treatment, for acetaminophen poisoning, is contraindicated in the presence of coma or vomiting or if activated charcoal has been given by mouth.

Individuals with cystinuria should avoid, or limit, their intake of cysteine supplements.

D-cysteine, D-cystine and 5-methyl cysteine are toxic forms that should not be used.

Interactions

Vitamin B6 is involved in the metabolism of the sulfur amino acids. Cysteine may increase iron absorption and may bind copper in the body. NAC may potentiate the antihypertensive effects of captopril.

References

Borowitz JD, et al. Combined use of nitroglycerin and N-acetylcysteine in the management of unstable angina pectoris. *Circulation*. Apr 1988; 77(4): 787–794.

Braverman ER, Pfeiffer CC. *The Healing Nutrients Within: Facts, Findings and New Research on Amino Acids*. New Canaan: Keats Publishing, Inc.; 1987: 87–119.

Budavari S, O'Neil MJ, Heckelman PE, Kinneary JF, eds. *The Merck Index*. 12th ed. Whitehouse Station: Merck & Co., Inc.; 1996.

Carter EA. Enhanced acetaminophen toxicity associated with prior alcohol consumption in mice; prevention by N-acetylcysteine. *Alcohol*. Jan-Feb 1987; 4(1): 69–71.

Christman BW, Bernard GR. Antilipid mediator and antioxidant therapy in adult respiratory distress syndrome. *New Horiz*. Nov 1993; 1(4): 623–630.

Davreux CJ, et al. N-acetylcysteine attenuates acute lung injury in the rat. *Shock*. Dec 1997; 8(6): 432–438.

Flanagan RJ, et al. Use of N-acetycysteine in clinical toxicology. *Am J Med*. Sep 30 1991; 91(3C): 131S–139S.

Franceschini G, et al. Dose-related increase in HDL-cholesterol levels after N-acetylcysteine in man. *Pharmacol Res*. Oct-Nov 1993; 28(3): 213–218.

Hultberg B, et al. Plasma homocysteine and thiol compound fractions after oral administration of N-acetylcysteine. *Scand J Clin Lab Invest*. Oct 1994; 54(6): 417–422.

Jackson IM, et al. Efficacy and tolerability of oral acetylcysteine (Fabrol) in chronic bronchitis: a double-blind placebo controlled study. *J Int Med Res*. 1984; 12(3): 198–206.

Marchetti G, et al. Use of N-acetylcysteine in the management of coronary artery diseases. *Cardiologia*. Jul 1999; 44(7): 633–637.

Murray MT, Pizzorno J. *Encyclopedia of Natural Medicine* 2nd ed. Rocklin: Prima Publishing; 1998: 455–458, 558–563, 818–825.

Orten JM, Neuhaus OW. *Human Biochemistry* 10th ed. St. Louis: The C.V Mosby Company; 1982: 721–723.

Pelle E, et al. Protection against cigarette smoke-induced damage to intact transformed rabbit corneal cells by N-acetyl-L-cysteine. *Cell Biol Toxicol*. Aug 1998; 14(4): 253–259.

Perry HE, Shannon MW. Efficacy of oral versus intravenous N-acetylcysteine in acetaminophen ovedose:results of an open-label, clinical trial. *J Pediatr*. Jan 1998;132(1): 149–152.

Roederer M, et al. N-acetylcysteine: a new approach to anti-HIV therapy. *AIDS Res Hum Retroviruses*. Feb 1992; 8(2): 209–217.

Ruiz FJ, et al. N-acetyl-L-cysteine potentiates depressor response to captopril and enalaprilat in SHRs. *Am J Physiol*. Sep 1994; 267 (3 Pt 2): R767–772.

Smilkstein MJ, et al. Efficacy of oral N-acetylcysteine in the treatment of acetaminophen overdose. Analysis of the national multicenter study (1976 to 1985).*N Engl J Med*. Dec 15 1988; 319(24): 1557–1562.

Stavem K. Anaphylactic reaction to N-acetylcysteine after poisoning with paracetamol. *Tidsskr Nor Laegeforen*. May 30 1997; 117(14): 2038–2039.

Walters MT, et al.. A double-blind, cross-over, study of oral N-acetylcysteine in Sjogren's syndrome. *Scand J Rheumatol Suppl*. 1986; 61: 253–258.

© Copyright Integrative Medicine Communications

Dehydroepiandrosterone — DHEA

Overview

Dehydroepiandrosterone (DHEA) is the most abundant androgen (15 to 30 mg/day) secreted by the adrenal glands and to some extent by the ovaries and testes. It is a precursor for other steroid hormones, such as testosterone and estrogen. Peak levels of DHEA occur at age 25. By age 80, DHEA levels have decreased to 10% to 20% of the peak level. DHEA has been called an antiaging hormone because deficiencies of DHEA in old age may make individuals more susceptible to cancer of the breast, prostate, bladder; atherosclerosis; hypertension; autoimmune diseases (e.g., diabetes, lupus erythematosus, rheumatoid arthritis); osteoporosis; high cholesterol; obesity; memory disturbances; chronic fatigue; and manifestations of aging (older persons with these conditions have been found to have low levels). When given to older patients, DHEA increased feelings of physical and psychological well-being; increased immune cell production; and enhanced mood, energy, and sleep. Older individuals with higher DHEA levels are often in better heath than individuals with lower levels. The two most important factors concerning DHEA are its decline in old age and its deficiency in several major disease states.

Sources

■ Dietary Sources

Most of the DHEA on the market is made in laboratories from sterols (especially diosgenin) extracted from wild yams found in Mexico. Some extracts from wild yams are marketed as "natural DHEA." These extracts of diosgenin are supposedly converted into DHEA by the body. However, because it takes several chemical reactions to covert diosgenin into DHEA, it is unlikely that the body can make this conversion. Thus, only pharmaceutical grade DHEA should be used.

■ Constituents/Composition

DHEA is a weak androgen synthesized in large quantities by the adrenal cortex. However, it can be converted into more potent androgens (testosterone and estrogen) throughout the body as needed. Only a small percentage of the body's DHEA (5%) is in the active form; the rest (95%) is attached to sulfur molecules (DHEA-S)—that is, it is sulfated by the liver—and serves as a reserve to be converted to the active form when needed. When blood levels of DHEA are measured, DHEAS is usually the measurement taken.

■ Commercial Preparations

DHEA is available in capsules, chewing gum, or drops that are placed under the tongue. DHEA is either natural or synthetic. However, it is debatable whether the body can process diosgenin into steroid hormones. Thus, it is recommended that only "pharmaceutical grade" DHEA be taken.

Therapeutic Uses

- Heart disease. Men with heart disease have low levels of DHEAS. In one study, healthy men with low levels of DHEAS were three times more likely to eventually die of heart disease than those with high levels of DHEAS.
- Obesity. Experimental animals given DHEA did not become obese, but a control group given no supplements did become obese when given the same amount of food. In human studies, DHEA has not demonstrated a beneficial effect on body composition, even at high doses.
- Aging. Significant positive changes (e.g., less muscle wasting, less memory loss, improved mood and energy) have been seen in elderly men given DHEA.
- Osteoporosis. DHEA given to postmenopausal women increases bone mass. However, supplementation is not recommended until more extensive human trials have been conducted.
- Cancer. Experimental animals bred for breast cancer did not develop cancer when given DHEA supplements. Also, women with breast cancer have low levels of DHEA.
- Autoimmune disease. Low levels of DHEA have been found in patients with autoimmune disorders (e.g., lupus erythematosus, rheumatoid arthritis, multiple sclerosis, ulcerative colitis, AIDS). DHEA supplements improved stamina and overall sense of well-being in patients with autoimmune disorders. Patients with lupus treated with DHEA have shown symptomatic improvement, especially of kidney function, often permitting a reduction of their corticosteroids.
- Depression. DHEA has been used experimentally, to treat depressed patients. Improvements in both depression and memory were observed.
- AIDS. DHEA treatment in AIDS patients may have promise since low DHEA levels have been correlated with decreased immune function. However, controlled trials have not been conducted to investigate this supposition.
- Performance enhancement. Because DHEA is thought to build muscle mass, reduce fat, and reduce recovery time following injury, it is popular with athletes. However, human studies are needed to verify these claims. DHEA is also used to enhance sexual performance.

Dosage Ranges and Duration of Administration

DHEA is available without a prescription. Dosages for men and women differ; men seem to tolerate higher doses. Men can safely take up to 50 mg/day; women should not take more than 25 mg/day. Positive effects have been noted at dosages as low as 5 mg/day. Because the long-term effects of DHEA supplementation have not been studied and data from clinical trials is virtually nonexistent, the safety and efficacy of DHEA has not been determined.

Cautions

■ Adverse Effects/Toxicology

High doses of DHEA are associated with negative side effects for both men and women. However, the administration of high doses may be appropriate when treating serious illness (e.g., autoimmune diseases). High doses may inhibit the body's natural ability to synthesize DHEA and may be heptatoxic. In addition, women should be alert for any signs of masculinization because the end products of DHEA in women are androgens (male hormones). Possible signs include loss of hair on the head, hair growth on the face, weight gain around the waist, and acne. Men should also be alert for signs of excess testosterone (e.g., sexual aggressiveness, testicular atrophy, aggressive tendencies, male pattern baldness, and high blood pressure). Blood levels of DHEA should be checked every six months.

■ Warnings/Contraindications/Precautions

Because DHEA is a precursor of estrogen and testosterone, patients with hormone-sensitive cancers (e.g., breast, prostate, ovarian, testicular) should avoid taking DHEA.

DHEA is not recommended for people under the age of 40, unless DHEA levels are known to be low (<130 mg/dL in women and <180 mg/dL in men).

The International Olympic Committee and the National Football League recently banned the use of DHEA by athletes because its effects are very similar to anabolic steroids.

Interactions

One study indicated that vitamin E may protect against the oxidative damage associated with DHEA treatment.

Alcohol can potentiate the effects of DHEA.

References

Balch JF, Balch PA. *Prescription for Nutritional Healing*. 2nd ed. Garden City Park, NY: Avery Publishing; 1997:544–555.

Mindell E, Hopkins V. *Prescriptions Alternatives*. New Canaan, Conn: Keats Publishing; 1998:473–476.

Reynolds JE. *Martindale: The Extra Pharmacopoeia*. 31st ed. London, England: Royal Pharmaceutical Society; 1996:1504.

Shealy CN. *The Illustrated Encyclopedia of Healing Remedies*. Shaftesbury, England: Element Books; 1998:273.

Thompson G. Doctors warn of dangers of muscle-building drugs. *The New York Times*. March 2, 1999.

© Copyright Integrative Medicine Communications

Flaxseed Oil

Overview

Flaxseed oil is a rich source of alpha-linolenic acid (ALA), an omega-3 fatty acid. Omega-3 fatty acids (n-3) constitute one of two major families of polyunsaturated fatty acids, the other family being omega-6 (n-6). ALA is the parent substance of the n-3 fatty acid family. Linoleic acid is the parent substance for the n-6 fatty acid family. These two families have very different biochemical roles in the body. ALA is an essential fatty acid and is necessary for the normal function of all tissues. Through a series of steps, it is metabolized to eicosapentaenoic acid (EPA), docosahexaenoic acid (DHA), and prostaglandins in the body. Prostaglandins are hormone-like compounds that help regulate blood pressure, blood clotting, heart rate, vascular dilation, lipolysis, and immune response.

American diets are typically high in n-6 fatty acids and low in n-3 fatty acids. The average diet supplies only 0.15 g of n-3 fatty acids per day. A high ratio of n-6:n-3 fatty acid may encourage production of proinflammatory metabolites (arachidonic acid, prostaglandin E1, and prostaglandin E2) and negatively affect the body's response to disease. Changing the intake of dietary fatty acids may modify the body's response to disease, injury, and infection. Clinical trials indicate that supplementation with n-3 fatty acids from plants such as flaxseed can encourage production of the anti-inflammatory metabolites and inhibit the production of proinflammatory metabolites.

ALA is used as a source of energy by the body and partly as a precursor of the metabolites. Most studies indicate that a certain amount of ALA is converted to EPA in the body but conversion to DHA is limited. Results of one study showed that with a diet high in saturated fat conversion to EPA and DHA is approximately 6% and 3.8%, respectively. With a diet rich in n-6 polyunsaturated fatty acids, conversion is reduced by 40% to 50%. Flaxseed oil raises tissue EPA levels comparably to fish oil when dietary linoleic acid is restricted. In one study, the degree of conversion was proportional to a weekly portion (50 to 100 g) of fatty fish depending on the fat content of the fish. In some instances, ALA may be an effective alternative to fish oil supplements. However, a high ratio of ALA:linoleic acid may be necessary to produce the effects demonstrated after feeding fish oils.

Deficiencies in essential fatty acid can reduce both primary and secondary immune responses and modify the inflammatory response in animals. Symptoms associated with a deficiency in n-3 fatty acids include neurological changes (parasthesias, weakness, pain in the legs, inability to walk) and impaired vision.

Sources

■ **Dietary Sources**
Ground flaxseed or flaxseed meal

■ **Constituents/Composition**
Flaxseed contains 55% to 65% essential fatty acids, beta-carotene, and mixed carotenoids. Some processors add vitamin E to increase the oil's stability and shelf life.

■ **Commercial Preparations**
- Flaxseed oil is easily destroyed by heat, light, and oxygen.
- For optimal stability, seeds should be fresh pressed at low temperatures in the absence of light, extreme heat, or oxygen.
- Flaxseed oil is available in liquid and softgel capsule form, and should be refrigerated to prevent rancidity.
- Liquids require bottling in nonreactive, opaque or dark containers to prevent transmission of light. Capsules require similar packaging.
- Flaxseed oil can be used on salads and cooked vegetables or added to foods after they have been cooked. Flaxseed oil should not be heated since this destroys its anti-inflammatory qualities.

Therapeutic Uses

- Inflammation. Arachidonic acid and its proinflammatory metabolites are released from membrane phospholipids during an inflammatory reaction. EPA and DHA decrease the production of proinflammatory prostaglandins and thromboxanes from arachidonic acid. EPA competes with liberated arachidonic acid and induces the production of less inflammatory and chemotactic derivatives. A 1:1 or 1.3:1 ratio of ALA:linoleic acid may be optimal for reducing arachidonic acid production. This gives flax oil a use in inflammatory conditions such as arthritis, asthma, allergies, and dysmenorrhea
- Skin disorders. A small amount of research indicates that n-3 fatty acids may be of value in alleviating certain skin diseases such as psoriasis.
- Immune system. Studies in humans and animals have demonstrated that flaxseed oil is as effective as EPA at inhibiting the autoimmune reaction. This may prove useful in such conditions as rheumatoid arthritis and ulcerative colitis.
- Hypertension. Fish oil or flaxseed oil appear to be very effective in lowering blood pressure. One tablespoon of flaxseed oil per day can lower both the systolic and diastolic readings by up to 9 mm Hg.
- Cardiovascular disease. n-3 fatty acids have been shown to improve lipid profiles in hundreds of studies. The majority of studies used fish oils, not flaxseed oil. The few studies conducted with flaxseed oil indicate that it is not equivalent to fish oil. Large quantities of flaxseed oil are required to induce similar effects seen with fish oils. Flaxseed may offer some cardiovascular protection by improving arterial circulation and arterial function in high-risk subjects.
- Diabetes. Flaxseed oil may be a safer alternative to fish oil supplements in diabetics with altered lipid metabolism. High doses of fish oils have been shown to increase blood lipids and worsen blood sugar control in some individuals. However, some Type II diabetics may have low delta-6-desaturase activity, which prevents them from efficiently converting ALA to EPA in the body; flaxseed oil may not be an effective therapy in these individuals.
- Nephritis. Flaxseed oil reduced glomerular filtration injury and declining renal function in a rat-5/6 renal ablation model. Blood pressure, plasma lipids, and urinary prostaglandins were also favorably affected by the flaxseed oil treatment.
- Drug resistance. ALA, gamma-linolenic acid, EPA, and DHA have been shown to reverse tumor cell drug resistance in vitro.

Dosage Ranges and Duration of Administration

One to three teaspoons liquid flaxseed oil per day, or 3,000 mg (capsules) bid, as a starting dose is most recommended.

Dosage for disease prevention and treatment will vary depending on fatty acid content of the diet, individual body physiology (ALA conversion to EPA), and the type of disorder.

Cautions

■ **Adverse Effects/Toxicology**
There are no side effects or toxicity associated with increased intake of flaxseed oil.

■ **Warnings/Contraindications/Precautions**
Flaxseed oil can add additional calories and fat to the diet if there is not a compensatory reduction in other fats.

Interactions

May increase vitamin E requirements. Reduced platelet aggregation due to lowered prostaglandin species may increase bleeding time. Begin with a lower dose for those on blood-thinning medication or with a bleeding disorder.

References

Allman-Farinelli MA, Hall D, Kingham K, Pang D, Petocz P, Favaloro EJ. Comparison of the effects of two low fat diets with different alpha-linolenic acid ratios on coagulation and fibrinolysis. *Atherosclerosis.* 1999;142:159–168.

Bierenbuam ML, Reichstein R, Watkins TR. Reducing atherogenic risk in hyperlipemic humans with flaxseed supplementation: a preliminary report. *J Am Coll Nutr.* 1993;12:501–504.

Clark WF, Parbtani A, Hugg MW, et al. Flaxseed: a potential treatment of lupus nephritis. *Kidney Int.* 1995;48:475–480.

Cunnane SC, Ganguli S, Menard C, et al. High alpha-linolenic acid flaxseed (Linum usitatissimum): some nutritional properties in humans. *Br J Nutr.* 1993;69:443–453.

Cunnane SC, Hamadeh MJ, Liede AC, Thompson LU, Wolever TM, Jenkins DJ. Nutritional attributes of traditional flaxseed in healthy-young adults. *Am J Clin Nutr.* 1995;61:62–68.

Das UN, Madhavi N, Sravan KG, Padma M, Sangeetha P. Can tumor cell drug resistance be reversed by essential fatty acids and their metabolites? *Prostaglandins Leukot Essent Fatty Acids.* 1998;58:39–54.

Dox IG, Melloni BJ, Eisner GM. *The HarperCollins Illustrated Medical Dictionary.* New York, NY: HarperCollins Publishers; 1993.

Gerster H. Can adults adequately convert alpha-linolenic acid (18:3n-3) to eicosapentaenoic acid (20:5n-3) and docosahexaenoic acid (22:6n-3)? *Int J Vitam Nutr Res.* 1998;68:159–173.

Harris WS. N-3 fatty acids and serum lipoproteins: human studies. *Am J Clin Nutr.* May 1997;65(5 suppl):1645S–1654S.

Heller A, Koch T, Schmeck J, Van Ackern K. Lipid mediators in inflammatory disorders. *Drugs.* 1998;55:487–496.

Ingram AJ, Parbtani A, Clark WF, Spanner E, Huff MW, Philbrick DJ, Holub BJ. Effects of flax oil diets in a rat-5/6 renal ablation model. *Am J Kidney Dis.* 1995;25:320–329.

Kaminskas A, Levaciov, Lupinovic V, Kuchinskene Z. The effect of linseed oil on the fatty acid composition of blood plasma low- and very low-density lipoproteins and cholesterol in diabetics [in Russian]. *Vopr Pitan.* 1992;5–6:13–14.

Leece EA, Allman MA. The relationships between dietary alpha-linolenic: linoleic acid and rat platelet eicosapentaenoic and arachidonic acids. *Br J Nutr.* 1996;76:447–452.

Mantzioris E, James MJ, Gibson RA, Cleland LG. Differences exist in the relationships between dietary linoleic and alph-linolenic acids and their respective long-chain metabolites. *Am J Clin Nutr.* 1995;61:320–324.

Mayser P, Mrowietz U, Arenberger P, et al. Omega-3 fatty acid-based lipid infusion in patients with chronic plaque psoriasis: results of a double-blind, randomized, placebo-controlled, multicenter trial. *J Am Acad Dermatol.* 1998;38:539–547

Murray MT, Pizzorno JE. *Encyclopedia of Natural Medicine.* 2nd ed. Rocklin, Calif: Prima Publishing; 1998.

Nestel PJ, et al. Arterial compliance in obese subjects is improved with dietary plant n-3 fatty acid from flaxseed oil despite increased LDL oxidizability. *Arterioscler Thromb Vasc Biol.* 1997;17:1163–1170.

Norman AW, Litwack G. *Hormones.* Orlando, Fla: Academic Press, Inc; 1987. Orten JM, Neuhaus OW, eds. *Human Biochemistry.* 10th ed. St. Louis, Mo: The C.V. Mosby Company; 1982.

Prasad K. Dietary flaxseed in prevention of hypercholesterolemic atherosclerosis. *Atherosclerosis.* 1997;132:69–76.

Shils ME, Olson JA, Shike M, eds. *Modern Nutrition in Health and Disease.* 8th ed. Media, Pa: Williams and Wilkins Co; 1994:1.

Schmidt MA. *Smart Fats: How Dietary Fats and Oils Affect Mental, Physical and Emotional Intelligence.* Berkeley, Calif: Frog, Ltd; 1997.

Valsta LM, Salminen I, Aro A, Mutanen M. Alpha-linolenic acid in rapeseed oil partly compensates for the effect of fish restriction on plasma long chain n-3 fatty acids. *Eur J Clin Nutr.* 1996;50:229–235.

© *Copyright Integrative Medicine Communications*

Gamma-Linolenic Acid GLA

Overview

Gamma-linolenic acid (GLA) is a polyunsaturated fatty acid (PUFA) in the omega-6 series. It is derived from linoleic acid, and it is the precursor of arachidonic acid and the prostaglandin E_1 series.

Direct supplementation of GLA is ordinarily in the form of evening primrose oil, black currant seed oil, and borage oil. These sources also provide linoleic acid. For example, evening primrose oil is 72% linoleic acid.

People who have diabetes are less able to convert linoleic acid to GLA than healthy individuals. Other conditions that appear to reduce the capacity to convert linoleic acid to GLA include aging, alcoholism, atopic dermatitis, premenstrual syndrome, rheumatoid arthritis, cancer, and cardiovascular disease.

GLA is of benefit to diabetics by improving nerve conduction and preventing diabetic neuropathy. One animal study suggests that the combination of GLA and ascorbate is particularly advantageous.

Upon ingestion, GLA is elongated rapidly to dihomo-gamma-linolenic acid (DGLA). DGLA is efficacious in vasodilation, lowering of blood pressure, and the prevention of atherosclerosis.

GLA has an anti-inflammatory effect in humans. The mechanism is not completely understood, but oral administration of GLA can help suppress T-cell proliferation; GLA and DGLA suppress T-cell activation. In at least one study, rheumatoid arthritis patients taking GLA for a year improved over time, suggesting that GLA can function as a slow-acting, disease-modifying antirheumatic drug. The hope is to establish a therapeutic GLA dose that will reduce the need for other medication in persons with rheumatoid arthritis. This would help reduce the gastrointestinal problems associated with the use of non-steroidal anti-inflammatory drugs (NSAIDs). Research results are, however, somewhat controversial. There is some evidence that the effect of long-term supplementation actually may be contrary to the desired results of reducing inflammation. Nevertheless, GLA supplementation is particularly popular with persons with rheumatoid arthritis.

Corroborated studies suggest that GLA is unique among the omega-6 PUFA series in suppressing tumor growth and metastasis. It inhibits both motility and invasiveness of human colon cancer, breast cancer, and melanoma cells. Whether DGLA and prostaglandin E are involved in the process remains to be determined.

Recent animal research has suggested that GLA, in combination with eicosapentaenoic acid (EPA), can be beneficial in senile osteoporosis because it enhances absorption and retention of calcium. In addition, a pilot study done on elderly women suggested that GLA and eicosapentaenoic acid (EPA) reduce bone turnover rates and have beneficial effects on bone density and calcium absorbtion.

A recent Japanese study showed that evening primrose oil may be beneficial for hemodialysis patients with uremic skin symptoms. Patients given evening primrose oil showed significant improvement in skin dryness, pruritis, and erythema; and an increase in plasma concentration of a wide variety of essential fatty acids, more than patients who were given linoleic acid.

The ratio of omega-6 oils to omega-3 oils should be 4:1. However, the American diet provides more than 10 times the needed amount of omega-6 oils in the form of linoleic acid. This is because they comprise the primary oil ingredient added to most processed foods and are found in commonly used cooking oils. The total intake of linoleic acid is approximately 100 times the GLA intake. Because GLA is not found in abundance in common foods, supplementation may be necessary to mimic clinical dosages.

Sources

■ Dietary Sources

In addition to the plant seed oils of evening primrose, black currant, borage, and fungal oils, GLA is found in human milk and, in small amounts, in a wide variety of common foods, particularly organ meats.

■ Constituents/Composition

Gamma-linolenic acid is a long-chain polyunsaturated fatty acid with 18 carbon atoms. It is derived from linoleic acid; it is elongated to dihomo-gamma-linolenic acid (DGLA), then desaturated to arachidonic acid, and then is converted to the prostaglandin E_1 series (PGE$_1$).

GLA is available directly from evening primrose oil (7% to 10% GLA), black currant seed oil (15% to 20% GLA), borage oil (18% to 26% GLA), and fungal oil (23% to 26% GLA). GLA bioavailability may be related to the precise triacylglycerol composition. Although the GLA concentration in borage oil appears to be twice as high as in evening primrose oil, research has shown that the GLA effects, such as formation of prostaglandin E_1, are comparable for both on a gram-for-gram basis.

The essential fatty acids are known as vitamin F. The Food and Drug Administration prohibits the term "vitamin F" for advertising purposes, because of problems with foods such as french fries being advertised as "vitamin enriched" because they were fried in oil.

■ Commercial Preparations

- Evening primrose oil
- Black currant seed oil
- Borage oil
- Borage oil capsules

Therapeutic Uses

- Rheumatoid arthritis: GLA may reduce inflammation by suppressing T-cell proliferation and activation.
- Diabetes: GLA supplementation assists nerve function and helps prevent nerve disease in diabetics.
- Cancer: GLA may suppress tumor growth and metastasis, particularly in colon cancer, breast cancer, and melanoma.
- Heart disease: GLA may prevent heart disease by inhibiting plaque formation, increasing vasodilation, and lowering blood pressure.
- Eyes: GLA is beneficial in Sjogren's syndrome and may be useful in other dry eye conditions.
- Supplementation may alleviate the symptoms of aging, alcoholism, atopic dermatitis, osteoporosis, and premenstrual syndrome.
- Menstrual problems (amenorrhea, dysmenorrhea): Essential fatty acids such as those found in flaxseed, evening primrose, and borage oils reduce inflammation and support hormone production. Dosage is 1,000 to 1,500 mg daily or bid.

Dosage Ranges and Duration of Administration

There is no recommended dietary allowance (RDA) for GLA.

A recommended dosage for rheumatoid arthritis is 1.4 g/day. As the cost of oils can be prohibitive, and lower doses are usually effective, an acceptable clinical dosage of evening primrose, black currant, or borage oil would be 1,500 mg daily or bid.

Studies have shown that up to 2.8 g of GLA/day is well tolerated.

Cautions

■ Adverse Effects/Toxicology

Dietary sources of GLA appear to be completely nontoxic. A healthy person eating a normal diet should consume fewer saturated fats and more polyunsaturated essential fatty acids.

■ Warnings/Contraindications/Precautions

N/A

Interactions

No significant interactions are noted.

References

Bolton-Smith C, Woodward M, Tavendale R. Evidence for age-related differences in the fatty acid composition of human adipose tissue, independent of diet. *Eur J Clin Nutr.* 1997;51:619–624.

Brzeski M, Madhok R, Capell HA. Evening primrose oil in patients with rheumatoid arthritis and side-effects of non-steroidal anti-inflammatory drugs. *Br J Rheumatol.* 1991;30:370–372.

Brown NA, Bron AJ, Harding JJ, Dewar HM. Nutrition supplements and the eye. *Eye.* 1998;12(pt 1):127–133.

Ensminger AH, Ensminger ME, Konlande JE, Robson JRK. *Foods & Nutrition Encyclopedia.* 2nd ed. Baton Rouge, Fla: CRC Press, Inc; 1994:1:684–708.

Fan YY, Chapkin RS. Importance of dietary gamma-linolenic acid in human health and nutrition. *J Nutr.* 1998;128:1411–1414.

Garrison RH Jr, Somer E. *The Nutrition Desk Reference.* 3rd ed. New Canaan, Conn: Keats Publishing, Inc; 1995:23–64.

Haas EM. *Staying Healthy with Nutrition.* Berkley, Calif: Celestial Arts Publishing; 1992:65–79.

Jamal GA, Carmichael H. The effects of gamma-linolenic acid on human diabetic peripheral neuropathy: a double-blind placebo-controlled trial. *Diabet Med.* 1990;7:319–323.

Jiang WG, Hiscox S, Bryce RP, Horrobin DF, Mansel RE. The effects of n-6 polyunsaturated fatty acids on the expression of nm-23 in human cancer cells. *Br J Cancer.* 1998;77:731–738.

Jiang WG, Hiscox S, Bryce RP, Horrobin DF, Mansel RE. Gamma linolenic acid regulates expression of maspin and the motility of cancer cells. *Biochem Biophys Res Commun.* 1997;237:639–644.

Kruger MC, Coetzer H, deWinter R, Gericke G, Papendorp DH. Calcium, gamma-linolenic acid and eicosapentaenoic acid supplementation in senile osteoporosis. *Aging (Milano).* 1998;10:385–394.

Leventhal LJ, Boyce EG, Zurier Rb. Treatment of rheumatoid arthritis with blackcurrant seed oil. *Br J Rheumatol.* 1994;33:847–852.

Murray MT. *Encyclopedia of Nutritional Supplements.* Rocklin, Calif: Prima Publishing; 1996:239–278.

Newstrom H. Nutrients Catalog. Jefferson, NC: McFarland & Co., Inc; 1993:103–105.

Puolakka J, Makarainen L, Viinikka L, Ylikorkala O. Biochemical and clinical effects of treating the premenstrual syndrome with prostaglandin synthesis precursors. *J Reprod Med.* 1985;30:149–153.

Shils ME, Olson JA, Shike M, Ross AC. *Modern Nutrition in Health and Disease.* 9th ed. Baltimore, Md: Williams & Wilkins; 1999:90–92; 1377–1378.

Wagner W, Nootbaar-Wagner U. Prophylactic treatment of migraine with gamma-linolenic and alpha-linolenic acids. *Cephalalgia.* 1997;17:127–130.

Werbach MR. *Nutritional Influences on Illness.* 2nd ed. Tarzana, Calif: Third Line Press; 1993:13–22; 655–671.

Zurier RB, Rossetti RG, Jacobson EW, et al. Gamma-Linolenic acid treatment of rheumatoid arthritis. A randomized, placebo-controlled trial. *Arthritis Rheum.* 1996;39:1808–1817.

© *Copyright Integrative Medicine Communications*

Glutamine

Overview

Glutamine is an amino acid, one of the building blocks of protein that are linked together by peptide bonds in specific chemical arrangements to form proteins. It is found in both plant and animal proteins and is available in a variety of supplemental forms. Glutamine helps the body maintain the correct acid-alkaline balance and is a necessary part of the synthesis of RNA and DNA. Glutamine also helps promote a healthy digestive tract.

Unlike other amino acids that have a single nitrogen atom, glutamine contains two nitrogen atoms that enable it to transfer nitrogen and remove ammonia from body tissues. Glutamine readily passes the blood-brain barrier and, within the brain, is converted to glutamic acid, which the brain needs to function properly. It also increases gamma-aminobutyric acid (GABA) in the brain, which is also needed for proper mental activity.

Glutamine is the most plentiful free amino acids in muscles. Its ability to help build and maintain muscle makes glutamine especially attractive to dieters and muscle-builders, but that same ability also helps prevent muscle-wasting associated with prolonged inactivity, disease, and stress. With sufficient glutamine in the bloodstream, muscle loss that would otherwise be caused by injury, surgery, trauma, prolonged illness, or stress can be prevented. The body uses glutamine and glucose to make glucosamine, an amino sugar that plays a key role in the formation of nails, tendons, skin, eyes, bones, ligaments, heart valves, and mucous secretions throughout the body.

Conditions that have been treated with L-glutamine supplements include fibrosis, autoimmune diseases, arthritis, intestinal ailments, peptic ulcers, diseases of the connective tissues, tissue damage caused by radiation treatment, developmental disabilities, epilepsy, schizophrenia, fatigue, and impotence.

Because L-glutamine possibly reduces sugar and alcohol cravings, it could be considered for treating recovering alcoholics. Suggested dose: 1,000 mg tid with 50 mg of vitamin B_6, on an empty stomach.

Sources

Dietary Sources

Glutamine is found in animal proteins and vegetable proteins. Natural sources of glutamine include soy proteins, milk, meats, raw spinach, raw parsley, and cabbage.

Nutrition experts recommend choosing supplements whose label describes the contents as USP pharmaceutical grade L-crystalline amino acids.

The purest form of amino acid supplements is called free-form and is available in powder or encapsulated powder. Free-form amino acids are readily absorbed and nonallergenic, and are stable at room temperature but destroyed by high temperatures (350° to 660° F) typical of cooking.

Constituents/Composition

Glutamine is available as an isolated amino acid or in combination amino acid and protein supplements.

L-forms of amino acid supplements such as L-glutamine are believed to be more compatible with human biochemistry than D-forms because the chemical structure spirals to the left.

Commercial Preparations

Glutamine is available in a variety of foods and food supplements, protein mixtures, amino acid formulas, and individual supplements in liquid, powder, tablets, and capsules. Supplemental forms of glutamine are sold in vitamin and mineral sections of most pharmacies and health food stores.

Therapeutic Uses

- Glutamine is not one of the nine essential amino acids (which must be ingested because the body cannot manufacture them). However, extreme stress and prolonged illness may cause glutamine to become an essential amino acid, and hence a valuable dietary component.
- Glutamine aids recovery after surgery, wounds or injury, hemorrhage, prolonged illness including AIDS and cancer, and chemotherapy.
- In one recent study, glutamine reduced mouth pain by 4.5 days compared to placebo users in 24 methotrexate chemotherapy patients suffering from mouth sores and difficulty swallowing.
- Glutamine speeds healing of peptic ulcers.
- Because glutamine is one of the primary fuels used by intestinal lining cells, supplementation with glutamine helps restore gastric mucosa and improves mucosa metabolism. Glutamine also helps repair the gastrointestinal lining after damage caused by radiation or leaky gut syndrome, and benefits chronic GI diseases such as colitis, AIDS, cancer, and Crohn's disease. Large doses (more than 1,000 mg tid) helped protect chemotherapy patients' stomach linings, according to a 1996 study.
- Glutamine helps suppress food cravings.

Dosage Ranges and Duration of Administration

- Glutamine supplements, like all amino acid supplements, should be taken on an empty stomach, preferably in the morning or between meals.
- For peptic ulcers, 500 mg daily, taken on an empty stomach, is recommended.
- To curb food cravings, 1,000 mg daily is recommended.
- To treat irritable bowel syndrome (IBS), eliminate foods that trigger symptoms and take glutamine (500 mg tid) and peppermint oil (1 capsule three to six times daily).
- For stasis ulcers (open sores on the leg that are caused by poor blood flow), take each day: glutamine (500 mg) with a basic nutritional supplement program and vitamin C (2,000 mg in divided doses with meals and at bedtime), vitamin A (10,000 IU), zinc (22.5 to 50 mg), and vitamin E (400 IU orally and additional vitamin E oil squeezed from capsules onto the wound to aid healing and prevent recurrence).
- To aid wound healing, take glutamine (500 mg) with a basic vitamin-mineral formula and vitamin C (2,000 mg divided at meals and bedtime), vitamin A (10,000 IU), zinc (22.5 to 50 mg), vitamin E (400 IU), and vitamin B_3 (100 mg) daily.

Cautions

Adverse Effects/Toxicology

Glutamine can worsen damage caused by any disease that allows ammonia to accumulate to excess in the blood. It is not recommended in patients who have Reye's syndrome, kidney disease, cirrhosis of the liver, or other illnesses that cause overload of ammonia in the body.

Proteins (taken as a source of amino acid glutamine) should not be overused. In healthy persons, protein is safely metabolized and broken down by the liver into glucose and ammonia, which is a toxin. If one consumes an excessive amount of protein or if digestion is poor or liver function is impaired, ammonia can accumulate in the body and cause damage. Strenuous exercise can also promote excess ammonia in the body. Too much ammonia can cause encephalopathy or hepatic coma, or it can pose serious health threats. As ammonia is broken down by the body into urea, the urea can cause kidney inflammation and back pain.

Warnings/Contraindications/Precautions

- Glutamine supplements must be kept completely dry because moisture causes glutamine powder to break down into ammonia and pyroglutamic acid.
- Glutamine in foods is readily destroyed by cooking.
- Despite the similarity of their names, the following substances are different and are not interchangeable: glutamine; glutamic acid, also called glutamate; glutathione; gluten; and monosodium glutamate.

Interactions

Glutamine is absorbed more readily when taken with vitamin B_6 and vitamin C.

References

Balch J, Balch P. *Prescription for Nutritional Healing*. 2nd ed. Garden City Park, NY: Avery Publishing Group; 1997.

Castell LM, Newsholme EA. The effects of oral glutamine supplementation on athletes after prolonged, exhaustive exercise. *Nutrition*. 1997;13:738–742.

Den Hond E. Hiele M, Peeters M, Ghoos Y, Rutgeerts P. Effect of long-term oral glutamine supplements on small intestinal permeability in patients with Crohn's disease. *J Parenter Enteral Nutr*. 1999;23:7–11.

Giller R, Matthews K. *Natural Prescriptions*. New York, NY: Carol Southern Books/Crown Publishers; 1994.

Gottlieb B. *New Choices in Natural Healing*. Emmaus, Pa.: Rodale Press, Inc.; 1995.

Haas R. *Eat Smart, Think Smart*. New York, NY: HarperCollins; 1994.

Glutamine SUPPLEMENTS

Kirschmann G, Kirschmann J. *Nutrition Almanac.* 4th ed. New York, NY: McGraw Hill; 1996.

LaValle J. Natural agents for a healthy GI tract. *Drug Store News.* January 12, 1998;20.

Li J, Langkamp-Henken B, Suzuki K, Stahlgren LH. Glutamine prevents paranteral nutrition-induced increases intestinal permeability. *J Parenter Enteral Nutr.* 1994;18:303–307.

Napoli M. Chemo effect alleviated. *Health Facts.* October 1998;23:6.

Noyer CM, Simon D, Borczuk A, Brandt LJ, Lee MJ, Nehra V. A double-blind placebo-controlled pilot study of glutamine therapy for abnormal intestintal permeability in patients with AIDS. *Am J Gastroenterol.* 1998;93:972–975.

Shabert JK, Wilmore DW. Glutamine deficiency as a cause of human immunodeficiency virus wasting. *Med Hypotheses.* March 1996;46:252–256.

Yoshida S, Matsui M, Shirouzu Y, Fujita H, Yamana H, Shirouzu K. Effects of glutamine supplements and radiochemotherapy on systemic immune and gut barrier function in patients with advanced esophageal cancer. *Ann Surg.* 1998;227:485–491.

© *Copyright Integrative Medicine Communications*

5-Hydroxytryptophan 5-HTP

Overview

5-hydroxytryptophan (5-HTP) is an amino acid that occurs in the body. It is the immediate precursor of the brain neurotransmitter serotonin. 5-HTP is well-absorbed with approximately 70% of an oral dose reaching the bloodstream. Some orally administered 5-HTP is rapidly decarboxylated to serotonin in the "peripheral vasculature" (before reaching the brain), and some crosses the blood-brain barrier and increases synthesis of serotonin. In the process of serotonin biosynthesis, tryptophan is hydroxylated to 5-HTP and then decarboxylated to serotonin (5-HT). The tryptophan hydroxylase enzyme catalyzes tryptophan's conversion to 5-HTP, and the 5-hydroxytryptophan decarboxylase enzyme catalyzes 5-HTP's conversion to 5-HT. The conversion of tryptophan to 5-HTP is the rate-limiting step in the production of serotonin from tryptophan.

The 5-HTP decarboxylase enzyme is widely distributed in the body with highest activity in the gut wall and liver. Peripheral serotonin does not cross the blood-brain barrier. 5-HTP Decarboxylase inhibitors are sometimes given in conjunction with 5-HTP to inhibit peripheral conversion and help insure that adequate levels of serotonin are produced in the brain. However, studies indicate that 5-HTP works as well, if not better, when used without decarboxylase inhibitors.

Sources

■ **Dietary Sources**
Griffonia simplicifolia seed

■ **Constituents/Composition**
Dietary supplements of 5-HTP should be manufactured to 99% or higher purity levels.

■ **Commercial Preparations**
5-HTP is extracted from the seeds of the African *Griffonia simplicifolia* plant using an alcoholic extraction process that produces an oily solid. The oily extract is then purified into a dry solid. Standard preparations available as 25, 50, and 100 mg capsules or tablets.

Therapeutic Uses

Bipolar (manic) depression: 5-HTP (200 mg tid) with lithium has proven helpful in the treatment of bipolar disorder.

Depression: 5-HTP has been shown to be effective in treating mild to moderate depression in 5-HT deficient individuals. Its effects are similar to those observed with the anti-depressant drugs Imipramine and Fluvoxamine. Treatment with 5-HTP (ranging from 150 to 300 mg per day for one to six weeks) improved depressed mood, anxiety, insomnia, and physical symptoms.

Fibromyalgia: Numerous clinical studies suggest that low serotonin levels cause symptoms of fibromyalgia. Treatment with 5-HTP enhances serotonin synthesis which increases pain tolerance and sleep quality. 5-HTP treatment (300 mg tid for 30 to 90 days) has been shown to improve symptoms of depression, anxiety, insomnia, and somatic pain (number of painful areas and morning stiffness) in patients with fibromylagia.

Insomnia: 5-HTP has been shown to reduce the time required to fall asleep and improve sleep quality in numerous double-blind, clinical trials.

Migraine Headache: 5-HTP (200 to 600 mg/day for two to six months), has been shown to reduce the frequency and severity of migraine headaches in several clinical trials. Significantly fewer side effects were observed with 5-HTP compared to other migraine headache drugs.

Obesity: 5-HTP treatment causes decreased carbohydrate intake and may result in weight loss in obese patients. It is hypothesized that 5-HTP may promote weight loss by promoting satiety. In one study, overweight persons were given 300 mg 5-HTP three times daily, for six weeks with no dietary restriction. For the second six weeks of the trial, they were placed on a 1,200 calorie-per-day diet in addition to the 5-HTP treatment. At the end of the 12 weeks, the 5-HTP group had lost an average of 11.63 pounds, while the placebo group had lost only 1.87 pounds. Early satiety was reported by 100% of the participants during the first six-week period, and by 90% of the participants on 5-HTP during the second six-week period. In another study, 5-HTP (750 mg per day for two weeks) administered to 25 overweight NIDDM patients caused a significant reduction in daily energy intake (from fat and carbohydrate) and body weight.

Headaches in children: Children with sleep disorder-related headaches have been shown to respond favorably to 5-HTP treatment.

Dosage Ranges and Duration of Administration

The therapeutic dose, and length of treatment, will depend on the condition being treated. In clinical trials, dosages ranged from 150 to 900 mg per day and lasted for two weeks to six months.

Cautions

■ **Adverse Effects/Toxicology**
Relatively few adverse effects are associated with its use in the treatment of depression. 5-HTP causes mild gastrointestinal disturbances in some people. These side effects include mild nausea, heartburn, flatulence, feelings of fullness, and rumbling sensations. Side effects are reduced after extended treatment (four to six weeks).

■ **Warnings/Contraindications/Precautions**
Individuals taking anti-depressant drugs, such as MAOIs or selective serotonin reuptake inhibitor (SSRIs), or other prescription drugs, should consult with their physician before taking 5-HTP. Excessive 5-HTP stimulation may cause "serotonin syndrome" (excess accumulation of serotonin in the synapses), characterized by altered mental states, autonomic dysfunction, and neuromuscular abnormalities.

Interactions

May potentiate the effects of St. John's wort.

Vitamin B_6, niacin, and magnesium serve as cofactors in the conversion of 5-HTP to serotonin.

References

Angst J, et al. The treatment of depression with L-5-hydroxytryptophan versus imipramine. Results of two open and one double-blind study. *Arch Psychiatr Nervenkr.* 1977;224:175–186.

Birdsall TC. 5-Hydroxytryptophan: a clinically-effective serotonin precursor. *Altern Med Rev.* 1998;3:271–280.

Byerley WF, et al. 5-Hydroxytryptophan: a review of its antidepressant efficacy and adverse effects. *J Clin Psychopharmacol.* 1987;7:127–137.

Cangiano C, et al. Effects of oral 5-hydroxy-tryptophan on energy intake and macronutrient selection in non-insulin dependent diabetic patients. *Int J Obes Relat Metab Disord.* 1998; 22:648–654.

Cangiano C, Ceci F, Cascino A, et al. Eating behavior and adherence to dietary prescriptions in obese adult subjects treated with 5-hydroxytryptophan. *J Clin Nutr.* 1992;56:863–867.

Caruso I, Sarzi Puttini P, Cazzola M, et al. Double-blind study of 5-hydroxytryptophan versus placebo in the treatment of primary fibromyalgia syndrome. *J Int Med Res.* 1990;18:201–209.

Ceci F, Cangiano C, Cairella M, Cascino A, et al. The effects of oral 5-hydroxytryptophan administration on feeding behavior in obese adult female subjects. *J Neural Transm.* 1989;76:109–117.

DeBenedittis G, Massei R. Serotonin precursors in chronic primary headache. A double-blind cross-over study with L-5-hydroxytryptophan vs. placebo. *J Neurosurg Sci.* 1985; 29:239–248.

DeGiorgis, G, et al. Headache in association with sleep disorders in children: a psychodiagnostic evaluation and controlled clinical study—L-5-HTP versus placebo. *Drugs Exp Clin Res.* 1987;13:425–433.

Ganong WF. *Review of Medical Physiology.* 13th ed. San Mateo, Calif: Appleton & Lange; 1987.

Juhl JH. Primary fibromyalgia syndrome and 5-hydroxy-L-tryptophan: a 90-day open study. *Altern Med Rev.* 1998;3:367–375.

Magnussen I, Nielson-Kudsk F. Bioavailability and related pharmacokinetics in man of orally administered L-5-Hydroxytryptophan in steady state. *Acta Pharmacol et Toxicol.* 1980;46:257–262.

Martin TG. Serotonin syndrome. *Ann Emerg Med.* 1996;28:520–526.

Murray MT, Pizzorno JE. *Encyclopedia of Natural Medicine.* 2nd ed. Rocklin, Calif: Prima Publishing; 1998.

Nicolodi M, Sicuteri F. Fibromyalgia and migraine, two faces of the same mechanism. Serotonin as the common clue for pathogenesis and thearpy. *Adv Exp Med Biol.* 1996;398:373–379.

Puttini PS, Caruso I. Primary fibromyalgia and 5-hydroxy-L-tryptophan: a 90-day open study. *J Int Med Res.*1992;20:182–189.

Reibring L, Agren H, Hartvig P, et al. Uptake and utilization of [beta-11c] 5-hydroxytryptophan (5-HTP) in human brain studied by positron emission tomography. *Pyschiatry Research.* 1992;45:215–225.

Shils ME, Olson JA, Shike M, eds. *Modern Nutrition in Health and Disease.* 8th ed. Media, Pa: Williams & Wilkins; 1994:1.

Takahashi S, et al. Measurement of 5-hydroxindole compounds during L-5-HTP treatment in depressed patients. Folia Psychiatr Neurol Jpn. 1976;30:461–473.

Van Hiele LJ. L-5-hydroxytryptophan in depression: the first substitution therapy in psychiatry? *Neuropsychobiology.* 1980; 6:230–240.

Van Praag HM. Management of depression with serotonin precursors. *Biol Psychiatry.* 1981;16:291–310.

Zmilacher K, et al. L-5-hydroxytryptophan alone and in combination with a peripheral decarboxylase inhibitor in the treatment of depression. *Neuropsychobiology.* 1988;20:28–33.

© *Copyright Integrative Medicine Communications*

Lipase

Overview

Lipases are one of three categories of enzymes manufactured by the pancreas. The pancreas also secretes the hormones insulin and glucagon, which are needed to metabolize sugar, into the bloodstream. The other two enzymes include amylases, which break starch molecules into more simple sugars, and proteases, which break protein molecules into single amino acids. The most common dietary fats, triglycerides, comprise 95% of all ingested fats and are comprised of a glycerol molecule combined with three fatty acid molecules. The lipases aid the digestion of fats by hydrolyzing the glycerol linkage within the chain to create more assimilable free fatty acids and monoglycerides. These components are then transported in the body by lipoproteins. Pancreatic lipase and bile salts are required for intestinal digestion and absorption.

Sources

■ Dietary Sources

This enzyme is manufactured by the pancreas. It does not come from diet, but may be supplemented by animal enzymes.

■ Constituents/Composition

Gastric and pharyngeal (salivary) lipases are different from pancreatic lipase. They have lower molecular weights, a lower pH optimum (4 to 6 vs. 6 to 8), and a greater stability at pH 3. Gastric lipase is produced in the stomach and cleaves triglycerides at Sn-3 position within the stomach and duodenum. Pharyngeal lipase is produced in the oral cavity, also cleaving triglycerides at Sn-3 position within the mouth, esophagus, and stomach. Pancreatic lipase is produced in the pancreas, splitting Sn-1 and Sn-3 positions within the duodenum.

These lipases are important in the hydrolysis of triglycerides in milk during infancy, when the secretion of pancreatic lipase is not fully developed. In adults, as much as 10% to 15% of ingested fat may be partially hydrolyzed in the stomach.

Hepatic lipase has also been shown to impact aspects of blood lipid metabolism. It facilitates the clearance of potentially artherogenic lipoproteins by the liver and impacts the levels of the protective high-density lipoproteins.

■ Commercial Preparations

Lipase tablets are available in units of 6,000 Lus, and 1 to 2 capsules are recommended daily, to be taken before meals.

Therapeutic Uses

Tablets or capsules of pancreatic enzyme extracts with meals can be used to treat impaired digestion, malabsorption, and subsequent nutrient deficiencies. Some consider pancreatic enzymes of value in treating autoimmune disorders, inflammatory diseases, and food allergies. They have been most studied in treating early diagnosed celiac disease by enhancing the benefit of a gluten-free diet.

A reduction in lipase activity is unlikely to induce malabsorption in an adult, because pancreatic lipase is usually secreted in abundant amounts. Deficiency of pancreatic lipase of clinical significance only when its secretion is below 10% to 15% of normal levels.

Dosage Ranges and Duration of Administration

Recommended treatment with lipase to aid fat digestion is 1 to 2 capsules of 6,000 LUs tid before meals. Lipase can also be found combined with protease and amylase.

Cautions

■ Adverse Effects/Toxicology
None reported

■ Warnings/Contraindications/Precautions

Lipase and other pancreatic enzyme supplements are not associated with side effects.

Interactions
None reported

References

Berkow R, ed. *The Merck Manual of Medical Information.* Home Ed. Whitehouse Station, NJ: Merck Research Laboratories; 1997.

Mahan KL, Marian A. *Krause's Food Nutrition and Diet Therapy.* 8th ed. Philadelphia, Pa: WB Saunders Co; 1993.

Murray MT. *Encyclopedia of Nutritional Supplements.* Rocklin, Calif: Prima Publishing; 1986.

Shils ME, Olson JA, Shike M, eds. *Modern Nutrition in Health and Disease.* 8th ed. Philadelphia, Pa.: Lea and Febiger; 1994.

© Copyright Integrative Medicine Communications

Lysine

Overview

Lysine is an essential amino acid that is not synthesized in adequate amounts by the body, so it must be obtained from dietary sources. Lysine furnishes the structural components for the synthesis of carnitine, which promotes fatty acid synthesis within the cell. It is particularly important for proper growth. Lysine also regulates calcium absorption and plays an important role in the formation of collagen.

A vegetarian diet may not provide sufficient lysine. Among protein sources, plants often contain insufficient sources of lysine. Lysine is the limiting amino acid of many cereals. In many areas of the world where diets are grain-based, this becomes important as a lysine deficiency can create a negative nitrogen balance and lead to kidney stones. Lysine deficiency may be characterized by fatigue, nausea, dizziness, appetite loss, emotional agitation, decreased antibody formation, decreased immunity, slow growth, anemia, reproductive disorders, pneumonia, acidosis, and bloodshot eyes.

Lysine has been used to treat herpes infections caused by both herpes simplex viruses and herpes zoster. Supplementation can improve recovery speed and suppress recurrences of infections. Some studies have found lysine of potential benefit in treating cardiovascular disease, osteoporosis, asthma, migraines, nasal polyps, and postepisiotomy pain.

Sources

Dietary Sources

Generally, lysine is found in the following foods:

- Meat, particularly red meats
- Cheeses
- Poultry
- Sardines
- Nuts
- Eggs
- Soybeans

The most concentrated sources are torula yeast, dried and salted cod, soybean protein isolate, soybean protein concentrate, Parmesan cheese, pork loin (excluding fat), dried and frozen tofu, freeze-dried parsley, defatted and low-fat soybean flour, fenugreek seed, and dried spirulina seaweed.

Constituents/Composition

Lysine is an essential amino acid. Chemically, lysine is unique among the amino acids in that it possesses two amino (NH_2) groups. The extra amino group can react with other substances, such as glucose or lactose, creating an amino-sugar complex that cannot be split by digestive enzymes, thus reducing the availability of lysine.

Lysine is also known as LYS, amino acid K, and 2-diamino-hexanoic acid. Its chemical composition is $C_6H_{13}NO_2$.

Commercial Preparations

- L-lysine acetylsalicylate (LAS)
- Lysine clonixinate (LC)
- L-lysine monohydrochlorine (LMH)

Therapeutic Uses

- Asthma: LAS, when administered by inhalation, has been shown to protect against histamine-induced bronchoconstriction.
- Herpes: Supplementation may improve recovery speed and suppress recurrences of infections.
- Migraine: Treatment with a combination of LAS and metoclopramide may be effective.
- Nasal polyps: Recent research suggests that LAS may prevent relapses of nasal polyps.
- Postepisiotomy pain: 125 mg/day of LC was found to reduce postepisiotomy pain in primiparous patients with moderate to severe postepisiotomy pain.

Dosage Ranges and Duration of Administration

The following are the recommended dietary allowances, according to the National Research Council.

- Birth to 4 months: 103 mg/kg/day
- 5 months to 2 years: 69 mg/kg/day
- 3 to 12 years: 44 mg/kg/day
- Adults and teenagers: 12 mg/kg/day

Based on obligatory amino acid losses (including data from amino acid tracer studies), it has been suggested that adults need 30 mg/kg/day.

Nutritional doses are 1 to 3 g per day.

Cautions

Adverse Effects/Toxicology

Lysine appears to be nontoxic.

Warnings/Contraindications/Precautions

L-lysine may increase cholesterol and triglyceride levels.

Interactions

Vitamin C aids lysine in collagen formation.

References

Bruzzese N, Sica G, Iacopino F, et al. Growth inhibition of fibroblasts from nasal polyps and normal skin by lysine acetylsalicylate. *Allergy.* 1998;53:431–434.

De los Santos AR, Marti MI, Espinosa D, Di Girolamo G, Vinacur JC, Casadei A. Lysine clonixinate vs. paracetamol/codeine in postepisiotomy pain. *Acta Physiol Pharmacol Ther Latinoam.* 1998;48(1):52–58.

Ensminger AH, Ensminger ME, Konlande JE, Robson JRK. *Foods & Nutrition Encyclopedia.* 2nd ed. Baton Rouge, Fla: CRC Press, Inc; 1994:1,2:60–64, 1,748.

Flodin NW. The metabolic roles, pharmacology, and toxicology of lysine. *J Am Coll Nutr.* 1997;16:7–21.

Garrison Jr RH, Somer E. *The Nutrition Desk Reference.* 3rd ed. New Canaan, Conn: Keats Publishing, Inc; 1995:39–52.

Haas EM. *Staying Healthy With Nutrition.* Berkeley, Calif: Celestial Arts Publishing; 1992.

Hugues FC, Lacoste JP, Danchot J, Joire JE. Repeated doses of combined oral lysine acetylsalicylate and metoclopramide in the acute treatment of migraine. *Headache.* 1997;37:452–454.

Newstrom H. *Nutrients Catalog.* Jefferson, NC: McFarland & Co; 1993:303–312.

Shils ME, Olson JA, Shike M, Ross AC. *Modern Nutrition in Health and Disease.* 9th ed. Baltimore, Md: Williams & Wilkins; 1999:41, 1,010.

Werbach MR. *Nutritional Influences on Illness.* 2nd ed. Tarzana, Calif: Third Line Press; 1993:159–160, 384, 434, 494–495, 506, 580, 613–614, 636.

© Copyright Integrative Medicine Communications

Manganese

Overview

Manganese is a trace element. It occurs widely in plant and animal tissues and is an essential element for many animal species. Manganese absorption occurs throughout the small intestine. The exact mechanism of absorption is unknown, although it is thought to occur by a two-step mechanism that involves an initial uptake from the lumen followed by active transport across the mucosal cells. A specific manganese-carrying plasma protein called transmanganin has been identified. Almost all absorbed manganese is excreted with the feces; only trace amounts are found in the urine. Absorption efficiency is estimated to be roughly 5% and may decline as dietary intake increases. The retention of manganese is estimated to be 10%, 14 days after feeding. The human body contains a mere 20 milligrams of manganese, mostly in cell mitochondria. Organs rich in mitochondria, such as liver, kidney, and pancreas have relatively high manganese concentrations. Bone has the highest concentration of manganese.

Manganese serves two primary biochemical functions in the body, (1) it activates specific enzymes, and (2) it is a constituent of several metalloenzymes. The enzymes manganese activates include hydrolases, decarboxylases, kinases, and transferases. Certain other ions (cobalt, magnesium) can replace its function in this capacity. The manganese metalloenzymes include arginase, pyruvate carboxylase, glutamine synthetase, and manganese superoxide dismutase.

Manganese participates in numerous biochemical functions in the body including steroid and sulfomucopolysacchride biosynthesis, carbohydrate and lipid metabolism, and bone, blood clot, and protein formation. It is also essential for normal brain function, possibly through its role in biogenic amine metabolism. Many of the precise biochemical roles of manganese have not been determined.

Manganese deficiency has been induced in several animal species, but not in humans. Deficiency symptoms in animals include skeletal abnormalities, impaired growth, disturbed or depressed reproductive function, ataxia of the newborn, and defects in lipid and carbohydrate metabolism. Although frank deficiency symptoms have not been observed in humans, biochemical evidence has established its essentiality in humans. Impaired fertility, growth retardation, birth defects, bone malformations, seizures, and general weakness may result from manganese deficiencies.

Sources

■ Dietary Sources

- Nuts (especially pecans, almonds)
- Wheat germ and whole grains
- Unrefined cereals
- Leafy vegetables
- Liver
- Kidney
- Legumes
- Dried fruits

Refined grains, meats, and dairy products contain only small amounts of manganese. Highly refined diets contain significantly less manganese (0.36 to 1.78 mg) than diets high in unrefined foods (8.3 mg).

■ Constituents/Composition

Mn^{2+} is the characteristic oxidative state of manganese in solution, in metal enzyme complexes, and in metalloenzymes. Mn^{3+} is the oxidative state in the enzyme manganese superoxide dismutase (MnSOD), and the form that binds to transferrin and interacts with Fe^{3+}.

■ Commercial Preparations

Manganese is available commercially in a wide variety of forms including manganese salts (sulfate and chloride) and manganese chelates (gluconate, picolinate, aspartate, fumarate, malate, succinate, citrate, and amino acid chelate). Preparation doses are typically between 2 and 20 mg.

Therapeutic Uses

- Diabetes: Type I and II diabetics have significantly less manganese than healthy individuals. Diabetics with liver disorders and those not on insulin therapy may excrete more manganese. Manganese appears to have a hypoglycemic effect and may decrease blood glucose levels in insulin-resistant diabetics.
- Rheumatoid Arthritis: RA, as well as other inflammation brought on by strains and sprains may respond well to manganese treatment. Levels of MnSOD may be significantly decreased in individuals with rheumatoid arthritis. Manganese supplementation increases MnSOD activity.
- Epilepsy: An important study in the early 1960s demonstrated that manganese-deficient rats were more susceptible to seizures, and had EEG tracings consistent with seizure activity. People who have schizophrenia may also respond well to magnesium supplementation.
- Osteoporosis: Manganese, and other trace elements, increase spinal bone mineral density in postmenopausal women.
- Immunocompetence and cancer: Adequate manganese is necessary for normal antibody production. Excessive or inadequate manganese intakes may affect neutrophil and macrophage function.
- Cadmium toxicity: Manganese reduces toxic effects of cadmium in rats.
- Other conditions: Manganese is also used to treat atherosclerosis, hypercholesterolemia, tinnitus, and hearing loss.
- Total parenteral nutrition (TPN): Bone changes may occur in patients given TPN solutions containing inadequate quantities of manganese. In contrast, cholestatic and nervous system disorders have been associated with high blood concentrations of manganese from long-term TPN treatment. Children's TPN solutions should contain low-dose manganese (0.018 mumol/kg per 24 hours).

Dosage Ranges and Duration of Administration

The exact amount of manganese required by the human body is not known. The Food and Nutrition Board (FNB) of the National Research Council (NRC) has established estimated safe and adequate daily intakes for manganese as follows:

- Infants 0 to 0.5 years: 0.3 to 0.6 mg
- Infants 0.5 to 1 year: 0.6 to 1.0 mg
- Children and adolescents 1 to 3 years: 1.0 to 1.5 mg
- Children and adolescents 4 to 6 years: 1.5 to 2.0 mg
- Children and adolescents 7 to 10 years: 2.0 to 3.0 mg
- Children and adolescents 11+ years: 2.0 to 5.0 mg
- Adults: 2.0 to 5.0 mg.

These estimates are based on the assumption that most dietary intakes fall in this range and do not result in deficiency or toxicity signs. The estimates may be modified as additional information becomes available. More manganese (10 mg/day) should be consumed if the diet contains high amounts of substances that inhibit manganese absorption. In therapeutic use for epilepsy, inflammation, or diarrhea, the dose may be increased three-to-sixfold.

Cautions

■ Adverse Effects/Toxicology

Manganese is one of the least toxic of the trace elements, though excessive intake may produce toxic effects. There are only a few reports of oral manganese poisoning in man. Manganese toxicity is more common in humans chronically exposed to manganese dust found in steel mills and mines and certain chemical industries. Toxicity principally affects the brain, causing severe psychiatric abnormalities, but may also increase blood pressure in the doses used to treat schizophrenia.

■ Warnings/Contraindications/Precautions

The FNB of the NRC recommends that the upper limits for the trace elements should not be habitually exceeded because the toxicity levels may be only several times usual intakes.

Interactions

Calcium, copper, iron, magnesium, and zinc compete for absorption in the small intestines. Excess intake of one can reduce absorption of the others. Excess manganese may produce iron-deficiency anemia.

References

Davis CD, Greger JL. Longitudinal changes of manganese-dependent superoxide dismutase and other indexes of manganese and iron status in women. *Am J Clin Nutr.* 1992;55:747–752.

el-Yazigi A, Hannan N, Raines DA. Urinary excretion of chromium, copper, and manganese in diabetes mellitus and associated disorders. *Diabetes Res.* 1991;18:129–134.

Fell JM, Reynolds AP, Meadows N, et al. Manganese toxicity in children receiving long-term parenteral nutrition. *Lancet.* 1996;347:1218–1221.

Friedman E, ed. *Biochemistry of the Essential Ultratrace Elements.* New York, NY: Plenum Press; 1984.

Goering PL, Haassen CD. Mechanism of manganese-induced tolerance to cadmium lethality and hepatotoxicity. *Biochem. Pharmacol.* 1985;34:1371–1379.

Itokawa Y. Trace elements in long-term total parenteral nutrition [in Japanese]. *Nippon Rinsho.* 1996;54:172–178.

Johnson MA, Smith MM, Edmonds JT. Copper, iron, zinc, and manganese in dietary supplements, infant formulas, and ready-to-eat breakfast cereals. *Am J Clin Nutr.* 1998;67(suppl):1035S–1040S.

Krause, MV., & Mahan, L.K. *Food, Nutrition, and Diet Therapy.* 7th ed. Philadelphia, Pa: WB Saunders Co., 1984.

Orten JM., Neuhaus OW, eds. *Human Biochemistry.* 10th ed. St. Louis, MO: The C.V. Mosby Co; 1982.

Pasquier C, Mach PS, Raichvarg D, Sarfati G, Amor B, Delbarre F. Manganese-containing superoxide-dismutase deficiency in polymorphonuclear leukocytes of adults with rheumatoid arthritis. *Inflammation.* 1984;8:27–32.

Saltman PD, Strause LG. The role of trace minerals in osteoporosis. *J Am Coll Nutr.* 1993;12:384–389.

Shils ME, Olsen JA, Shike M, eds. *Modern Nutrition in Health and Disease.* 8th ed. Media, Pa: Williams and Wilkins Co; 1994:1.

Shvets NV, Kramarenko LD, Vydyborets SV, Gaidukova SN. Disordered trace element content of the erythrocytes in diabetes mellitus [in Russian]. *Lik Sprava.* 1994;1:52–55.

Somer E. *The Essential Guide to Vitamins & Minerals.* New York, NY: HarperCollins Publishers; 1992.

Whitney EN, Hamilton EN. *Understanding Nutrition.* 3rd ed. St. Paul, Minn: West Publishing Co; 1984.

© *Copyright Integrative Medicine Communications*

Melatonin

Overview

Melatonin is an important hormone that is secreted by the pineal gland in the brain. Since its identification in 1958, studies have shown that melatonin plays a crucial role in ordering the complex hormone secretion patterns that regulate the body's circadian rhythm. Melatonin also helps control sleeping and waking periods, because its release is stimulated by darkness and suppressed by light. It also controls the timing and release of female reproductive hormones, affecting menstrual cycles, menarche, and menopause.

Overall levels of melatonin in the body also contribute to the process of aging. The standard rhythmic pattern of melatonin levels are absent until about 3 months of age. After that, the nocturnal levels of melatonin are at their highest for the first few years and then begin to decline as puberty begins. After puberty, nocturnal melatonin levels are relatively stable throughout adulthood and then fall as people age. In old age, the nocturnal rise in melatonin may be barely detectable. Because melatonin opposes the degeneration caused by high levels of corticosteroids (i.e. protein catabolism, suppressed immune function, and altered blood glucose metabolism), higher melatonin levels may help promote health and extend life-span.

Studies show that jet lag is most likely caused by a disrupted circadian rhythm that can be effectively adjusted by using melatonin. Insomnia that is seen in the elderly and in some children with sleeping disorders is usually caused by low melatonin levels. That, too, can be treated with the proper supplementation. Childhood diseases that may cause melatonin-related sleep disorders include autism, epilepsy, Down syndrome, and cerebral palsy. Melatonin supplementation can also benefit blind people whose sleeping rhythms are disturbed. Melatonin is not effective as a sleeping aid for persons with normal melatonin levels.

Several studies have shown how melatonin levels shift during monthly menstrual cycles. Nocturnal melatonin is highest during the premenstrual period and lowest during the midmenstrual period. It is thought that rising melatonin levels may bring on menstruation and lowering ones may bring on a surge of luteinizing hormone and ovulation. Administering melatonin prior to the midcycle surge of luteinizing hormone appears to block ovulation, leading to speculation about the use of melatonin as a natural contraceptive.

Melatonin also has antioxidant, antiestrogenic, and oncostatic properties, which may produce some of its anticancer effects. As an antioxidant, melatonin appears to be able to neutralize hydroxyl, the most damaging of all oxygen-based free radicals. Studies show that melatonin can help prevent and treat some hormonally related cancers, such as breast cancer and prostate cancer. The most promising results are seen when melatonin is used in conjunction with interferon or interleukin-2, anticancer agents that are much less effective without melatonin. Melatonin not only enhances the use of interleukin-2, an important immune cytokine, but it also reduces the numerous side effects often associated with it.

Many studies have shown that some patients suffering from depression have lower-than-normal melatonin levels. Seasonal affective disorder (SAD) is often effectively treated with phototherapy, and research has shown that SAD patients often have delayed melatonin rhythms in the winter. While some forms of depression may have direct links to melatonin levels, other types of depression have not responded well to melatonin treatment. Exaggerated depressive symptoms have been reported in some cases of depressed patients receiving daytime melatonin supplements. Melatonin has increased psychotic behavior in some schizophrenic patients.

Sources

■ Dietary Sources
N/A

■ Constituents/Composition
Melatonin is a hormone manufactured by serotonin and secreted by the pineal gland. It is an indole, like the simple amino acid, tryptophan.

■ Commercial Preparations
Melatonin can be taken in tablet, capsule, and sublingual tablet form.

Therapeutic Uses

- Used to restore sleeping patterns and fatigue caused by jet lag
- As a sleeping aid for those who suffer from insomnia as a result of low melatonin levels (i.e. elderly and some children with sleep disorders)
- Inhibits initiation and growth of some hormonally related cancers and non-small cell lung cancer, particularly in conjunction with interferon or interleukin 2 treatment
- May be beneficial for treatment of depression related to low melatonin levels (i.e. SAD)
- Preliminary studies show it may be useful in multiple sclerosis, SIDS, coronary heart disease, epilepsy and post-menopausal osteoporosis.

Dosage Ranges and Duration of Administration

Official dosage ranges have not yet been set for melatonin supplementation. Sensitivity to melatonin may vary from individual to individual. For those especially sensitive to it, lower doses may work more effectively than the standard amount. Higher doses could cause anxiety or irritability.

For treatment of insomnia, a dose of 3 mg taken an hour before bedtime is usually effective, although dosages as low as 0.1 to 0.3 mg may improve sleep for some people. If 3 mg a night is not effective after three days, try 6 mg one hour before bedtime. An individually effective dose should produce restful sleep and no daytime irritability or fatigue. For treatment of jet lag, take 5 mg of melatonin one hour before bedtime upon arrival at new location; repeat for the first five days. Dosages for anticancer treatment may be much higher (i.e. 10 to 50 mg per day). Long-term melatonin supplementation should not be carried out without a health care provider's supervision.

Cautions

■ Adverse Effects/Toxicology
There are no known serious side effects to regulated melatonin supplementation. Some people may experience vivid dreams or nightmares. Overuse or incorrect use of melatonin could disrupt circadian rhythms. Long term effects have not been well studied. In rats, melatonin decreases T_4 and T_3 uptake levels.

■ Warnings/Contraindications/Precautions
Melatonin can cause drowsiness if taken during the day. If morning drowsiness is experienced after taking melatonin at night, reduce dosage levels. In some cases of depression, daytime doses of melatonin can increase depression. May be contraindicated for those with autoimmune disorders and immune system cancers (i.e. lymphoma, leukemia). Because melatonin suppresses corticosteroid activity, those who are taking corticosteroids for anti-inflammatory or immune suppressive purposes (i.e. transplant patients) should exercise caution with melatonin supplementation. Melatonin could interfere with fertility. It is also contraindicated during pregnancy and lactation. Lack of sleep and insufficient exposure to darkness may suppress natural production of melatonin.

Interactions

- Vitamin B_{12} influences melatonin secretion in the body. Low levels of melatonin will often reflect low vitamin B_{12} levels as well. Taking vitamin B_{12} (1.5 mg of methylcobalamin per day) can improve sleeping disorders.
- Protein, vitamin B_6, niacinamide, and acetyl carnitine all support melatonin production.
- Nonsteroidal anti-inflammatory drugs (NSAIDs) reduce melatonin secretion in the body.
- Beta blockers inhibit the nocturnal rise of melatonin levels
- Tricyclics, monoamine oxidase inhibitors, and some antidepressants increase the levels of brain melatonin.
- Benzodiazepines, like Xanax and Valium, interfere with melatonin production.
- Alcohol and caffeine can interfere with melatonin production.
- Diuretics and calcium channel blockers can interfere with melatonin production.

References

Atkins R. *Dr. Atkin's Vita-Nutrient Solution.* New York, NY: Simon and Schuster. 1998.

Balch J and Balch P. *Prescription for Nutritional Healing.* Garden City Park, NY: Avery Publishing Group; 1997.

Lissoni, P, Vigore L, Rescaldani R, et al. Neuroimmunotherapy with low-dose subcutaneous interleukin-2 plus melatonin in AIDS patients with CD4 cell number below 200/mm3: a biological phase-II study. *J Biol Regul Homeost Agents.* 1995;9:155–158.

MacIntosh A. Melatonin: clinical monograph. *Q Rev Nat Med.* 1996; 47–60.

Mindell E and Hopkins V. *Prescription Alternatives.* New Canaan, Conn: Keats Publishing, Inc.; 1998.

Murphy P, Myers B, Badia P. NSAIDs suppress human melatonin levels. *Am J Nat Med.* 1997; iv: 25.

Murray, M. *Encyclopedia of Nutritional Supplements.* Rocklin, Calif: Prima Publishing; 1996.

Petrie K, Conaglen JV, Thompson L, Chamberlain K. Effect of melatonin on jet lag after long haul flights. *BMJ.* 1989;298:705–707.

Rosenfeld, I. *Dr. Rosenfeld's Guide to Alternative Medicine.* New York, NY: Random House; 1996.

Tzischinsky O, Lavie P. Melatonin possesses time-dependent hypnotic effects. *Sleep.* 1994;17:638–645.

Zhdanova IV, Wurtman RJ, Morabito C, Piotrovska VR, Lynch HJ. Effects of low oral doses of melatonin, given 2-4 hours before habitual bedtime, on sleep in normal young humans. *Sleep.* 1996;19:423–431.

Zhdanova IV, Wurtman RJ, Lynch HJ, et al. Sleep-inducing effects of low doses of melatonin ingested in the evening. *Clin Pharmacol Ther.* 1995; 57:552–558.

© *Copyright Integrative Medicine Communications*

Omega-3 Fatty Acids

Overview

The omega-3 fatty acids include alpha-linolenic acid (ALA), eicosapentaenoic acid (EPA), and docosahexaenoic acid (DHA). These are long-chain, polyunsaturated fatty acids. Omega-3 fatty acids have been established as essential for optimum tissue formation. Intense research is studying the optimum amounts of omega-3 fatty acids in the diet and their role in the central nervous system.

ALA is found in plant products; EPA and DHA are obtained from fish oils. Additionally, ALA is converted in the human body to EPA and DHA. ALA is found in unhydrogenated oils, such as rapeseed (canola), flaxseed, and soybean oil, and in margarines and other fats containing such oils. Note that many commercial margarines contain high amounts of trans-fatty acids, which probably outweigh the beneficial effects of the omega-3 oils they contain. EPA and DHA can be introduced into the body directly from cold-water fish such as salmon, mackerel, halibut, and herring.

The beneficial effects of the omega-3 series oils include: lowering cholesterol and triglyceride levels, reducing the risk of heart disease, lowering blood pressure, improving rheumatoid arthritis, and protecting myelin formation and function. There is evidence to suggest that omega-3 oils can be helpful in treating asthma, glaucoma, multiple sclerosis, and diabetes, and in preventing cancer.

Recent research indicates that ALA may have a beneficial effect on coronary heart disease, including the inhibition of atherosclerosis. In one small study of 15 obese persons on daily intakes of 20 g of ALA from margarine products based on flaxseed oil, there was improvement in arterial compliance and thus decreased cardiovascular risk, despite a rise in LDL oxidizability. At the same time, insulin sensitivity and HDL cholesterol diminished.

Another study found that the omega-3 fatty acids, whether ALA supplements from vegetable oil or EPA and DHA supplements from marine sources, have largely parallel effects on hemostatic factors.

Other research has indicated that ALA acts equivalently to n-6 fatty acids with respect to lipid and lipoprotein effects, but that very large amounts of ALA, which is plant-based, is needed to have the effect of reducing tricylgycerol concentrations, which is the hallmark effect of the marine-based omega-3 fatty acids. The study concludes that in terms of effects on lipoprotein metabolism, the plant-derived ALA is not equivalent to the marine-based acids. One area of general agreement is that the interrelationship among the fatty acids and the ratio of ALA to linoleic acid in the diet is an important area for further study.

The omega-3 fatty acids have anti-inflammatory and immunoregulatory effects. Successful treatment of migraines and alleviation of depression with omega-3 fatty acids have been reported. A recent study demonstrated that omega-3 fatty acids improved the short-term course of illness in patients with bipolar disorder. One study showed that patients with panic attacks or a history of agoraphobia may benefit from ALA supplementation.

Sources

■ **Dietary Sources**

ALA: flax seeds, flaxseed oil, linseed oil, rapeseed oil, canola oil, soybean oil, pumpkin, and walnuts

EPA and DHA: fish oils, particularly from cold-water fish such as salmon, mackerel, halibut, and herring

■ **Constituents/Composition**

The parent fatty acid in the omega-3 series, alpha-linolenic acid (ALA), is converted to eicosapentaenoic acid (EPA), then to docosahexaenoic acid (DHA), then to the prostaglandin E_3 series (PGE_3). Marine products can introduce EPA and DHA directly into the body.

The essential fatty acids are vitamin F, yet the Food and Drug Administration prohibits the term "vitamin F" for advertising purposes, because of problems with foods such as french fries being advertised as "vitamin enriched" because they were fried in oil.

■ **Commercial Preparations**

There are essentially two types of commercial preparations:

- Cooking oils (canola, soybean, and margarines made from these oils; hydrogenated products are not preferred)
- Medicinal oil (flaxseed)

Several manufacturing methods can destroy the nutrient value of the products. Some preferred methods use proprietary names for their process, generically known as modified atmospheric packing methods. Bio-Electron Process, Spectra-Vac, and Omegaflo are some examples. Generally, a high-quality oil will be certified as organic by a reputable third party, will be found in light-resistant containers, may be refrigerated, and will be dated. These oils have been extracted by expeller presses at relatively low temperatures.

Therapeutic Uses

The primary uses of omega-3 oils include the following.

- Cardiovascular disease: reducing cholesterol levels and lowering blood pressure
- Allergic and inflammatory conditions, including psoriasis and eczema listItem
- Autoimmune diseases, including multiple sclerosis, lupus, and cancer listItem

Health conditions that may reflect deficiencies in, or which can be improved by supplementation of, omega-3 oils include: acne, AIDS, allergies, Alzheimer's, angina, arthritis, atherosclerosis, autoimmune diseases, behavioral disorders, breast cysts, breast pain, breast tenderness, cancer, cartilage destruction, coronary bypass, cystic fibrosis, dementia, diabetes, *E. coli* infection, eczema, heart disease, hyperactivity, hypertension, hypoxia, ichthyosis, immune disorders, infant nutrition, inflammatory conditions, intestinal disorders, kidney function, learning, leprosy, leukemia, lupus, mastalgia, menopause, mental illness, metastasis, multiple sclerosis, myopathy neurological diseases, obesity, osteoarthritis, postviral fatigue, pregnancy malnutrition, psoriasis, Refsum's syndrome, Reye's syndrome, rheumatoid arthritis, schizophrenia, sepsis, Sjogren-Larsson syndrome, stroke, vascular disease, vision.

Dosage Ranges and Duration of Administration

- There is no Recommended Dietary Allowance (RDA), yet one or two tablespoons of flaxseed oil daily (or equivalent capsule) is considered optimal for a healthy individual. Capsule doses are 3,000 mg per day for prevention and 6,000 mg per day for treatment.
- A diet that gets 1% to 2% of its calories from linoleic acid has been shown to give maximum tissue levels of DHA, avoiding any apparent deficiency symptoms.
- For rheumatoid arthritis, the estimated therapeutic dose of ALA is 5 g/day, while the estimated therapeutic dose of EPA is 1.8 g/day.
- For agoraphobia: 2 to 6 tablespoons of flaxseed oil daily, in divided doses.
- A healthy person eating a typical diet should reduce consumption of saturated fats and increase consumption of the polyunsaturated essential fatty acids.

Cautions

■ **Adverse Effects/Toxicology**

Excessive amounts of omega-3 oils may reduce blood-clotting time.

■ **Warnings/Contraindications/Precautions**

Total fat intake should be considered. The ratio of omega-3 fatty acids to other essential fatty acids may be important in treating some conditions, and the balance of omega-3 to omega-6 oils is essential to the metabolism of prostaglandins. Omega-3 oils should be used with caution in patients who bruise easily, have bleeding disorders, or are on blood-thinning medication.

Interactions

The omega-3 fatty acids interact with other fatty acids. The optimal ratio of omega-3 to omega-6 fatty acids is 1:4.

References

Ando H, Ryu A, Hashimoto A, Oka M, Ichihashi M. Linoleic acid and alpha-linolenic acid lightens ultraviolet-induced hyperpigmentation of the skin. *Arch Dermatol Res*. July 1998;290(7):375–381.

Billeaud C, Bougle D, Sarda P, et al. Effects of preterm infant formula supplementation with alpha-linolenic acid with a linoleate/alpha-linoleate ration of 6. *Eur J Clin Nutr*. 1997;51(8):520–527.

DeDeckere EA, Korver O, Verschuren PM, Katan MB. Health aspects of fish and n-3 polyunsaturated fatty acids from plant and marine origin. *Eur J Clin Nutr*. 1998;52(10):749–753.

Edwards R, Peet M, Shay J, Horrobin D. Omega-3 polyunsaturated fatty acid levels in the diet and in red blood cell membranes of depressed patients. *J Affect Disord*. 1998;48(2–3):149–155.

Ensminger AH, Ensminger ME, Konlande JE, Robson JRK. *Foods & Nutrition Encyclopedia*. 2nd ed. Vol 2. Boca Raton, Fla: CRC Press, Inc; 1994:684–708.

Garrison RH Jr, Somer E. *The Nutrition Desk Reference*. 3rd ed. New Canaan, Conn: Keats Publishing, Inc; 1995:23–64.

Haas EM. *Staying Healthy with Nutrition*. Berkley, Calif: Celestial Arts Publishing; 1992:65–79.

Harris WS. N-3 fatty acids and serum lipoproteins: human studies. *Am J Clin Nutr*. 1997;65(5):1645S (10).

Murray MT. *Encyclopedia of Nutritional Supplements*. Rocklin, Calif: Prima Publishing; 1996:239–278.

Murray MT, Pizzorno JE. *Encyclopedia of Natural Medicine*. 2nd ed. Rocklin, Calif: Prima Publishing; 1996:49–52, 255, 266, 487, 533–34, 765–66, 779–781.

Nestel PJ, Pomeroy SE, Sasahara T, et al. Arterial compliance in obese subjects is improved with dietary plant n-3 fatty acid from flaxseed oil despite increased LDL oxidizability. *Arterioscler Thromb Vasc Biol*. July 1997;17(6):1163–1170.

Newstrom H. *Nutrients Catalog*. Jefferson, NC: McFarland & Co., Inc.; 1993:103–105.

Shils ME, Olson JA, Shike M, Ross AC. *Modern Nutrition in Health and Disease*. 9th ed. Baltimore, Md: Williams & Wilkins; 1999:90-92, 1377–1378.

Stoll AL, Severus WE, Freeman MP, et al. Omega 3 fatty acids in bipolar disorder: a preliminary double-blind placebo-controlled trial. *Arch Gen Psychiatry*. 1999:56(5):407–412.

Von Schacky C, Angerer P, Kothny W, et al. The effect of dietary omega-3 fatty acids on coronary atherosclerosis. A randomized, double-blind, placebo-controlled trial. *Ann Intern Med*. 1999;107(7):554–562.

Voskuil DW, Feskens EJM, Katan MB, Kromhout D. Intake and sources of alpha-linolenic acid in Dutch elderly men. *Euro J Clin Nutr*. 1996;50(12):784–787.

Wagner W, Nootbaar-Wagner U. Prophylactic treatment of migraine with gamma-linolenic and alpha-linolenic acids. *Cephalalgia*. 1997;17(2):127–130.

Werbach MR. *Nutritional Influences on Illness*. 2nd ed. Tarzana, Calif: Third Line Press; 1993:13-22, 655–671.

Yehuda S, Rabinovitz S, Carasso RL, Mostofsky DI. Fatty acids and brain peptides. *Peptides*. 1998;19(2):407–419.

© Copyright Integrative Medicine Communications

Omega-6 Fatty Acids

Overview

As essential fatty acids, the omega-6 series are generally necessary for stimulation of growth, maintenance of skin and hair growth, regulation of metabolism, lipotropic activity, and maintenance of reproductive performance. The omega-6 oil linoleic acid is specifically required to maintain the integrity of the epidermal water barrier of the skin. Researchers believe they play an important role in reducing the risk of many chronic degenerative diseases such as heart disease, cancer, and stroke. Yet experts estimate that up to 80% of Americans consume an insufficient quantity of essential fatty acids.

The omega-6 fatty acids have been shown to improve nerve conduction and prevent neuropathy in diabetics. One animal study has suggested that the combination of gamma-linolenic acid (GLA) of the omega-6 series and ascorbate is particularly advantageous.

GLA has been shown to have an anti-inflammatory effect in humans and may play a role in treating conditions such as rheumatoid arthritis. Corroborated studies suggest that GLA is unique among the omega-6 series in suppressing tumor growth and metastasis. It has been shown to inhibit both motility and invasiveness of human colon cancer, breast cancer, and melanoma cells.

Recent animal research has suggested that omega-6 fatty acids can be beneficial in senile osteoporosis because it enhances absorption and retention of calcium. They also can be efficacious in vasodilation, lowering of blood pressure, and the prevention of atherosclerosis. Arachidonic acid of the omega-6 series is particularly important in normal brain function.

The optimal ratio of omega-6 oils to omega-3 oils should be 4:1. However, the American diet provides more than 10 times the needed amount of omega-6 fatty acids. This is because they are the primary fatty acids added to most processed foods and are commonly used cooking oils. However, consumption of refined and adulterated fats and oils inhibit the body's ability to use the essential fatty acids it consumes.

Sources

■ Dietary Sources

Sources of omega-6 fatty acids are plant seed oils, including evening primrose, black currant, borage, and fungal oils. Gamma-linolenic acid (GLA) is found in human milk and, in small amounts, in a wide variety of common foods, particularly organ meats. Linoleic acid is found in polyunsaturated vegetable oils, particularly sunflower oil, safflower oil, corn oil, and soybean oil. Arachidonic acid is found in egg yolk, organ meats, and other animal-based foods.

■ Constituents/Composition

The omega-6 essential, polyunsaturated fatty acids are derived from linoleic acid and include gamma-linoleic acid, dihomo-gamma-linolenic acid (which converts to the desirable prostaglandin E_1 series) and arachidonic acid (which converts to the unfavorable series 2 prostaglandin).

The essential fatty acids are vitamin F, yet the Food and Drug Administration prohibits the term "vitamin F" for advertising purposes because of problems with foods such as french fries being advertised as "vitamin enriched" because they were fried in oil.

■ Commercial Preparations

Evening primrose oil, black currant seed oil, borage oil, borage oil capsules, soybean oil, safflower oil, sunflower oil, corn oil

Therapeutic Uses

- Rheumatoid arthritis: GLA may reduce inflammation by suppressing T-cell proliferation and activation.
- Diabetes: Omega-6 fatty acid supplementation assists nerve function and helps prevent nerve disease in diabetics.
- Cancer: GLA may suppress tumor growth and metastasis, particularly in colon cancer, breast cancer, and melanoma.
- Heart disease: GLA may prevent heart disease by inhibiting plaque formation, vasodilation, and lowering blood pressure.
- Eyes: GLA is beneficial in Sjogren's syndrome and may be useful in other dry-eye conditions.

Supplementation may alleviate some of the symptoms of aging, alcoholism, atopic dermatitis, osteoporosis, and premenstrual syndrome.

Dosage Ranges and Duration of Administration

- There is no Recommended Dietary Allowance (RDA).
- The recommended dosage for rheumatoid arthritis is 1.4 g per day of GLA.
- Supplementation with 480 mg of GLA per day for diabetes is recommended.
- Studies have shown that up to 2.8 g of GLA per day is well tolerated.

Cautions

■ Adverse Effects/Toxicology

Dietary sources of omega-6 acids appear to be completely nontoxic.

■ Warnings/Contraindications/Precautions

A healthy person eating a typical diet should reduce consumption of refined fats and increase consumption of the essential fatty acids. Omega-6 oils are far more available through dietary sources than omega-3 oils.

Interactions

There are no significant interactions noted with supplemental omega-6 acids.

References

Bolton-Smith C, Woodward M, Tavendale R. Evidence for age-related differences in the fatty acid composition of human adipose tissue, independent of diet. *Eur J Clin Nutr*. 1997;51(9):619–624.

Brown NA, Bron AJ, Harding JJ, Dewar HM. Nutrition supplements and the eye. *Eye*. 1998; 12(pt. 1): 127–133.

Ensminger AH, Ensminger ME, Konlande JE, Robson JRK. *Foods & Nutrition Encyclopedia*, 2nd ed. Boca Raton, Fla: CRC Press, Inc.;1994:684–708.

Fan YY, Chapkin RS. Importance of dietary gamma-linolenic acid in human health and nutrition. *J Nutr*. 1998; 128(9): 1411–1414.

Garrison RH Jr, Somer E. *The Nutrition Desk Reference*. 3rd ed. New Canaan, Conn: Keats Publishing, Inc.; 1995:23–64.

Haas EM. *Staying Healthy with Nutrition*. Berkley, Calif: Celestial Arts Publishing; 1992:65–79.

Jiang WG, Hiscox S, Bryce RP, Horrobin DF, Mansel RE. The effects of n-6 polyunsaturated fatty acids on the expression of nm-23 in human cancer cells. *Br J Cancer*. 1998;77(5):731–738.

Jiang WG, Hiscox S, Horrobin DF, Bryce RP, Mansel RE. Gamma linolenic acid regulates expression of maspin and the motility of cancer cells. Biochem *Biophys Res Commun*. 1997;237(3): 639–644.

Kruger MC, Coetzer H, DeWinter R, Gericke G, Papendorp DH. Calcium, gamma-linolenic acid and eicosapentaenoic acid supplementation in senile osteoporosis. *Aging (Milano)*. 1998;10(5):385–394.

Murray MT. *Encyclopedia of Nutritional Supplements*. Rocklin, Calif: Prima Publishing; 1996:239–278.

Newstrom H. *Nutrients Catalog*. Jefferson, NC: McFarland & Co. Inc; 1993:103–105.

Shils ME, Olson JA, Shike M, Ross AC. *Modern Nutrition in Health and Disease*. 9th ed. Baltimore, Md: Williams & Wilkins; 1999:90-92, 1377–1378.

Wagner W, Nootbaar-Wagner U. Prophylactic treatment of migraine with gamma-linolenic and alpha-linolenic acids. *Cephalalgia*. 1997;17(2):127–130.

Werbach MR. *Nutritional Influences on Illness*. 2nd ed. Tarzana, Calif: Third Line Press; 1993:13–22, 655–671.

Ziegler EE, Filer LJ, eds. *Present Knowledge in Nutrition*. 7th ed. Washington, DC: ILSI Press; 1996:58–64.

© Copyright Integrative Medicine Communications

Phenylalanine

Overview

Phenylalanine is an essential amino acid that is not synthesized in adequate amounts by the body, so it must be obtained from dietary sources. In healthy individuals, phenylalanine is converted by the body into tyrosine. Tyrosine is the parent compound for the manufacturing of the hormones norepinephrine and epinephrine by the adrenal medulla and of the hormones thyroxine and triiodothyronine by the thyroid gland. In adults, approximately 90% of the recommended dietary allowance (RDA) of phenylalanine is hydroxylated to form tyrosine. The remaining 10% is used for tissue protein synthesis. In children, 60% of the RDA is used for tissue protein synthesis, and the remaining 40% is hydroxylated to form tyrosine.

The inability to convert excess phenylalanine to tyrosine is the underlying cause of phenylketonuria (PKU), the most common metabolic genetic defect. PKU is actually a group of inherited disorders involving phenylalanine metabolism. Patients with PKU have one or more of a number of enzyme defects associated with a corresponding recessive gene. The disease appears in infants 3 to 6 months old. As it must be treated before 3 months of age, PKU screening is done during the first 48 hours of life. The incidence of PKU is approximately 1 in 10,000 Caucasian infants and 1 in 132,000 black infants. Mental retardation, usually severe, is the primary manifestation of untreated PKU. Other manifestations may include seizures, muscular hypertonicity, exaggerated tendon reflexes, tremors, and hyperactivity. A skin condition similar to eczema occurs in 15% to 20% of untreated patients.

Treatment for PKU-positive patients is a phenylalanine-restricted, tyrosine-supplemented diet to maintain adequate blood phenylalanine levels for optimum brain development and growth. There is some disagreement about whether these diets can be discontinued without adverse effect and, if so, at what age. Some studies have shown significant differences in mental functioning, in both performance and intelligence, between those who have discontinued the diet and those who have maintained the diet. In adults who have discontinued the diet, severe agoraphobia has been reported, which is reversible with a return to the phenylalanine-restricted diet.

Pregnant women with PKU that is untreated at the time of conception and during gestation give birth to infants with poor intrauterine growth, microcephaly, and congenital abnormalities that are often severe.

Symptoms of phenylalanine deficiency may include confusion, emotional agitation, depression, decreased alertness, decreased memory, behavioral changes, decreased sexual interest, bloodshot eyes, and cataracts. If not corrected by supplemental dietary phenylalanine and tyrosine, the deficiency may lead to restricted weight gain and stunted growth, osteopenia, anemia, alopecia, and even death.

Aspartame (Nutrasweet®), the synthetic sweetener, is formed by combining phenylalanine and aspartic acid. The FDA maintains that it is safe; however, there continues to be controversy over its use, and relatively little is known about its effect during pregnancy in the general population.

Sources

Dietary Sources

Generally, phenylalanine is found in cheeses; nuts and seeds; milk chocolate; meat (excluding fat), particularly organ meats; poultry (excluding skin); fish, including shellfish; milk; and eggs. The most concentrated sources are torula yeast, soybean protein isolate, soybean protein concentrate, peanut flour, dried spirulina seaweed, defatted and low-fat soybean flour, dried and salted cod, defatted soy meal, dried and frozen tofu, Parmesan cheese, almond meal, dry roasted soybean nuts, dried watermelon seeds, and fenugreek seeds.

Constituents/Composition

Phenylalanine is an essential amino acid. It is also known as PHA, PHE, amino acid F, and 2-amino-3-phenyl propanoic acid. Its chemical composition is $C_9H_{11}NO_2$.

Commercial Preparations

- D-phenylalanine capsules
- L-phenylalanine capsules
- D,L-phenylalanine capsules (50/50 blend of D-phenylalanine and L-phenylalanine)
- Topical creams

Therapeutic Uses

- Cancer: Restriction of phenylalanine and tyrosine may help decrease tumor growth and metastasis, particularly in malignant melanoma.
- Depression: L-phenylalanine has been used in treating bipolar disorders with both manic and depressive states combined with vitamins B_6; and D.
- Inflammation: Supplementation in the form of D-phenylalanine may be beneficial.
- Multiple sclerosis: Supplementation has been shown to improve bladder control, increase mobility, and ameliorate depression.
- Pain: Supplementation has been effective for chronic pain, particularly for osteoarthritis; use in doses of 250 mg 15 to 30 minutes before meals tid for a period of at least two days and up to three weeks.
- Parkinson's disease: Supplementation in the form of D-phenylalanine may reduce rigidity, walking disabilities, and speech difficulties.
- Rheumatoid arthritis: Supplementation in the form of D,L-phenylalanine was shown to be beneficial in one study.
- Vitiligo: Beneficial effects have been shown given treatment with oral L-phenylalanine, topical cream containing 10% phenylalanine, and ultraviolet-A radiation.

Dosage Ranges and Duration of Administration

The following are the recommended dietary allowances for phenylalanine plus tyrosine, according to the National Research Council.

- Birth to 4 months: 125 mg/kg/day
- 5 months to 2 years: 69 mg/kg/day
- 3 to 12 years: 22 mg/kg/day
- Adults and teenagers: 14 mg/kg/day

Based on obligatory amino acid losses (including data from amino acid tracer studies), it has been suggested that adults need 39 mg/kg/day.

Nutritional doses are 0.75 to 2 g per day; therapeutic doses are 2 to 3 g per day; experimental doses are 4 to 5 g per day.

Cautions

Adverse Effects/Toxicology

See "Warnings/Contraindications/Precautions".

Warnings/Contraindications/Precautions

- Anxiety, headaches, and hypertension are possible side effects of supplementation.
- Individuals with PKU and women who are lactating or pregnant should avoid supplementation.
- L-dopa competes with phenylalanine and should not be taken at the same time of day.
- Little is known about the use of aspartame (Nutrasweet) during pregnancy.

Interactions

- Vitamins B_6 and C help the body absorb phenylalanine.
- Increased amounts of other amino acids will inhibit phenylalanine.

References

Bugard P, Bremer HJ, Buhrdel P, et al. Rationale for the German recommendations for phenylalanine level control in phenylketonuria 1997. *Eur J Pediatr.* 1999;158:46–54.

Ensminger AH, Ensminger ME, Konlande JE, Robson JRK. *Foods & Nutrition Encyclopedia.* 2nd ed. Baton Rouge, Fla: CRC Press, Inc; 1994:1,2:60–64, 1,748

Garrison Jr RH, Somer E. *The Nutrition Desk Reference.* 3rd ed. New Canaan, Conn: Keats Publishing, Inc; 1995:39–52.

Haas EM. Staying Healthy With Nutrition. Berkeley, Calif: Celestial Arts Publishing; 1992.

Herbert V, Subak-Sharpe GJ, eds. *Total Nutrition (Mount Sinai School of Medicine).* New York, NY: St. Martin's Press; 1995:318–320.

Newstrom H. *Nutrients Catalog.* Jefferson, NC: McFarland & Co; 1993:303–312.

Pietz J. Neurological aspects of adult phenylketonuria. *Curr Opin Neurol.* 1998;11:679–688.

Pietz J, Dunckelmann R, Rupp A, et al. Neurological outcome in adult patients with early-treated phenylketonuria. *Eur J Pediatr.* 1998;157:824–830.

Shils ME, Olson JA, Shike M, Ross AC. *Modern Nutrition in Health and Disease.* 9th ed. Baltimore, Md: Williams & Wilkins; 1999:41, 1,010.

Start K. Treating phenylketonuria by a phenylalanine-free diet. *Prof Care Mother Child.* 1998;8:109–110.

Werbach MR. *Nutritional Influences on Illness.* 2nd ed. Tarzana, Calif: Third Line Press; 1993:159–160, 384, 434, 494–495, 506, 580, 613–614, 636.

© Copyright Integrative Medicine Communications

Phosphorus

Overview

Next to calcium, phosphorus is the most abundant mineral in the body, making up about 1% of total body weight. Most of it is found in bones and teeth. Phosphorus is present in the body as phosphates and, in addition to its role in bone formation, it is vital to energy production and exchange. Phosphorus helps in muscle contraction and nerve conduction. It aids kidney function and helps maintain the body's pH balance. Phospholipids are fat molecules that play a role in the maintenance of cell membranes. As a component of adenosine triphosphate (ATP), phosphorus is involved in the body's primary metabolic cycles and in protein synthesis for growth, maintenance, and repair of all body tissues and cells, as well as in the production of the nucleic acids in DNA and RNA. It is also necessary for the absorption of many vitamins and minerals, including vitamin D, calcium, iodine, magnesium, and zinc.

The parathyroid hormone (PTH) regulates the metabolism of phosphorus and calcium in the body. About two-thirds of phosphorus is absorbed from the intestine, the rate depending to some extent on levels of calcium and vitamin D, as well as the activity of PTH. While 85% of phosphorus is deposited in bones and teeth, the remainder is found in cells and other body tissues. The blood contains about 3.5 mg of phosphorus per 100 ml of plasma; total blood phosphorus is between 30 and 40 mg. Together, calcium and phosphorus assure the formation and maintenance of strong bones. The ideal dietary ratio of Ca/P is 1:1. A low Ca/P ratio can lead to bone resorption as the body draws upon existing calcium stores in the bone to pair with excess phosphorus. Not only is phosphorus absorbed more efficiently than calcium, but people are likely to get more phosphorus from their diets. The typical American diet has Ca/P ratios ranging from 1:2 to 1:4. The growing consumption of soft drinks, which are buffered with phosphates (as much as 500 mg in one serving), and high consumption of red meat and poultry, which contain 10 to 20 times as much phosphorus as calcium, are largely responsible for this imbalance. Decreased Ca/P ratios due to excess dietary phosphorus impair calcium absorption, which contributes to bone loss, osteoporosis, and periodontal disease. Low Ca/P ratios have also been associated with an increased incidence of hypertension and elevated risk for colon-rectal cancer.

Phosphorus deficiency, or hypophosphatemia, is rare except in people affected by certain diseases, in those receiving parenteral nutrition, or in those who have received phosphate-binding agents that contain aluminum for extended periods. It has been associated with anorexia, anxiety, apprehension, bone pain, bone fragility, stiffness in the joints, fatigue, irregular breathing, irritability, numbness, paresthesias, weakness, and weight change. In children, decreased growth, poor bone and tooth development, and symptoms of rickets may be signs of phosphorus deficiency. A greater concern for physicians is hyperphosphatemia, or an excess of phosphorus. This is most often the result of dietary imbalance. This has a negative result in terms of bone density and is of particular concern to women. Acute or chronic renal failure may also lead to hyperphosphatemia; in these cases restricting phosphorus intake to 800 to 1,000 mg is indicated.

Sources

■ Dietary Sources

Dietary sources of phosphorus include the following.

- Red meat and poultry
- Dried milk and milk products
- Wheat germ
- Yeast
- Grains
- Hard cheeses
- Canned fish
- Nuts
- Potatoes
- Eggs
- Soft drinks

■ Constituents/Composition

Elemental phosphorus, a white or yellow waxy substance that burns on contact with air (thus the term phosphorescent), is used in some homeopathic remedies. However, because it is highly toxic, it is no longer used in medicine. Instead, inorganic phosphates are used to treat phosphate deficiency. The following forms are used.

- Dibasic potassium phosphate
- Monobasic potassium phosphate
- Dibasic sodium phosphate
- Monobasic sodium phosphate
- Tribasic sodium phosphate

■ Commercial Preparations

Phosphorus is available over-the-counter in capsules. Because it is readily available in a variety of foods, phosphorus supplementation is usually confined to athletes who take it to reduce muscle pain and fatigue.

Therapeutic Uses

Phosphorus, by itself, is used in the treatment of only a few medical conditions. Along with calcium, however, it can help in healing bone fractures and in the treatment of osteomalacia, osteoporosis, and rickets. Regulating the ratio of calcium/phosphorus intake through dietary sources can reduce stress and alleviate problems like arthritis, which are related to calcium metabolism.

Hypophosphatemia can cause an impaired response to insulin for which supplementation with dibasic calcium phosphate (2 g tid with meals) has shown good results. Phosphate supplementation is also used in the treatment of diabetic ketoacidosis (DKA), and in constipation due to hypercalcemia. Mono- and dibasic sodium phosphates may be used as mild laxatives administered by mouth or rectally. Elemental phosphorus is used in homeopathic treatments for coughs and some types of acute gastroenteritus.

Dosage Ranges and Duration of Administration

The U.S. RDA for phosphorus is 800 to 1,200 mg daily. The RDA for those up to age 24 and during pregnancy and lactation is 1,200 mg daily.

Cautions

■ Adverse Effects/Toxicology

Phosphates can be toxic at levels over 1 g/day, leading to diarrhea, calcification of organs and soft tissue, and preventing the absorption of iron, calcium, magnesium, and zinc. High levels of phosphorus can promote the loss of calcium through nutritional hyperparathyroidism.

■ Warnings/Contraindications/Precautions

The overconsumption of foods high in phosphorus can drain calcium resources and lead to reduced bone mass. American dietary habits, particularly the high consumption of meat and soft drinks, makes low Ca/P ratios quite common. This imbalance may be the source of the high incidence of osteoporosis in the U.S. and other affluent nations where similar dietary habits prevail. Some researchers have identified this as the likely mechanism contributing to low bone mass in American women. Further retrospective studies are needed to investigate this hypothesis. Low ratios of dietary Ca/P also reduce the efficacy of treatments for osteoporosis. A 1986 experimental study of 158 females, aged 20 to 75, found that treatment of osteoporosis may in fact be fruitless when dietary Ca/P ratios exceed 1:1.25. Patients need to be aware of the dietary sources of both calcium and phosphorus so that they can take a more active role in balancing these two elements in their diet.

Interactions

Overuse of aluminum-containing antacids can result in phosphorus deficiency. Iron and magnesium interfere with phosphorus absorption, and caffeine increases phosphorus excretion by the kidneys. Low vitamin D intake can also contribute to phosphorus deficiency.

References

Anderson JJB. Calcium, phosphorus, and human bone development. *J Nutr.* 1996;126:1153S–1158S.

Berner YN, Shike M. Consequences of phosphate imbalance. *Annu Rev Nutr.* 1988;8: 121–148.

Carey CF, Lee HH, Woeltje KF, eds. *The Washington Manual of Medical Therapeutics.* 29th ed. New York, NY: Lippincott-Raven; 1998:230–237,444–448.

da Cunha DF, dos Santos VM, Monterio JP, de Carvalho da Cunha SF. *Miner Electrolyte Metab.* 1998;24:337–340.

Kuntziger H, Altman JJ. Hyperphosphoremia and hypophosphoremia [in French]. *Rev Prat.* 1989;39:949–953.

Metz JA, Anderson JJB, Gallagher Jr PN. Intakes of calcium, phosphorus, and protein, and physical activity level are related to radial bone mass in young adult women. *Am J Clin Nutr.* 1993;58: 537–542.

Mindell E, Hopkins V. *Prescription Alternatives.* Canaan, Conn: Keats Publishing Inc; 1998:495–496.

Reynolds JEF, ed. *Martindale: The Extra Pharmacopoeia.* 31st ed. London, Great Britain: Royal Pharmaceutical Society; 1996:1181–1182, 1741.

Shires R, Kessler GM. The absorption of tricalcium phosphate and its acute metabolic effects. *Calcif Tissue Int.* 1990;47:142–144.

Villa ML, Packer E, Cheema M, et al. Effects of aluminum hydroxide on the parathyroid-vitamin D axis of postmenopausal women. *J Clin Endocrinol Metab.* 1991;73:1256–1261.

Walker LP, Brown EH. *The Alternative Pharmacy.* NJ: Prentice-Hall; 1998:97.

Werbach MR. *Nutritional Influences on Illness: A Sourcebook of Clinical Research.* Canaan, Conn: Keats Publishing Inc; 1987.

© Copyright Integrative Medicine Communications

Quercetin

Overview

Quercetin is a flavonoid, a substance found in fruits, flowers, and vegetables that, among other functions, gives them their color. The average daily intake of flavonoids in the United States is between 150 and 200 mg. In general, flavonoids have been found to have both antioxidant and anti-inflammatory properties, useful in preventing or treating many health conditions. The thousands of flavonoid compounds can be placed into a handful of categories—one of which is quercetin. Quercetin can decrease allergic reactions and may be beneficial in treating other inflammatory responses, such as canker sores, hives, asthma, and arthritis. Other conditions for which quercetin may be beneficial include diabetes mellitus, dysentery, gout, heart disease, infections, inflammatory bowel disease, cataracts, atopic dermatitis, and psoriasis.

Recently, research has focused on prevention of carcinogenesis. Quercetin has been found to be effective in the prevention of skin carcinogenesis. In one study, antitumor activity was found in patients with ovarian cancer and hepatoma.

Sources

Dietary Sources

Fruits and vegetables, particularly citrus fruits, apples, onions, parsley, tea, and red wine.

Constituents/Composition

Quercetin is a flavonoid. Flavonoids are found in fruits and vegetables, are ascorbic-acid-related substances, and are compounds that are in human diets as glycosides. Research suggests, however, that many of the biologic effects are associated with aglycone, a substance that is released in the intestine, rather than with the compound bound in the glycoside.

Commercial Preparations

- Quercetin is available commercially in several strengths in powder or capsule form.
- Quercetin is often packaged with bromelain as an anti-inflammatory agent.
- Flavonoid-rich extracts include those from grape seed, bilberry, *Ginkgo biloba*, and green tea. Quercetin is one of the many flavonoids these substances contain.

Therapeutic Uses

- Allergies and hives: Research shows that quercetin inhibits histamine release from basophils and mast cells.
- Asthma: Quercetin has been shown to inhibit histamine release, as with allergies.
- Cancer: Recent research suggests that quercetin may be beneficial in the treatment of cancer, particularly skin cancer, and may have anti-tumor effects in other cancers, such as ovarian cancer.
- Canker sores: Quercetin may be beneficial in the treatment of canker sores by increasing the number of ulcer-free days and by producing mild symptomatic relief.
- Diabetes mellitus: Quercetin can reduce the accumulation of sorbitol in lens tissues, and thus may be beneficial in preventing cataracts, retinopathy, neuropathy, and other complications of diabetes mellitus. Flavonoids, including quercetin, promote insulin secretion, increase intracellular vitamin C levels, protect blood vessels, prevent easy bruising, and support the immune system, all of which are beneficial to individuals with diabetes.
- Dysentery: Quercetin and tocopherol in combination were found to restore the immune homeostasis and to normalize clinical indices in patients with dysentery.
- Gout: Quercetin inhibits uric acid production, as well as the manufacture and release of inflammatory compounds.
- Heart disease: Although studies are not conclusive on the benefits of quercetin in the treatment of coronary disease, it has been shown that individuals with very low intakes of flavonoids are at higher risk.
- Infection: Quercetin inhibits infectiousness and/or replication of such viruses as herpes simplex type 1, polio virus type 1, parainfluenza virus type 3, and respiratory syncytial virus.
- Psoriasis: Quercetin inhibits lipoxygenase.
- Rheumatoid arthritis: Quercetin may be beneficial by inhibiting mast cell degranulation, thus reducing tissue destruction.

Dosage Ranges and Duration of Administration

- 100 to 250 mg tid is thought to be an effective general supplementation dose.
- 250 to 600 mg per day, divided in several doses, is effective in reducing histamine levels and allergy symptoms.
- 200 to 400 mg of quercetin should be taken with bromelain between meals tid for the treatment of gout. (Bromelain both enhances the absorption of quercetin and provides anti-inflammatory effects of its own.)
- 200 to 400 mg of quercetin should be taken approximately 20 minutes before each meal for the treatment of chronic hives. Acute symptoms of allergies or outbreaks of hives can be treated with 800 mg qid.

Cautions

Adverse Effects/Toxicology

No side effects have been associated with quercetin.

Warnings/Contraindications/Precautions

No problems with quercetin have been demonstrated.

Interactions

There do not appear to be any adverse interactions. Quercetin may be beneficial to vitamin C use and efficacy. Quercetin and bromelain in combination are more effective as an anti-inflammatory than either taken alone, as each apparently enhances the absorption of the other.

References

Duthie SJ, Collins AR, Duthie GG, Dobson VL. Quercetin and myricetin protect against hydrogen peroxide-induced DNA damage (strand breaks and oxidised pyrimidines) in human lymphocytes *Mutat Res*. 1997;393(3):223–231.

Ferry DR, Smith A, Malkhandi J, et al. Phase I clinical trial of the flavonoid quercetin pharmacokinetics and evidence for in vivo tyrosine kinase inhibition. *Clin Cancer Res*. 1996;2(4):659–668.

Frolov VM, Peresadin NA, Khomutianskaia NI, Pshenichnyi I. The efficacy of quercetin and tocopherol acetate in treating patients with Flexner's dysentery [in Ukrainian]. *Lik Sprava*. 1993;4:84–86

Gross M, Pfeiffer M, Martini M, Campbell D, Slavin J, Potter J. The quantitation of metabolites of quercetin flavonols in human urine. *Cancer Epidemiol Biomarkers Prevent*. 1996;5(9):711–720.

Haas EM. *Staying Healthy with Nutrition*. Berkley, Calif: Celestial Arts Publishing; 1992:272, 882–884.

Hollman PC, Van Trijp JM, Mengelers MJ, De Vries JH, Katan, MB. Bioavailability of the dietary antioxidant flavonol quercetin in man.*Cancer Lett*. 1997;114(1-2):139–140.

Knekt P, Jarvinen R, Reunanen A, Maatela J. Flavonoid intake and coronary mortality in Finland: a cohort study. *BMJ (Clinical Research Ed.)*. 1996;312(7029):478–481.

Murray MT. *Encyclopedia of Nutritional Supplements*. Rocklin, Calif: Prima Publishing; 1996: 320–321.

Murray MT, Pizzorno JE. *Encyclopedia of Natural Medicine*. 2nd ed. Rocklin, Calif: Prima Publishing; 1996:268, 314, 422, 494, 546–47, 766.

Shils ME, Olson JA, Shike M, Ross AC. *Modern Nutrition in Health and Disease*. 9th ed. Baltimore, Md: Williams & Wilkins; 1999:1274–1277.

Werbach MR. *Nutritional Influences on Illness*. 2nd ed. Tarzana, Calif: Third Line Press; 1993:179, 259, 267, 389.

Young JF, Nielsen SE, Haraldsdottir J, et al. Effect of fruit juice intake on urinary quercetin excretion and biomarkers of oxidative status. *Am J Clin Nutr*. 1999; 69(1):87–94.

© Copyright Integrative Medicine Communications

Selenium

Overview

Selenium is a trace mineral and an important part of the enzyme glutathione peroxidase. It is an effective antioxidant, especially when combined with vitamin E. Working as part of this enzyme, selenium or, more specifically, the organic complex selenocysteine, helps protect intracellular structures by preventing the formation of damaging free radicals. Like other antioxidant supplements, selenium slows chemical aging and helps maintain elasticity of bodily tissues, organs, and the cardiovascular system.

Extreme selenium deficiency can lead to a rare heart disorder known as Keshan disease, which results in congestive heart failure and is most evident in parts of China where soil-selenium levels are low. More commonly, though, selenium deficiency is indicated in high rates of cancer, heart disease, and immunodepression. Selenium is frequently lacking in Western diets, again due to mineral-poor farmland. Typical consumption in the U.S. is estimated at 100 mcg/day. Many of selenium's antioxidant and anti-carcinogenic functions require much greater augmentation (>200 mcg/day).

Numerous animal and human studies conclude that fortifying the diet with added selenium, vitamin E, and other vital antioxidants boosts the immune system by stimulating white blood cell development and thymus function. In this way, selenium significantly challenges cancerous tumor incidence and development, and contributes to myriad other immune system benefits. Conversely, research finds low levels of selenium and glutathione peroxidase in cancer patients.

Selenium also plays a crucial role in preventing or managing coronary heart disease, stroke, and cardiovascular disease both before and after heart attacks, especially for patients who smoke, due to its antioxidant mechanisms and its role in lowering LDL cholesterol levels. Selenium also appears to inhibit platelet aggregation, increasing its significance in cardiovascular health.

Other studies have determined that selenium improves liver and metabolic function, even in extreme cases of alcoholic cirrhosis of the liver, and enhances pancreatic function. Additionally, sufficient selenium intake has been indicated in prostrate health and sperm motility, plays a prominent role in skin health and elasticity, and protects against cataract formation. Selenium acts as an antagonist to heavy metals.

Sources

Dietary Sources

Brewer's yeast and wheat germ, liver, butter, fish and shellfish, garlic, grains, sunflower seeds, and Brazil nuts are all food sources for naturally occurring selenium. Herbal sources include alfalfa, burdock root, catnip, fennel seed, ginseng, raspberry leaf, and yarrow.

The amount of selenium in foodstuffs corresponds directly to selenium levels in soil. Deficiencies are noted in parts of China and the U.S. where soil-selenium ratios are low.

Food-source selenium is destroyed during processing. Therefore, a varied diet of whole foods is recommended. (Whole foods are those eaten in their original form, rather than canned, frozen, or otherwise commercially processed or prepared.)

Constituents/Composition

Selenium occurs most commonly in nature as inorganic sodium selenite. Other, more absorbable and active forms include selenomethione or selenocysteine and selenium-rich yeast.

Commercial Preparations

Selenium is available as part of many vitamin-mineral supplements, all nutritional antioxidant formulas, and, increasingly, as an independent supplement. Suggested intake is between 50 and 200 mcg per day for adults. Men apparently require more than women, because stores are lost with ejaculation. Selenium should be taken with vitamin E, as the two act synergistically, and without vitamin C, which decreases absorbability and is likely to increase risk of selenium toxicity.

Therapeutic Uses

Clinical trials suggest that supplemental selenium well beyond daily dietary intake (>100 mcg) is necessary to support at least some of the following functions. Selenium deficiency is most evident in a positive response to supplemental selenium therapy. Blood and urinary levels are inadequate indicators of selenium intake and tissue levels.

- Cancer. Acts as an anti-cancer antioxidant, protecting against or reducing the incidence of breast, colon, liver, skin, and respiratory tumors and cancers.
- Heart disease. Prevents and manages coronary heart disease, cardiovascular disease, and stroke by helping to lower LDL cholesterol and reduce platelet aggregation. Reduces post-heart attack mortality. Successful in treatment of Keshan disease.
- Immunodepression. Boosts immune function and white blood cell development. Suggested in the treatment of depressed immune disorders such as lupus. Contributes to body's ability to fight bactericidal action of phagocytes. Counters heavy metal toxicity such as lead, mercury, and cadmium poisoning. Stimulates antibody formation in response to vaccinations.
- Liver disease. Effective against alcohol-induced cirrhosis of the liver and alcoholic cardiomyopathy. Promotes proper liver and metabolic function.
- Skin disorders. Indicated for treatment of acne, eczema, psoriasis, vasculitis, and other skin disorders. Responds to vitamin E deficiencies in combination with vitamin E supplementation. Prevents premature aging.
- Muscular and inflammatory illness. Effective in treating all major symptoms of myotonic dystrophy. Suggested in the treatment of inflammatory conditions such as rheumatoid arthritis.
- Eyesight. Required for the antioxidant protection of the lens; helps prevent cataract formation.
- Reproductive Health. May assist in male fertility, prostate function, and sperm motility.
- Promotes healthy fetal development and may help in prevention of SIDS.

Dosage Ranges and Duration of Administration

A minimum RDA for selenium is as follows.

- Neonates to 6 months: 10 mcg.
- Infants 6 months to 1 year: 15 mcg
- Children 1 to 6 years: 20 mcg
- Children 7 to 10 years: 30 mcg
- Males 11 to 14 years: 40 mcg
- Males 15 to 18 years: 50 mcg
- Males over 19 years: 70 mcg
- Females 11 to 14 years: 45 mcg
- Females 15 to 18 years: 50 mcg
- Females over 19 years: 55 mcg
- Pregnant females: 65 mcg
- Lactating females: 75 mcg
- Usual dosage for children: 30 to 150 mcg or 1.5 mcg per pound of body weight. For adults: 50 to 200 mcg/day.

Cautions

Adverse Effects/Toxicology

Long-term ingestion of excessive levels of selenium (>1,000 mcg/day) may produce fatigue, depression, arthritis, hair or fingernail loss, garlicky breath or body odor, gastrointestinal disorders, or irritability. Such high intakes and chronic toxicity are rare.

Warnings/Contraindications/Precautions

Studies found high hair selenium levels in children with learning disabilities and behavioral problems. Extremely high doses may cause cumulatively toxic effects over time.

Interactions

Vitamin E and other antioxidant nutrients increase selenium's effectiveness in promoting glutathione peroxidase activity. Use and absorption of selenium are hampered by high doses of vitamin C, heavy metals and, possibly, high intakes of zinc and other trace minerals. Vitamin C may also increase risk of selenium toxicity. Chemotherapy drugs may increase selenium requirements.

References

Balch JF, Balch PA. *Prescription for Nutritional Healing*. 2nd ed. Garden City Park, NY: Avery Publishing Group; 1997:28.

Clark LC, Combs GF Jr, Turnbull BW, et al. Effects of selenium supplementation for cancer prevention in patients with carcinoma of the skin. *JAMA*. 1996;276:1957–1963.

Combs GF, Clark LC. Can dietary selenium modify cancer risk? *Nutr Rev*. 1985;43:325–331.

Dworkin BM. Selenium deficiency in HIV infection and the acquired immunodeficiency syndrome (AIDS). *Chem Biol Interact.* 1994;91:181–186.

Garland M, Morris JS, Stampfer MJ, et al. Prospective study of toenail selenium levels and cancer among women. *J Natl Cancer Inst.* 1995;8:497–505.

Haas EM. *Staying Healthy with Nutrition: The Complete Guide to Diet and Nutritional Medicine.* Berkeley, Calif: Celestial Arts; 1992:211–216.

Murray MT. *Encyclopedia of Nutritional Supplements: The Essential Guide for Improving Your Health Naturally.* Rocklin, Calif: Prima Publishing; 1996:1013, 222–228.

National Research Council, Diet and Health. *Implications for Reducing Chronic Disease Risk.* Washington, DC: National Academy Press; 1989:376–379.

Prasad K, ed. *Vitamins, Nutrition and Cancer.* New York, NY: Karger; 1984.

Walker LP, Hodgson Brown E. *The Alternative Pharmacy.* Paramus, NJ: Prentice Hall Press; 1998:313.

Wasowicz W. Selenium concentration and glutathione peroxidase activity in blood of children with cancer. *J Trace Elem Electrolytes Health Dis.* 1994;8:53–57.

Werbach MR. *Nutritional Influences on Illness: A Sourcebook of Clinical Research.* New Canaan, Conn: Keats Publishing; 1988.

Yang GQ, Xia YM. Studies on human dietary requirements and safe range of dietary intakes of selenium in China and their application in the prevention of related endemic diseases. *Biomed Environ Sci.* 1995;8:187–201.

Yoshizawa K, Willett WC, Morris SJ, et al. Studies of prediagnostic selenium level in toenails and the risk of advanced prostrate cancer. *J Natl Cancer Inst.* 1998;90:1219–1224.

© *Copyright Integrative Medicine Communications*

Spirulina

Overview

Spirulina is a type of blue-green algae of which there are several species. It grows best in a warm climate and in warm alkaline water. Spirulina was historically used by the Mexican (Aztec, Mayan), African, and Asian peoples, who consumed it as a staple for thousands of years.

Spirulina is a rich source of nutrients, especially protein. Its antiviral and anticancer properties are a result of its being rich in phycocyanin, a blue polypeptide that gives spirulina its blue-green color. Phycocyanin has the ability to stimulate the production and activity of both white and red blood cells and to increase the production of antibodies and cytokines, which help fight foreign invasions. Because of these properties, spirulina has been used extensively in Russia to treat the victims, especially children, of the nuclear disaster at Chernobyl. In these children whose bone marrow had been damaged from radiation exposure, spirulina promoted the evacuation of radionucleotides and stimulated T-cell production, which boosted the immune system of these patients.

Sources

■ Dietary Sources

Spirulina is a microalgae that flourishes in warm climates and warm alkaline water. It is available dried and freeze-dried.

■ Constituents/Composition

Spirulina is a complete protein—62% of it is made up of essential and nonessential amino acids. It is also thought to provide the entire B complex of vitamins, though its vitamin B_{12} content has been called into question. It is also rich in phycocyanin, chlorophyll, beta-carotene and other carotenoids, vitamin E, minerals (e.g., zinc, manganese, copper, iron), trace minerals (e.g., selenium), and essential fatty acids (e.g., gamma-linolenic acid). Because the cell walls of spirulina are made of complex proteins and sugars (unlike other species of blue-green algae whose walls are made up of cellulose), it is very easily digested. The exact nutrient profile depends on the species.

■ Commercial Preparations

Most spirulina consumed in the United States is cultivated scientifically. There are many different spirulina species, only some of which are identified on commercial preparations. *Spirulina maxima* (cultivated in Mexico) and *Spirulina platensis* (cultivated in California) are the most popular.

Therapeutic Uses

Currently, spirulina has the following uses:

- AIDS and other viruses (e.g., herpes simplex, human cytomegalovirus, influenza virus, mumps, measles). Spirulina has the ability to inhibit viral replication as well as strengthen the immune system by stimulating T-cell, macrophage, bone marrow stem cell, and natural-killer-cell production and activity. Data from one study indicate that calcium spirulina (Ca-Sp), a component of spirulina, is a powerful antiviral agent against HIV-1 and HSV-1.
- Cancer. Spirulina causes regression and inhibition of some cancers in experimental animals by stimulating enzyme activity (e.g. endonuclease), which is responsible for repairing damaged DNA. A study performed in India showed that *Spirulina fusiformis* supplementation reversed oral leukoplakia in tobacco chewers.
- Anemia. Spirulina promotes hematopoiesis (formation and development of blood cells).
- Skin disorders. Because spirulina is rich in gamma-linolenic acid, it helps to maintain healthy skin and treat several skin disorders (such as eczema and psoriasis).
- Vitamin A deficiency. Studies in India determined that *Spirulina fusiformis* is an effective source of dietary vitamin A.
- Colitis. One study showed that a component of spirulina, C-phycocyanin, reduced inflammation caused by acetic acid-induced colitis in rats. It also showed some reduction in colonic damage.
- Clinical applications of spirulina include malabsorption syndrom with gas and bloating, general immune support, and as an easily absorbed protein supplement for people with a lack of appetite. It is also used in the treatment of Candida and hypogylcemia. It is often used by weight lifters as a protein source.

Dosage Ranges and Duration of Administration

Patients should consult their health care providers for the correct dosage of spirulina. However, a standard dose of spirulina is 4 to 6 500 mg tablets per day.

Cautions

■ Adverse Effects/Toxicology

No adverse effects were found after high-dose experiments in animals.

■ Warnings/Contraindications/Precautions

No fetotoxicity nor teratogenicity was found when high-doses of spirulina were administered to pregnant animals.

Interactions

None reported

References

Annapurna VV, Deosthale YG, Bamji MS. Spirulina as a source of vitamin A. *Plant Foods Hum Nutr.* 1991;41:125–34.

Chamorro G, Salazar M, Favila L, Bourges H. Pharmacology and toxicology of Spirulina alga. *Rev Invest Clin.* 1996;48:389–399. Abstract.

Chamorro G, Salazar M. Teratogenic study of spirulina in mice. *Arch Latinoam Nutr.* 1990;40:86–94.

Spirulina: good source of beta-carotene, but no miracle food. *Environ Nutr.* 1995;18:7.

Gonzalez R, Rodriguez S, Romay C, et al. Anti-inflammatory activity of phycocyanin extract in acetic acid-induced colitis in rats. *Pharmacol Res.* 1999;39:1055–1059.

Hayashi K, Hayashi T, Kojima I. A natural sulfated polysaccharide, calcium spirulan, isolated from *Spirulina platensis*: in vitro and ex vivo evaluation of anti-herpes simplex virus and anti-human immunodeficiency virus activities. AIDS Res Hum Retroviruses. 1996;12:1463–1471.

Mathew B, Sankaranarayanan R, Nair PP, et al. Evaluation of chemoprevention of oral cancer with *Spirulina fusiformis. Nutr Cancer.* 1995;24:197–202.

Qureshi MA, Garlich JD, Kidd MT. Dietary *Spirulina platensis* enhances humoral and cell-mediated immune functions in chickens. *Immunopharmacol Immunotoxicol.* 1996;18:465–476.

Romay C, Armesto J, Remirez D, Gonzalez R, Ledon N, Garcia I. Antioxidant and anti-inflammatory properties of C-phycocyanin from blue-green algae. *Inflamm Res.* 1998;47:36–41

Salazar M, Martinez E, Madrigal E, Ruiz LE, Chamorro GA. Subchronic toxicity study in mice fed *Spirulina maxima. J Ethnopharmacol.* 1998;62:235–241.

Shealy NC. *The Illustrated Encyclopedia of Healing Remedies.* Boston, Mass: Element Books; 1998:277.

Walker LP, Brown EH. *The Alternative Pharmacy.* Paramus, NJ: Prentice Hall Press; 1998:51–53.

© Copyright Integrative Medicine Communications

Sulfur

Overview

The mineral sulfur has been used medicinally for more than 2,000 years. In *The Odyssey,* Homer describes burning sulfur to purify the air. This same practice was used during times of plague in Europe to disinfect contaminated areas. It is a constituent of the amino acids cystine, cysteine, and methionine, present in all cells of the body. It is considered non-toxic as any excess not used by the body is excreted in the urine and feces. Recognized as a "macromineral," it is found in significant amounts (>5g) in the body. About 0.25% of our body weight is sulfur. It is most prevalent in the keratin of skin, hair, and nails. It also is found as a component of the anti-coagulant heparin, and as chondriotin sulfate found in healthy bones and cartilage. Known as "nature's beauty mineral" it is fundamental for the synthesis of collagen which keeps the skin elastic and young-looking. Today, it is primarily used as a treatment for skin ailments such as eczema and other itchy skin conditions. It also aids oxidation reactions and protects the body against toxins which are increasingly present in our environment.

Arthritis sufferers flock to therapeutic sulfur hot springs to benefit from their pain-reducing effect, whether it be solely through the sulfur content, or through some action of other minerals. A 1992 Russian study determined that sulfur baths significantly lowered the pain sensitivity of patients with rheumatic diseases. An early study determined that taking sulfur baths raises the body's blood level of sulfur, in effect acting as a supplement, while other research indicates that sulfur is a desensitizing agent for the pain and discomfort experienced by cancer patients undergoing radiation therapy. Recent research suggests the reported beneficial effects of garlic (such as lowering cholesterol, blood pressure, and blood sugar) are at least partly due to the sulfur it contains.

Sources

■ Dietary Sources

Because sulfur is a constituent of the amino acids cystine, cysteine, and methionine, it is found in protein-rich foods such as meat, organ meats, poultry, fish, eggs, cooked dried beans and peas, and milk and milk products. Other good sources include garlic, onions, brussel sprouts, asparagus, kale, and wheat germ.

■ Constituents/Composition

Sulfur in its elemental form is a mineral found in rock beside hot springs and volcanic craters. It is found sparsely in elemental form, but is widely seen combined with other metals. The sulfur used in homeopathic treatment is a yellow-green powder extracted from the mineral. The characteristic "rotten egg" smell is caused from sulfur dioxide gas.

■ Commercial Preparations

Supplementation of sulfur is usually not necessary because most people get the required amount from dietary protein, but certain commercial preparations are available. To ease skin rashes, ointments, creams, lotions and dusting powders containing sulfur as the active ingredient are available. Organic sulfur in the form of MSM (metylsulfonylmethane) is available as a dietary supplement in tablets and capsules.

Therapeutic Uses

- Used to ease the red, itchy rash of eczema, candidiasis, dry scalp, diaper rash, hemorrhoids, and similar conditions
- Aids in digestive disorders, especially regurgitation of food, indigestion made worse by milk, and chronic diarrhea and vomiting in the morning
- To help gynecological complaints such as PMS and menopausal symptoms
- To ease the symptoms of rheumatism, osteoarthritis, rheumatoid arthritis
- Can help acne; used as a topical antiseptic similar to benzoyl peroxide, but not as potent or irritating to the skin
- May aid mental stress such as depression, irritability, forgetfulness, disturbed sleep
- Good for eye health
- Can help treat offensive body odors
- Reported to reduce reaction to radiation therapy used in cancer treatment

Dosage Ranges and Duration of Administration

There is no specific RDA established for sulfur. It is thought that approximately 850 mg/day is needed, considering the daily turnover of sulfur in the body.

For arthritis patients, 500 to 1,000 mg/day is the pharmacologic dosage range.

Cautions

■ Adverse Effects/Toxicology

No toxicity symptoms have been reported for elemental sulfur specifically since all excesses are excreted. However, some people are highly allergic to relatives of sulfur such as sulfites and sulfa drugs. Sulfites, sulfur-containing food preservatives, can trigger asthma and other allergic reactions in susceptible individuals. The major side effect of sulfa drugs is hypoglycemia, although other reactions include skin rashes, headache, fever, fatigue, and gastric distress. Sulfur-sensitive patients should avoid these drugs.

■ Warnings/Contraindications/Precautions

- Regarding sulfa drugs: Do not use during long-term corticosteroid use or pregnancy.
- Persons who are allergic to various sulfur containing compounds such as sulfites, sulfates and sulfa drugs, should probably avoid sulfur supplements as a precaution.
- Use sulfa drugs with caution in those who are elderly, alcoholic, or have impaired kidney or liver function.

Interactions

- Sulfur is a component of vitamin B_1, biotin, and the active form of pantothenic acid (also called co-enzyme A), which are required for metabolism and nerve health.
- Too much selenium can compete with sulfur. It can substitute itself for sulfur in the proteins of some enzymes, altering their functions.
- Arsenic poisoning is a result of arsenic's ability to bind with the sulfur portion of some amino acids, thus inactivating them.

References

Balch J, Balch P. *Prescription for Nutritional Healing.* 2nd ed. Garden City, NY: Avery Publishing Group; 1997.

Eades MD. *The Doctor's Complete Guide to Vitamins and Minerals.* New York, NY: Dell Publishing; 1994.

Haas EM. *Staying Healthy with Nutrition.* Berkeley, Calif: Celestial Arts; 1992.

Lockie A. Geddes N. *The Complete Guide to Homeopathy.* New York, NY: DK Publishing; 1995.

Lester MR. Sulfite sensitivity: significance in human health. *J Am Coll Nutr.* 1995;14(3):229–32.

Mahan LK, Arlin MT. *Krause's Food, Nutrition and Diet Therapy.* 8th ed. Philadelphia, Pa: WB Saunders Company (Harcourt, Brace, Jovanovich, Inc.); 1992.

Martensson J. The effect of fasting on leucocyte and plasma glutathione and sulfur amino acid concentrations. *Metabolism.* 1986;35:118–121.

Midell E, Hopkins V. *Prescription Alternatives.* New Canaan, Conn: Keats Publishing; 1998.

The Mineral Connection website. MSM, Biologicial Sulfur supplements. Accessed at *www.mineralconnection.com/msm.htm* on March 5, 1999.

Murray MT; Pizzorno JE. *Encyclopedia of Natural Medicine.* Rev. 2nd edition. Rocklin, Calif: Prima Publishing; 1998.

Nutrition Search, Inc.. *Nutrition Almanac.* Rev. ed. New York, NY: McGraw-Hill; 1979.

Pratsel HG, Eigner UM, Weinert D, Limbach B. The analgesic efficacy of sulfur mud baths in treating rheumatic diseases of the soft tissues [In Russian]. *Vopr Kurortol Fizioter Lech Fiz Kult.* 1992;(3):37–41.

Roediger WE, Moore J, Babidge W. Colonic sulfide in pathogenesis and treatment of ulcerative colitis. *Dig Dis Sci.* 1997;42:1571–1579.

Rossi A, Kaitila I, Wilcox WR, et al. Proteoglycan sulfation in cartilage and cell cultures from patients with sulfate transporter chondrodysplasias: relationship to clinical severity and indications on the role of intracellular sulfate production. *Matrix Biol.* 1998;17:361–369.

Shealy CN. *The Illustrated Encyclopedia of Healing Remedies.* Boston, Mass: Element Books, Inc; 1998.

Smith SM, McDonald A, Webb D. *Complete Book of Vitamins and Minerals.* Lincolnwood, Ill: Publications International, Ltd; 1998.

Smirnova OV, Saliev VP, Klemparskaia NN, Dobronravova NN. Purified sulfur as an agent to relieve the side effects in the radiation therapy of cervical cancer [In Russian]. *Med Radiol Mosk.* 1991;36:16–19.

Somer E. *The Essential Guide to Vitamins and Minerals.* New York, NY: Harper Collins Publishers Inc; 1995.

Sukenik S, Giryes H, Halevy, et al. Treatment of psoriatic arthritis at the Dead Sea. *J Rheumatol.* 1994;21:1305–1309.

Weiner M. *The Complete Book of Homeopathy.* New York, NY: MJF Books; 1989.

Werbach MR. *Nutritional Influences on Illness: A Sourcebook of Clinical Research.* New Canaan, Conn: Keats Publishing, Inc; 1988.

© *Copyright Integrative Medicine Communications*

Tyrosine

Overview

Tyrosine is a nonessential amino acid. It is synthesized in the body from phyenylalanine and is a precursor of adrenaline (epinephrine), norepinephrine, dopamine, thyroid hormones, and some types of estrogen. In order for tyrosine to metabolize into these substance, folic acid, niacin, vitamin C, and copper are needed. Low levels of tyrosine can lead to deficiencies in norepinephrine and dopamine—neurotransmitters that regulate mood. Depression can result. Animal studies have demonstrated that stressed animals have reduced levels of norepinephrine; however, administration of tyrosine prevented a norepinephrine deficiency. Tyrosine deficiency is also associated with low blood pressure, low body temperature, and restless leg syndrome.

Tyrosine aids in the the production of melanin (pigment responsible for hair and skin color) and in the functions of the adrenal, thryroid, and pituitary glands. A deficiency of tyrosine has been associated with hypothyroidism.

Because tyrosine binds unstable molecules that can potentially cause damage to the cells and tissues, it is considered a mild antioxidant. Thus, it may be useful in heavy smokers and in individuals exposed to chemicals and radiation.

Sources

■ **Dietary Sources**

Although tyrosine is found in soy products, chicken, fish, almonds, avocados, bananas, dairy products, lima beans, pumpkin seeds, and sesame seeds, it is difficult to get therapeutic amounts of it from food. It is also produced from phenylalanine in the body.

■ **Constituents/Composition**
N/A

■ **Commercial Preparations**
Many tyrosine supplements are available.

Therapeutic Uses

- Depression. Tyrosine appears to be a safe and effective treatment for depression; however, symptoms of depression recur when tyrosine is discontinued. Most data regarding tyrosine's efficacy in treating depression are anecdotal.
- Stress. Tyrosine seems to relieve the physical symptoms of stress if administered before the stressful situation, though limited human studies have been performed.
- Premenstrual syndrome (PMS). Though most data are anecdotal, tyrosine appears to help reduce the irritability, depression, and fatigue associated with PMS.
- Low sex drive. Tyrosine appears to stimulate the libido.
- Parkinson's disease. Parkinson's disease is treated with L-dopa, which is made from tyrosine; thus, the effects of tyrosine supplementation is being studied in Parkinson's disease patients.
- Weight loss. Tyrosine is an appetite suppressant and helps to reduce body fat.
- Chronic fatigue and narcolepsy. Tyrosine appears to have a mild stimulatory effect on the central nervous system.
- Drug detoxification. Tyrosine appears to be a successful adjunct for the treatment of cocaine abuse and withdrawal. It is often used in conjunction with tryptophan and imipramine (an antidepressant). In one study, 75% to 80% of patients treated with tyrosine stopped cocaine use completely or decreased usage by 50%. Successful withdrawal from caffeine and nicotine has also been anecdotally reported.
- Phenylketonuria (PKU). Tyrosine supplementation is advocated in patients with PKU; however, it is necessary to control plasma tyrosine levels (normal: 45 micromole/L) before tyrosine supplementation is considered.

Dosage Ranges and Duration of Administration

- For depression, premenstrual syndrome, and chronic fatigue, a 500 to 1,000 mg dose before each of three meals is recommended.
- For stress, 1500 mg/day is recommended.
- For low sex drive, Parkinson's disease, drug detoxification, and weight loss, 1 to 2 g/day in divided doses is recommended.
- It appears that up to 12 g/day of tyrosine can be ingested safely. However, high-dose therapy should be monitored by a health care provider.

Cautions

■ **Adverse Effects/Toxicology**

- Migraine headache
- High blood pressure
- Mild gastric upset
- Promotes cancer cell division

■ **Warnings/Contraindications/Precautions**

Tyrosine should not be given to patients who are taking monoamine oxidase (MAO) inhibitors for depression or to patients with high blood pressure because it can cause dangerously high blood pressure elevations. Tyrosine may also promote the growth of malignant melanoma by promoting the division of cancer cells.

Amino acids should not be taken regularly; ingestion may inhibit the body's natural production of these chemicals.

Interactions

Some researchers feel that tyrosine is more effective if it is taken with up to 25 mg of vitamin B_6. It should be taken 30 minutes before meals three times a day on an empty stomach (with juice or water). Tyrosine should not be taken with other amino acids or proteins such as milk.

References

Balch JF, Balch PA. *Prescriptions for Nutritional Healing*. 2nd ed. Garden City Park, NY: Avery Publishing; 1997:42.

Haas EM. *Staying Healthy with Nutrition*. Berkeley, Calif: Celestial Arts; 1992:51.

Mindell E, Hopkins V. Prescription Alternatives. New Canaan, Conn: Keats Publishing; 1998:398.

Shealy CN. *The Illustrated Encyclopedia of Healing Remedies*. Shaftesbury, England: Element; 1998:269.

Werbach MR. *Nutritional Influences on Illness*. New Canaan, Conn: Keats Publishing, 1987:162.

© Copyright Integrative Medicine Communications

Vanadium

Overview

Vanadium is an essential trace mineral. Although scientists know very little about how vanadium functions in humans, they believe that at the very least it is necessary for bone and tooth formation. One hundred years ago, vanadium was administered as a cure for various diseases, but it was toxic at the high doses that were prescribed. Based on animal studies, scientists believe that a lack of vanadium may result in high cholesterol and triglyceride levels, poor blood sugar control (e.g., diabetes or hypoglycemia), and cardiovascular and kidney disease.

Some experts believe that most American diets provide from 20 to 60 mcg of vanadium per day; others believe that the amount is many times that. At any given time, the body contains 25 to 100 mg of vanadium. It is present in varying amounts in the soil and in many foods. It can also be inhaled from the air as a result of burning petroleum or petroleum products. Deficiency states in humans have not been described, and no RDA has been established. Vanadium is poorly absorbed by the body once ingested, with as much as 95% eliminated.

Recently, a derivative of vanadium, peroxovanadium, has been used in experimental animals. It was 50 times more potent than vanadate in normalizing blood sugar without the toxicity shown by vanadium. Tests in humans have not been completed.

Sources

Dietary Sources

While vanadium is found in many foods, the best sources are sunflower, safflower, corn, and olive oils, as well as buckwheat, parsley, oats, rice, green beans, carrots, cabbage, pepper, and dill. It is also found in shellfish. Vanadium supplementation for a healthy person is rarely necessary. Eating any of the above foods should supply a sufficient quantity.

Constituents/Composition

Vanadium exists in several forms including vanadyl or vanadate. Vanadyl sulfate is most commonly found in nutritional supplements. There are at least three other forms of vanadium less biologically significant.

Commercial Preparations

Over-the-counter doses of vanadium are 30 to 60 mg/day in pill form.

Therapeutic Uses

- Diabetes (15 to 100 mg/day). Vanadium improves insulin sensitivity and glucose tolerance in type I and type II diabetes mellitus in experimental animals; however, supporting data on humans are not available.
- Bones and teeth. Vanadium improves the mineralization of bones and teeth in experimental animals.
- Body building (0.5 mg/kg/day). Studies have been unable to determine definitively any performance-enhancing effects of vanadium.
- High cholesterol. Vanadium seems to have the ability to reduce cholesterol in experimental animals.
- Heart disease. Rates of heart disease are low in areas of the world (e.g., South America) where the soil contains high levels of vanadium.

Dosage Ranges and Duration of Administration

Taking 50 to 100 mcg/day of vanadium is enough to meet or exceed nutritional requirements, without risking toxicity. Some manufacturers promote high dosages (15 to 100 mg) of vanadyl sulfate per day, but clinical data do not warrant such dosages at this time. Because deficiency states have not been described and nontoxic therapeutic dosages have not been determined, caution should be taken when using vanadium as a nutritional supplement. Bodybuilders and persons with diabetes are tempted to take high doses because of its purported ability to improve or mimic insulin action.

Cautions

Adverse Effects/Toxicology

Animal studies have not been successful in proving the efficacy and safety of vanadium. Death rates for laboratory animals are high when doses required to reduce blood sugar are administered. In lower doses, high blood pressure elevation and tremor have also been reported. High levels of vanadium may also contribute to some bone and kidney diseases. Additional problems reported include:

- Gastrointestinal upset with low doses
- Manic depression with high doses
- Inhibition of protein synthesis
- Pulmonary irritation from inhaled vanadium dust (e.g., petroleum workers)
- Oxidative damage to beta cells

Warnings/Contraindications/Precautions

Although vanadium is inhaled wherever petroleum is burned, it is not usually a cause for concern. However, extremely high doses (e.g., in workers who clean petroleum storage tanks) appear to irritate the lungs and may turn the tongue green, but neither symptom appears to cause any long-term or serious problem. High levels of vanadium may cause manic depression.

Interactions

- The effects of vanadium are reduced by some psychiatric medications (e.g., phenothiazines, monoamine oxidase inhibitors).
- Vanadium inhibits sodium-potassium pump activity; however, lithium, which is used in the treatment of manic depression, can reverse or reduce this inhibition.
- Ascorbic acid, ethylenediaminetetraacetic acid (EDTA), and methylene blue decrease vanadium levels in the body and thus are effective in treating manic depression in which vanadium levels are high.
- Tobacco decreases vanadium uptake.
- Vanadium and chromium should not be taken together.

References

Balch JF, Balch PA. *Prescription for Nutritional Healing.* Garden City Park, NY: Avery Publishing; 1997:29.

Bender DA, Bender AE. *Nutrition: A Reference Handbook.* New York, NY: Oxford University Press; 1997:424.

Murray MT. *Encyclopedia of Nutritional Supplements.* Rocklin, Calif: Prima Publishing; 1996:232–234.

Murray MT, Pizzorno JE. *Encyclopedia of Natural Medicine.* 2nd ed. Rocklin, Calif: Prima Publishing; 1998:283–284.

Shealy CN. *The Illustrated Encyclopedia of Healing Remedies.* Boston, Mass: Element Books; 1998:268.

Role of vanadium as a mimic of insulin. *Nutri Res Newslett.* 1998;17:11.

Werbach MR. *Nutritional Influences on Illness.* New Canaan, Conn: Keats Publishing; 1987:87–88, 159.

Yale J-F, Lachance D, Bevan AP. Hypoglycemic effects of peroxovanadium compounds in Sprague-Dawley and diabetic BB rats. *Diabetes.* 1995;44:1274–1276.

© Copyright Integrative Medicine Communications

Vitamin H — Biotin

Overview

Biotin is a water-soluble vitamin whose primary function is as a coenzyme in carbohydrate, amino acid, and lipid metabolism. Biotin is essential for cell growth and replication through its role in the manufacturing of DNA and RNA. Biotin has been shown to improve blood glucose control in diabetes by enhancing insulin sensitivity and increasing the activity of glucokinase, the enzyme responsible for the first step in the utilization of glucose by the liver. Studies have observed improvements with doses from 9 mcg to 16 mcg. High doses of biotin may also be useful in the treatment of diabetic neuropathy. Healthy hair and nails require biotin. Supplementation (up to 2,500 mcg/day) has been effective in treating frail, splitting, or thin toenails or fingernails and in improving hair health (through its action on the metabolism of scalp oils). Biotin has also been used to combat premature graying of hair, though it's likely to be useful only for those with a biotin deficiency.

Biotin is synthesized in the intestinal microflora. For this reason, deficiency states are rare. A vegetarian diet enhances the synthesis and absorption of biotin. Those at risk for biotin deficiency include infants with inherited deficiency disorders, babies fed biotin-deficient formula, people who eat large amounts of raw egg whites, which inactivate biotin, and people who are fed intravenously. Symptoms include hair loss, a dry, scaly dermatitis, anorexia, nausea, and depression. Biotin deficiency can exacerbate seborrheic dermatitis (cradle cap) in infants. Several case histories reveal the successful treatment of cradle cap in infants with biotin through direct supplementation to either the infant or the mother if she is breast-feeding. In adults with seborrheic dermatitis, biotin supplementation in conjunction with vitamin B-complex supplementation is necessary. Biotin deficiency also impacts the immune system.

Sources

■ Dietary Sources

- Liver
- Nuts
- Kidney
- Egg yolks
- Brewer's yeast
- Chocolate
- Whole grains and whole grain breads
- Beans
- Fish

Food-processing techniques can destroy biotin, therefore less-processed products will have a greater percentage of their biotin intact.

■ Constituents/Composition

Biotin is available as isolated biotin or as biocytin, a complex in brewer's yeast, composed of 65.6% biotin.

■ Commercial Preparations

Biotin is available in multivitamin and vitamin B complexes, and in individual supplements.

Standard preparations are available in 10 mcg, 50 mcg, 100 mcg, and 500 mcg tablets.

Therapeutic Uses

Biotin can be used to treat:

- Infants with a potentially fatal genetic abnormality, which leads to an inability to utilize biotin
- Some skin disorders, such as seborrheic dermatitis (cradle cap)
- Blood glucose control in diabetics
- Diabetic neuropathy
- Frail, splitting, or thin nails
- Hair loss due to deficiency
- Gray hair (in some instances)
- Metabolic abnormalities in Duchenne muscular dystrophy
- Fat metabolism in weight-loss programs (normalizes)
- Intestinal candidiasis

Dosage Ranges and Duration of Administration

Due to biotin's synthesis in the gut, an RDA has not been set. The adequate intake for biotin has been estimated at 30 to 100 mcg per day. Average daily biotin intake in the American diet has been estimated to be 28 to 42 mcg.

Cautions

■ Adverse Effects/Toxicology

There have been no reported toxic effects, even at high doses.

■ Warnings/Contraindications/Precautions

No contraindications have been identified.

Interactions

- Biotin works closely with folic acid, pantothenic acid, vitamin B12, and coenzyme Q10—all must be present for activity.
- Biotin lessens the symptoms of pantothenic acid and zinc deficiencies.
- Raw egg white contains a protein called avidin that prevents biotin absorption.
- Sulfa drugs, estrogen, and alcohol may raise biotin requirements.
- Prolonged use of anticonvulsant drugs may lead to biotin deficiency.
- Long-term use of antibiotics can affect the balance of the digestive system and reduce or stop the manufacturing of biotin by bacteria.

References

Bendich A, Deckelbaum R. *Preventive Nutrition: The Comprehensive Guide for Health Professionals.* Totowa, NJ: Humana Press; 1997.

Houchman LG, et al. Brittle nails: response to biotin supplementation. *Cutis.* 1993;51:303–307.

Jung U, Helbich-Endermann M, Bitsch R, et al. Are patients with chronic renal failure (CRF) deficient in biotin and is regular biotin supplementation required? *Z Ernahrungswiss.* 1998;37:363–367.

Koutsikos D, Agroyannis B, Tzanatos-Exarchou H. Biotin for diabetic peripheral neuropathy. *Biomed Pharmacother.* 1990;44:511–514.

Koutsikos D, Fourtounas C, Kapetanaki A, et al. Oral glucose tolerance test after high-dose i.v. biotin administration in normoglucemic hemodialysis patients. *Ren Fail.* 1996;18:131–137.

Messina M. *The Dietitian's Guide to Vegetarian Diets: Issues and Applications.* Gaithersburg, Md: Aspen Publishers, Inc; 1996.

Murray M. *Encyclopedia of Nutritional Supplements.* Rocklin, Calif: Prima Publishing; 1997.

Reavley N. *Vitamins etc.* Melbourne, Australia: Bookman Press; 1998.

Ringer DL. *Physicians Guide to Nutraceuticals.* Omaha, Neb: Nutritional Data Resources; 1998.

Schulpis KH, Nyalala JO, Papakonstantinou ED, et al. Biotin recycling impairment in phenylketonuric children with seborrheic dermatitis. *Int J Dermatol.* 1998;37:918–921.

Zempleni J, Mock DM. Advanced analysis of biotin metabolites in body fluids allows a more accurate measurement of biotin bioavailability and metabolism in humans. *J Nutr.* 1999;129:494–497.

© *Copyright Integrative Medicine Communications*

Zinc

Overview

Zinc is an essential trace mineral, which, next to iron, is the second most abundant trace mineral in the body. It is a component in over 200 enzymes. Zinc is stored primarily in muscle but high concentrations are also found in red and white blood cells, and the retina. It is also found in bones, skin, kidney, liver, and pancreas. In men, the prostate gland contains more zinc than any other organ.

Zinc is a part of some important antioxidant compounds, including superoxide dismutase (SOD) and zinc monomethionine. It protects the liver from chemical damage, helping with detoxification of the body. It is required for a healthy immune system. Taking zinc supplements has been shown to reduce infection and speed wound healing. Studies have shown it helps treat and prevent acne. It is essential for proper growth and development, especially early in life. It is necessary to maintain proper vision, taste, and smell.

Zinc deficiency may be a more common problem than previously thought, especially as people age. In clinical studies on the effects of zinc supplementation in the elderly, zinc improved immune system function, reduced the incidence of illness, and decreased the incidence of anorexia.

Recent research has been conducted to determine the true value of zinc lozenges in preventing or reducing cold symptoms.

Sources

■ Dietary Sources

Zinc absorption from foods varies from 20% to 40% of ingested zinc. Zinc from animal foods is the best-absorbed form. When bound with the phytates or oxalates in vegetable sources, zinc is less available, and vegetable fiber itself impedes the absorption of zinc. Dairy products and eggs contain fair amounts of zinc, but again, it may be poorly absorbed from these sources.

The following foods contain high amounts of zinc in the most absorbable form.

- Oysters (richest source)
- Red meats
- Shrimp, crab, and other shellfish

Other good sources, but which may be less absorbable, include legumes (especially lima beans, black-eyed peas, pinto beans, soybeans, peanuts) whole grains, miso, tofu, brewer's yeast, cooked greens, mushrooms, green beans, and pumpkin seeds.

■ Constituents/Composition

Zinc is a metallic element present in soil.

■ Commercial Preparations

The most commonly used zinc supplement has been zinc sulfate. This is the least expensive form, but it may cause gastric irritation and is less absorbable than other forms. It is usually prescribed as 220 mg zinc sulfate, which provides approximately 55 mg of elemental zinc. More absorbable forms such as the following are available.

- Zinc picolinate
- Zinc citrate
- Zinc acetate
- Zinc glycerate
- Zinc monomethionine

These forms come in capsules supplying 30 or 50 mg of elemental zinc. The amount in milligrams per capsule of these other zinc compounds can vary, according to the percentage of elemental zinc contained. Zinc lozenges are also available which supply varying amounts of zinc and used for treating colds.

Therapeutic Uses

Benefits of zinc include the following.

- Treats depressed immunity
- Improves wound healing
- Treats and may prevent acne
- May prevent macular degeneration
- Treats anorexia nervosa (anorexia is a symptom of zinc deficiency, and the teenage population is at higher risk for zinc deficiency due to dietary habits)
- Improves male fertility and sexual function, especially among smokers
- Treats rheumatoid arthritis
- Treats Wilson's disease (a disorder of excess copper storage)
- Decreases taste alteration during cancer treatments
- Improves sense of taste and smell

Some conditions may impair zinc absorption, or increase the need for zinc. Individuals with the following conditions may benefit from zinc supplementation.

- Acrodermatitis eteropathica (the inherited disease of zinc malabsorption)
- Pregnancy, lactation
- Alcoholism
- Diabetes
- Kidney disease, dialysis
- Celiac disease
- Inflammatory bowel disease, ulcerative colitis
- Chronic diarrhea
- Pancreatic insufficiency
- Oral contraceptive use
- Prostate problems (BPH, prostatitis, cancer)

Dosage Ranges and Duration of Administration

The RDA for zinc is as follows.

- Infants to 1 year: 5 mg
- 1 to 10 years: 10 mg
- Males over 10 years: 15 mg
- Females over 10 years: 12 mg
- Pregnant females: 15 mg
- Lactating females: (0 to 6 months) 19 mg, (6 to 12 months) 16 mg

Therapeutic ranges (elemental zinc):

- Men: 30 to 60 mg daily
- Women: 30 to 45 mg daily

Doses over this amount should be limited to only a few months under the supervision of a health care professional.

Cautions

■ Adverse Effects/Toxicology

Zinc is the least toxic trace mineral. Symptoms of toxicity are GI irritation and vomiting, usually occurring after a dose of 2,000 mg or more has been ingested. Studies have confirmed that up to 10 times the RDA (150 mg) taken even over time was not toxic. Doses this high are unnecessary and interfere with the assimilation of other trace minerals such as copper and iron.

Too much zinc (over 150 mg/day over time) lowers HDL cholesterol and raises LDL cholesterol, an undesirable affect. Megadoses of zinc are reported to depress immune function. Studies on this have been inconclusive, and further research is needed.

Zinc sulfate can cause gastric irritation, but another form can be used instead if this occurs. Other reported side effects of zinc toxicity are dizziness, headache, drowsiness, increased sweating, muscular incoordination, alcohol intolerance, hallucinations, and anemia.

■ Warnings/Contraindications/Precautions

Because of the multiple interactions zinc has with other nutrients, it is advisable to take a balanced multiple vitamin/mineral preparation that contains zinc as well as copper, iron, and folate, to help prevent deficiencies of these nutrients.

Interactions

- Excess zinc can interfere with copper absorption and cause a copper deficiency which indirectly affects iron status and can lead to anemia.
- Excess copper intake interferes with zinc absorption.
- Iron supplements can impair zinc absorption. Optimally, zinc supplements should be taken at a separate time from iron-containing supplements.
- Calcium may interfere with zinc absorption at high doses.
- Zinc interferes with folate absorption.
- Dietary fiber (present in vegetables and, to a lesser degree, fruit) interferes with the absorption of zinc.

References

Eby GA. Zinc ion availability—the determinant of efficacy in zinc lozenge treatment of common colds. *J Antimicrob Chemother.* 1997;40:483-493.

Feltman J. *Prevention's Food & Nutrition.* Emmaus, Pa: Rodale Press; 1993.

Fortes C, Forastiere F, Agabiti N, et al. The effect of zinc and vitamin A supplementation on immune response in an older population. *J Am Geriatr Soc.* 1998;46:19-26.

Garland ML, Hagmeyer KO. The role of zinc lozenges in treatment of the common cold. *Ann Pharmacother.* 1998;32:63-69.

Golik A, Zaidenstein R, Dishi V, et al. Effects of captopril and enalapril on zinc metabolism in hypertensive patients. *J Am Coll Nutr.* 1998;17:75-78.

Haas E. *Staying Healthy with Nutrition, The Complete Guide to Diet and Nutritional Medicine.* Berkeley, Calif: Celestial Arts Publishing; 1992.

Hendler SS. *The Doctors' Vitamin and Mineral Encyclopedia.* New York, NY: Fireside Press; 1991.

Lieberman S, Bruning N. *The Real Vitamin & Mineral Book.* 2nd ed. New York, NY: Avery Publishing Group; 1997.

Murray M. *Encyclopedia of Nutritional Supplements.* Rocklin, Calif: Prima Publishing; 1996.

Pronsky Z. *Food-Medication Interactions.* 9th ed. Pottstown, Pa: Food-Medicine Interactions; 1995.

Sazawal S, Black RE, Jalla S, et al. Zinc supplementation reduces the incidence of acute lower respiratory infections in infants and preschool children: a double-blind, controlled trial. *Pediatrics.* 1998;102(part 1):1-5.

Shealy CN. *The Illustrated Encyclopedia of Healing Remedies.* Boston, Mass: Element Books Inc.; 1998.

Somer E. *The Essential Guide to Vitamins and Minerals.* New York, NY: HarperCollins Publishers, Inc.; 1995.

Whitney E, Cataldo C, Rolfes S. *Understanding Normal and Clinical Nutrition.* St. Paul, Minn: West Publishing Co.; 1987.

© *Copyright Integrative Medicine Communications*

INDEX

A

Acanthopanax senticosus, *see* **Ginseng, Siberian,** *p. 51*
Achillea millefolium, *see* **Yarrow,** *p. 105*
Allii sativi bulbus, *see* **Garlic,** *p. 41*
Allium sativum, *see* **Garlic,** *p. 41*
Aloe, *p. 3*
Aloe barbadensis, *see* **Aloe,** *p. 3*
Aloe ferox, *see* **Aloe,** *p. 3*
Aloe vera, *see* **Aloe,** *p. 3*
Alpha-Linolenic Acid (ALA), *p. 109*
Alpha-Lipoic Acid, *p. 111*
Althaea, *see* **Marshmallow,** *p. 77*
Althaea officinalis, *see* **Marshmallow,** *p. 77*
American ginseng, *see* **Ginseng, American,** *p. 47*
Apii fructus, *see* **Celery Seed,** *p. 19*
Apium graveolens, *see* **Celery Seed,** *p. 19*
Arctium lappa, *see* **Burdock,** *p. 11*
Arctium minus, *see* **Burdock,** *p. 11*
Arctium tomentosum, *see* **Burdock,** *p. 11*
Asian ginseng, *see* **Ginseng, Asian,** *p. 49*

B

Barberry, *p. 5*
Barberry bark, *see* **Barberry,** *p. 5*
Barberry root, *see* **Barberry,** *p. 5*
Barberry root bark, *see* **Barberry,** *p. 5*
Bardanae radix, *see* **Burdock,** *p. 11*
Berberidis cortex, *see* **Barberry,** *p. 5*
Berberidis radicis cortex, *see* **Barberry,** *p. 5*
Berberidis radix, *see* **Barberry,** *p. 5*
Berberis vulgaris, *see* **Barberry,** *p. 5*
Betaine, *p. 113*
Bilberry, *p. 7*
Black Cohosh, *p. 9*
Brewer's Yeast, *p. 115*
Bromelain, *p. 117*
Burdock, *p. 11*

C

Calcium Salts, *see Section 40:12 in AHFS Drug Information*
Calendula flower, *see* **Calendula (Pot Marigold),** *p. 13*
Calendula herb, *see* **Calendula (Pot Marigold),** *p. 13*
Calendula officinalis, *see* **Calendula (Pot Marigold),** *p. 13*
Calendula (Pot Marigold), *p. 13*
Calendulae flos, *see* **Calendula (Pot Marigold),** *p. 13*
Calendulae herba, *see* **Calendula (Pot Marigold),** *p. 13*
Camellia sinensis, *see* **Green Tea,** *p. 57*
capensis, *see* **Aloe,** *p. 3*
Capsicum, *see* **Cayenne,** *p. 17*
Capsicum frutescens, *see* **Cayenne,** *p. 17*
Capsicum spp., *see* **Cayenne,** *p. 17*

Cardui mariae fructus, *see* **Milk Thistle,** *p. 79*
Cardui mariae herba, *see* **Milk Thistle,** *p. 79*
Carnitine (L-Carnitine), *p. 119*
Cartilage, *p. 121*
Cat's Claw, *p. 15*
Cayenne (Paprika), *p 17*
Celery Seed, *p. 19*
Chamaemelum nobile, *see* **Chamomile, Roman,** *p. 23*
Chamomile, German, *p. 21*
Chamomile, Roman, *p. 23*
Chamomillae romanae flos, *see* **Chamomile, Roman,** *p. 23*
Chromium, *p. 123*
Chrysanthemum parthenium, *see* **Feverfew,** *p. 37*
Cimicifuga racemosa, *see* **Black Cohosh,** *p. 9*
Cimicifugae racemosae rhizoma, *see* **Black Cohosh,** *p. 9*
Coenzyme Q10, *p. 125*
Comfrey, *p. 25*
Comfrey leaf, *see* **Comfrey,** *p. 25*
Comfrey root, *see* **Comfrey,** *p. 25*
Copper, *p. 127*
crataegi flos, *see* **Hawthorn,** *p. 59*
crataegi folium, *see* **Hawthorn,** *p. 59*
crataegi folium cum flore, *see* **Hawthorn,** *p. 59*
Crataegi fructus, *see* **Hawthorn,** *p. 59*
Crataegus monogyna, *see* **Hawthorn,** *p. 59*
Crataegus laevigata, *see* **Hawthorn,** *p. 59*
Creatine, *p. 129*
Curcuma longa, *see* **Turmeric,** *p. 99*
Curcumae longae rhizoma, *see* **Turmeric,** *p. 99*
Cysteine, *p. 131*

D

Dandelion, *p. 27*
Dandelion Herb, *see* **Dandelion,** *p. 27*
Dandelion Root With Herb, *see* **Dandelion,** *p. 27*
Dehydroepiandrosterone (DHEA), *p. 133*
Devil's Claw, *p. 29*
Devil's claw root, *see* **Devil's Claw,** *p. 29*
Dioscorea villosa, *see* **Wild Yam,** *p. 103*
Dioscoreae villosae rhizoma, *see* **Wild Yam,** *p. 103*

E

Echinacea, *p. 31*
Echinacea angustifolia, *see* **Echinacea,** *p. 31*
Echinacea Angustifolia herb-root, *see* **Echinacea,** *p. 31*
Echinacea angustofoliae herba-radix, *see* **Echinacea,** *p. 31*
Echinacea pallida, *see* **Echinacea,** *p. 31*
Echinacea Pallida herb-root, *see* **Echinacea,** *p. 31*
Echinacea pallidae herba-radix, *see* **Echinacea,** *p. 31*
Echinacea purpurea, *see* **Echinacea,** *p. 31*
Echinacea Purpurea herb-root, *see* **Echinacea,** *p. 31*
Echinacea purpureae herba-radix, *see* **Echinacea,** *p. 31*
Eleutherococci radix, *see* **Ginseng, Siberian,** *p. 51*

Eleutherococcus senticosus, *see* **Ginseng, Siberian,** *p. 51*
Equiseti herba, *see* **Horsetail,** *p. 61*
Equisetum arvense, *see* **Horsetail,** *p. 61*
Eucalypti aetheroleum, *see* **Eucalyptus,** *p. 33*
Eucalypti folium, *see* **Eucalyptus,** *p. 33*
Eucalyptus, *p. 31*
Eucalyptus fructicetorum, *see* **Eucalyptus,** *p. 33*
Eucalyptus globulus, *see* **Eucalyptus,** *p. 33*
Eucalyptus polybractea, *see* **Eucalyptus,** *p. 33*
Eucalyptus smithii, *see* **Eucalyptus,** *p. 33*
Eucalyptus leaf, *see* **Eucalyptus,** *p. 33*
Eucalyptus oil, *see* **Eucalyptus,** *p. 33*
Evening Primrose, *p. 35*

F

Feverfew, *p. 37*
Flaxseed, *p. 39*
Flaxseed Oil, *p. 135*
Folic Acid, *see Section 88:08 in AHFS Drug Information*

G

Gamma-Linolenic Acid (GLA), *p. 137*
Garlic, *p. 41*
Ginger, *p. 43*
Ginger root, *see* **Ginger,** *p. 43*
Ginkgo Biloba, *p. 45*
Ginkgo biloba, *see* **Ginkgo Biloba,** *p. 45*
Ginkgo folium, *see* **Ginkgo Biloba,** *p. 45*
Ginseng, American, *p. 47*
Ginseng, Asian, *p. 49*
Ginseng, Siberian, *p. 51*
Ginseng radix, *see* **Ginseng, American,** *p. 47*
Ginseng radix, *see* **Ginseng, Asian,** *p. 49*
Glutamine, *p. 139*
Glycyrrhiza glabra, *see* **Licorice,** *p. 71*
Goldenseal, *p. 53*
Grape Seed, *see* **Grape Seed Extract,** *p. 55*
Grape Seed Extract, *p. 55*
Green Tea, *p. 57*

H

Harpagophyti radix, *see* **Devil's Claw,** *p. 29*
Harpagophytum procumbens, *see* **Devil's Claw,** *p. 29*
Hawthorn, *p. 59*
Hawthorn berry, *see* **Hawthorn,** *p. 59*
Hawthorn flower, *see* **Hawthorn,** *p. 59*
Hawthorn leaf, *see* **Hawthorn,** *p. 59*
Hawthorn leaf with flower, *see* **Hawthorn,** *p. 59*
Horsetail, *p. 61*
Hydrastis canadensis, *see* **Goldenseal,** *p. 53*
Hydrastis rhizoma, *see* **Goldenseal,** *p. 53*
5-Hydroxytryptophan (5-HTP), *p. 141*
Hyperici herba, *see* **St. John's Wort,** *p. 97*
Hypericum perforatum, *see* **St. John's Wort,** *p. 97*

I

Iodine, *see Section 84:04.16 in AHFS Drug Information*
Iron Preparations, Oral, *see Section 20:04.04 in AHFS Drug Information*

J

Jamaica Dogwood, *p. 63*

K

Kava Kava, *p. 65*

L

Lactobacillus Acidophilus, *see Section 56:08 in AHFS Drug Information*
Lavandula angustifolia, *see* **Lavender,** *p. 67*
Lavandulae, *see* **Lavender,** *p. 67*
Lavender, *p. 67*
Lemon Balm, *p. 69*
Licorice, *p. 71*
Linden, *p. 73*
Linden charcoal, *see* **Linden,** *p. 73*
Linden Flower, *see* **Linden,** *p. 73*
Linden Leaf, *see* **Linden,** *p. 73*
Linden Wood, *see* **Linden,** *p. 73*
Lini semen, *see* **Flaxseed,** *p. 39*
Linum usitatissimum, *see* **Flaxseed,** *p. 39*
Lipase, *p. 143*
Liquiritiae radix, *see* **Licorice,** *p. 71*
Lobelia, *p. 75*
Lobelia inflata, *see* **Lobelia,** *p. 75*
Lysine, *p. 145*

M

Magnesium Sulfate, *see Section 28:12.92 in AHFS Drug Information*
Manganese, *p. 147*
Marshmallow, *p. 77*
Matricaria recutita, *see* **Chamomile, German,** *p. 21*
Matricariae flos, *see* **Chamomile, German,** *p. 21*
Melatonin, *p. 149*
Melissa officinalis, *see* **Lemon Balm,** *p. 69*
Melissae folium, *see* **Lemon Balm,** *p. 69*
Menthae piperitae aetheroleum, *see* **Peppermint,** *p. 85*
Menthae piperitae folium, *see* **Peppermint,** *p. 85*
Mentha X piperita, *see* **Peppermint,** *p. 85*
Milk Thistle, *p. 79*
Milk thistle fruit, *see* **Milk Thistle,** *p. 79*
milk thistle herb, *see* **Milk Thistle,** *p. 79*
Millefolii flos, *see* **Yarrow,** *p. 105*
Millefolii herba, *see* **Yarrow,** *p. 105*
Myrtilli folium, *see* **Bilberry,** *p. 7*
Myrtilli fructus, *see* **Bilberry,** *p. 7*

O

Oenothera biennis, *see* **Evening Primrose,** *p. 35*
Omega-3 Fatty Acids, *p. 151*
Omega-6 Fatty Acids, *p. 153*

P

Panax ginseng, *see* **Ginseng, Asian,** *p. 49*
Panax quinquefolium, *see* **Ginseng, American,** *p. 47*
Passiflora incarnata, *see* **Passionflower,** *p. 81*
Passiflorae herba, *see* **Passionflower,** *p. 81*
Passionflower, *p. 81*
Pau d'Arco, *p. 83*
Peppermint, *p. 85*
Phenylalanine, *p. 155*
Phosphorus, *p. 157*
Piper methysticum, *see* **Kava Kava,** *p. 65*
Piperis methystici rhizoma, *see* **Kava Kava,** *p. 65*
Piscidia erythrina, *see* **Jamaica Dogwood,** *p. 63*
Piscidia piscipula, *see* **Jamaica Dogwood,** *p. 63*
Piscidiae radicis cortex, *see* **Jamaica Dogwood,** *p. 63*
Potassium supplements, *see Section 40:12 in AHFS Drug Information*
Psyllium, *see Section 56:12 in AHFS Drug Information*

Q

Quercetin, *p. 159*

R

Roman chamomile, *see* **Chamomile, Roman,** *p. 23*
Rosemary, *p. 87*
Rosemary, *see* **Rosemary,** *p. 87*
Rosmarini, *see* **Rosemary,** *p. 87*
Rosmarinus officinalis, *see* **Rosemary,** *p. 87*

S

Sabal fructus, *see* **Saw Palmetto,** *p. 89*
Sabal serrulata, *see* **Saw Palmetto,** *p. 89*
Saw Palmetto, *p. 89*
Saw Palmetto Berry, *see* **Saw Palmetto,** *p. 89*
Scutellaria lateriflora, *see* **Skullcap,** *p. 91*
Scutellariae herba, *see* **Skullcap,** *p. 91*
Selenium, *p. 161*
Serenoa repens, *see* **Saw Palmetto,** *p. 89*
Siberian ginseng, *see* **Ginseng, Siberian,** *p. 51*
Silybum marianum, *see* **Milk Thistle,** *p. 79*
Skullcap, *p. 91*
Slippery elm, *p. 93*
Slippery Elm, *see* **Slippery elm,** *p. 93*
Spirulina, *p. 163*
St. John's Wort, *p. 97*
Stinging Nettle, *p. 95*
Stinging nettle herb, *see* **Stinging Nettle,** *p. 95*
stinging nettle leaf, *see* **Stinging Nettle,** *p. 95*
stinging nettle root, *see* **Stinging Nettle,** *p. 95*

Sulfur, *p. 165*
Symphyti folium, *see* **Comfrey,** *p. 25*
Symphyti radix, *see* **Comfrey,** *p. 25*
Symphytum officinale, *see* **Comfrey,** *p. 25*

T

Tabebuia avellanedae, *see* **Pau d'Arco,** *p. 83*
Tanaceti parthenii herba, *see* **Feverfew,** *p. 37*
Tanacetum parthenium, *see* **Feverfew,** *p. 37*
Taraxaci herba, *see* **Dandelion,** *p. 27*
Taraxaci radix cum herba, *see* **Dandelion,** *p. 27*
Taraxacum officinale, *see* **Dandelion,** *p. 27*
Tilia cordata, *see* **Linden,** *p. 73*
Tilia platyphyllos, *see* **Linden,** *p. 73*
Tiliae carbo, *see* **Linden,** *p. 73*
Tiliae flos, Tiliae folium, *see* **Linden,** *p. 73*
Tiliae lignum, *see* **Linden,** *p. 73*
Turmeric, *p. 99*
Tyrosine, *p. 167*

U

Ulmi rubrae, *see* **Slippery elm,** *p. 93*
Ulmus fulva, *see* **Slippery elm,** *p. 93*
Uncaria tomentosa, *see* **Cat's Claw,** *p. 15*
Urtica dioica, *see* **Stinging Nettle,** *p. 95*
Urtica urens, *see* **Stinging Nettle,** *p. 95*
Urticae folium, *see* **Stinging Nettle,** *p. 95*
Urticae herba, *see* **Stinging Nettle,** *p. 95*
Urticae radix, *see* **Stinging Nettle,** *p. 95*

V

Vaccinium myrtillus, *see* **Bilberry,** *p. 7*
Valerian, *p. 101*
Valerian root, *see* **Valerian,** *p. 101*
Valeriana officinalis, *see* **Valerian,** *p. 101*
Valerianae radix, *see* **Valerian,** *p. 101*
Vanadium, *p. 169*
Vitamin A, *see Section 88:04 in AHFS Drug Information*
Vitamin B_1, *see Section 88:08 in AHFS Drug Information*
Vitamin B_2, *see Section 88:08 in AHFS Drug Information*
Vitamin B_6, *see Section 88:08 in AHFS Drug Information*
Vitamin B_{12}, *see Section 88:08 in AHFS Drug Information*
Vitamin H (Biotin), *p. 171*
Vitamin K, *see Section 88:24 in AHFS Drug Information*
Vitis vinifera, *see* **Grape Seed Extract,** *p. 55*

W

Wild Yam, *p. 103*

Y

Yarrow, *p. 105*
Yarrow Flower, *see* **Yarrow,** *p. 105*
Yarrow Herb, *see* **Yarrow,** *p. 105*

Z

Zinc, *p. 173*
Zingiber officinale, *see* **Ginger,** *p. 43*
Zingiberis rhizoma, *see* **Ginger,** *p. 43*